Literate Thought
Understanding Comprehension and Literacy

Peter V. Paul, PhD
Professor
School of Teaching and Learning
The Ohio State University
Columbus, Ohio

Ye Wang, PhD
Assistant Professor
Department of Communication Sciences and Disorders
Missouri State University
Springfield, Missouri

TOURO COLLEGE LIBRARY
Kings Hwy

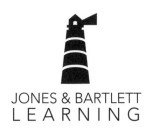

JONES & BARTLETT
LEARNING

KH

World Headquarters

Jones & Bartlett Learning
40 Tall Pine Drive
Sudbury, MA 01776
978-443-5000
info@jblearning.com
www.jblearning.com

Jones & Bartlett Learning
Canada
6339 Ormindale Way
Mississauga, Ontario L5V 1J2
Canada

Jones & Bartlett Learning
International
Barb House, Barb Mews
London W6 7PA
United Kingdom

Jones & Bartlett Learning books and products are available through most bookstores and online booksellers. To contact Jones & Bartlett Learning directly, call 800-832-0034, fax 978-443-8000, or visit our website, www.jblearning.com.

Substantial discounts on bulk quantities of Jones & Bartlett Learning publications are available to corporations, professional associations, and other qualified organizations. For details and specific discount information, contact the special sales department at Jones & Bartlett Learning via the above contact information or send an email to specialsales@jblearning.com.

Production Credits
Publisher: David D. Cella
Associate Editor: Maro Gartside
Editorial Assistant: Teresa Reilly
Senior Production Editor: Renée Sekerak
Production Assistant: Sean Coombs
Marketing Manager: Grace Richards
Manufacturing and Inventory Control Supervisor: Amy Bacus
Cover Design: Kristin E. Parker
Cover Image: Book © Arosoft/Dreamstime.com; Brain © Linda Bucklin/Dreamstime.com;
    Keyboard © Janaka Dharmasena/Dreamstime.com; Screen © Seesea/Dreamstime.com;
    Sound © Vladimirdreams/Dreamstime.com
Composition: DataStream Content Solutions, LLC
Printing and Binding: Malloy, Inc.
Cover Printing: Malloy, Inc.

Library of Congress Cataloging-in-Publication Data
Paul, Peter V.
    Literate thought : understanding comprehension and literacy / Peter V. Paul, Ye Wang.
        p. ; cm.
    Includes bibliographical references and index.
    ISBN-13: 978-0-7637-7852-1 (casebound)
    ISBN-10: 0-7637-7852-4 (casebound)
    1. Comprehension 2. Developmentally disabled children. 3. Special education. I. Wang, Ye,
1977- II. Title.
    [DNLM: 1. Comprehension. 2. Child. 3. Developmental Disabilities. 4. Education, Special.
5. Language Disorders. 6. Learning Disorders. 7. Reading. BF 325]
    BF325.P38 2012
    153.4—dc22

                                                                                        2010053635
6048

Printed in the United States of America
15 14 13 12 11   10 9 8 7 6 5 4 3 2 1

9/2/11

Contents

Preface

But any true understanding of Einstein's imagination and intuition will not come from poking around at his patterns of glia and grooves. The relevant question was how his mind worked, not his brain.

The explanation that Einstein himself most often gave for his mental accomplishments was his curiosity. As he put it near the end of his life, "I have no special talents, I am only passionately curious."

Isaacson, 2007, p. 548

Thus far, understanding how the *mind* works has eluded scholars and philosophers, despite their passionate endeavors and rigorous methods. Part of the difficulty is that we cannot actually observe the workings of the mind. We cannot see the *imagination, intuition,* or *curiosity* of the individual. As implied by the above passage, examining the structures and actions of the brain may not reveal much about the intricate processes that take place in the mind.

Social forces—that is, events, structures, and practices that occur *outside-the-head*—certainly contribute to mental development; nevertheless, thinking is a mental activity. Thinking is a process that culminates in products such as thoughts, art, mathematics, and written language. These products do provide some insights into the nature of thinking—but not necessarily the entire picture.

Although adopting a completely *internalist* position is not tenable, our goal is still to describe what is going on *inside-the-head* when individuals engage in science, mathematics, reading, and, in our case, the development of literate thought. As such, literate thought may be a metaphor for cognition; however, we have just begun the journey, especially with this book, of exploring the possible processes and components associated with this metaphor.

The journey begins with an introduction in Chapter 1 of the multi-faceted concept of literate thought, defined as the ability to think creatively, logically, rationally, and reflectively. We explore the influence of writing on the use of oral (through-the-air) language and as an external aid in the development of thought. We also attempt to clarify the nature of the demands and constraints associated with the use of orality or the oral tradition for an internal representation of reality. More important, it is suggested that other external forms of captured information might be equivalent to or can provide similar benefits as does writing. In the rest of the chapter, we connect literate thought to other diverse domains such as the New and Multiple Literacies, cognitive or disciplinary models, and critico-creative thinking skills.

Chapter 2 explores the notion of comprehension and relates it to the development of literate thought, particularly with respect to the different types of literacy. We argue that additional research is needed on non-print forms of captured information and the manner in which these forms are affected by skills associated with general listening or language comprehension. A portion of the chapter is devoted to delineating a few major processes and components of literate thought. Although it is admitted that literate thought is not an inside-the-head entity only, we maintain that social practices or environmental enrichment activities will not contribute much to its development (or any other cognitive activity) if individuals do not possess the ability to access and interpret these realms of experiences.

Chapter 3 provides insights into the *brave new world* of the New and Multiple Literacies and the impact on our understanding of literate thought and knowledge. The word *literacy* now means more than the ability to read and write given the multitude of terms that have emerged in recent years. Nevertheless, we emphasize a recurring theme—namely that *literacy* should be defined broadly as a form of captured information. We assert that a few print literacy skills are required in certain New and Multiple Literacies activities whereas other New and Multiple Literacies activities do not involve any basic print literacy skills. The chapter concludes with the effects of the New and Multiple Literacies on children with disabilities and those who have traditional language/literacy problems such as English Language Learners (ELLs).

In Chapters 4 and 5, we complete our discussion of the multifaceted concept of literate thought. The focus of Chapter 4 is on the nature of two broad themes and their interactions: cognitive models and discipline structures. After providing a brief introduction to models, structures, processes, and products, we discuss the contributions of cognitive psychology to the acquisition of discipline knowledge in three areas: literacy, mathematics, and science. We emphasize what it means to operate like a literacy expert or to think like a mathematician or scientist. In fact, we are convinced of the need for a better understanding of the structures of the disciplines and the capabilities of individuals to acquire and develop their knowledge in a specific discipline.

The murky, but interesting, world of critico-creative thinking is examined in Chapter 5. The term *critico-creative* combines the concepts of critical thinking and that of creative thinking. There should be a few surprises in this chapter when readers grapple with the various problems and challenges associated with generalizability and evaluation. Regardless of whether one believes in general aspects (i.e., generalizations across domains or subjects) or in specific, disciplinary or domain aspects, we maintain that the underlying values and attitudes associated with critico-creative thinking remain constant across content areas or subjects. Finally, the chapter provides a few examples of instructional exercises ranging from simple to complex. These activities can be developed to be used in through-the-air and captured modes.

Chapters 6 to 8 provide highlights on the challenges of developing literate language in various groups of children with disabilities. The types of disabilities we cover include children with language and/or learning disabilities (Chapter 6), children with sensory disabilities such as visual and hearing impairments (Chapter 7), and children with cognitive and developmental disabilities, including mental retardation and autism (Chapter 8). In each chapter, it is important to describe the characteristics of the population, especially those associated with various subgroups.

A considerable portion of each chapter (6 to 8) is devoted to a synthesis of the literature on the development of English language and literacy to illustrate, in part, the range and depth of these difficulties. Much of the attention is devoted to the development of and problems with reading or script literacy skills because reading has received much emphasis in the schools. Finally, we demonstrate the application of the concepts of the New and Multiple Literacies and conclude with specific implications for developing literate thought.

One of the fastest growing groups of children in K to 12th grade settings is that of children who are English Language Learners (ELLs), as discussed in Chapter 9. These children present enormous challenges for teachers and clinicians. After explaining various terms associated with this population, we synthesize the research on the development and teaching of English focusing on word recognition skills, written language comprehension skills, and motivational factors. We provide highlights on issues such as instruction, programs, and assessment, and we examine the need to consider the effects of sociocultural contexts on literacy achievement. Finally, we conclude with implications for developing literate thought, emphasizing that technology can and should play a major role.

Historically, many educators and scholars have inquired: What is or should be the goal of education? What is or should be the goal of language and literacy programs? Fast forward to the beginning of the twenty-first century. Are we preparing students and others to live in a *brave new world*? It is possible that our students—adolescents and young adults—may turn out to be the *dumbest generation* (Bauerlein, 2008). Even with technological advances and accessibility to information, students expend much of their time and energy on social networking and discovering shortcuts with respect to obtaining and understanding knowledge. In fact, several scholars remarked that most of today's youth (and even a number of adults) exhibit a blatant disregard for deep, serious reading and reflective, rational thinking (Bauerlein; Blackburn, 2005; Specter, 2009).

In our view, the goal of education is to develop literate thought as we remark repeatedly throughout the book and, again, in Chapter 10. We warn about the shortcomings associated with concepts such as functional literacy and the vocationalization of education. With the proliferation of ideas about virtual realities, multiple realities, and possible realities, educators and clinicians need to extend their techniques so that students can handle these different types of realities. This is important for the further development of imagination, intuition, creativity, and, of course, literate thought. In essence, literate thought might be mandatory for survival in a *brave new world*.

REFERENCES

Bauerlein, M. (2008). *The dumbest generation: How the digital age stupefies young Americans and jeopardizes our future (or, don't trust anyone under 30)*. New York: Penguin.

Blackburn, S. (2005). *Truth: A guide*. New York: Oxford University Press.

Isaacson, W. (2007). *Einstein: His life and universe*. New York: Simon & Schuster.

Specter, M. (2009). *Denialism: How irrational thinking hinders scientific progress, harms the planet, and threatens our lives*. New York: Penguin Press.

Acknowledgments

We are indebted to the researchers who provided the findings on which this book is based. We are grateful to both our reviewers for their valuable comments on earlier drafts and Ms. Sara Hann, a graduate student at Missouri State University, for assisting us with the index and literature search. The contributions of the staff at Jones & Bartlett Learning, especially Sean Coombs, Maro Gartside, and David Cella, are also appreciated. Thanks to our spouses and children, who helped to maintain our sanity. The first author would like to acknowledge (again) the guidance of his mentor (now retired), Dr. Stephen P. Quigley. The contributions of a mentor leave a lasting imprint and become even more prominent in one's subsequent scholarly works.

About the Authors

Peter V. Paul, PhD, is a Professor in the School of Teaching and Learning in the College of Education & Human Ecology at the Ohio State University. One of his major responsibilities is teacher education for individuals interested in the education of d/Deaf or hard of hearing students. Dr. Paul's research interests involve the areas of vocabulary, language, and literacy. He has published extensively on language and literacy development. His scholarly texts include *Education and Deafness* (1990), *Toward a Psychology of Deafness* (1993), *Literacy and Deafness* (1998), *Language and Deafness* (2009, 4th ed.), *Reading and Deafness* (2010; with B. Trezek and Y. Wang), and *Hearing and Deafness* (2011). Dr. Paul has conducted workshops for educators and parents on an international, national, state, and local level on topics in literacy and literate thought. He is the current Editor of the *American Annals of the Deaf* (established in 1847), the oldest professional journal in the field of deafness. Dr. Paul has received the College of Education Senior Research Award (2000) and the Richard and Laura Kretschmer National Leadership Award in Hearing Impairment (2010; Ohio School Speech Pathology Educational Audiology Coalition [OSSPEAC]).

Ye Wang, PhD, is an Assistant Professor and Program Coordinator for Education of the Deaf and Hard of Hearing Program in the Department of Communication Sciences and Disorders, Missouri State University. Dr. Wang is a teacher educator preparing teachers of the d/Deaf and hard of hearing students as well as a researcher. Dr. Wang's primary research interest is the language and literacy development of students who are d/Deaf or hard of hearing. Her other research and scholarly interests include multiple literacies, technology and literacy instruction, inclusive education, research methodology, and early childhood education. She has numerous scholarly publications including books, chapters, and peer-reviewed academic journal articles. Dr. Wang has been active as a guest reviewer for several journals as well as a member of the Editorial Board and a guest editor of a special issue for the *American Annals of the Deaf.*

Reviewers

Martha Dunkelberger, PhD, CCC-SLP
Assistant Clinical Professor
Communication Sciences and Disorders
The University of Houston
Houston, TX

Renee Fabus, PhD, CCC-SLP, TSHH
Assistant Professor
Department of Speech Communication Arts and Sciences
Brooklyn College
Brooklyn, NY

Monica Gordon Pershey, EdD, CCC-SLP
Associate Professor and Program Director
Speech and Hearing Program
Department of Health Sciences
Cleveland State University
Cleveland, OH

Deborah M. Haydon, EdD
Associate Professor
Education of the Deaf and Hard of Hearing Program
Eastern Kentucky University
Richmond, KY

Karole Howland, PhD
Clinical Assistant Professor
Speech, Language, and Hearing Sciences
Boston University
Boston, MA

Thomas L. Layton, PhD
ASHA Fellow
Professor
Department of Communications Disorders
North Carolina Central University
Durham, NC

Colleen McAleer, PhD
Department of Communication Sciences and Disorders
Clarion University
Clarion, PA

Wendy McCarty, EdD
Associate Professor
Department of Education
Illinois College
Jacksonville, IL

Johanna Price, PhD, CCC-SLP
Assistant Professor
Department of Speech-Language Pathology
Mississippi University for Women
Columbus, MS

Susan M. Schultz, EdD
Graduate Program Director
Special Education
St. John Fisher College
Rochester, NY

Mary Shea, PhD
Director of Graduate Literacy Programs
Canisius College
Buffalo, NY

CHAPTER 1

Introduction to Literate Thought

Much of modern culture, science and technology would not have been developed without the thought and memory aid of writing. Consider learning or teaching the basics of physics, chemistry, biology, or mathematics without a pencil or blackboard. Worse still, imagine trying to discover the principles involved in these or other subjects from a mass of data that had to be stored and manipulated using only human memory.
Rubin, 1995, p. 308

Many students have difficulty accessing academic content information that, traditionally, has been presented in print. Because much of the information that reflects school knowledge is obtained through printed texts, these students will lag in their knowledge development and not have ample opportunities to develop a high level of literate thought—that is, the ability to reflect upon information, solve problems, or develop other higher-level critical thinking skills. Students need opportunities to think about complex information through a captured mode other than print . . .
Paul & Wang, 2006a, p. 304

The main goal of this book is to introduce professionals and students to the multifaceted concept of literate thought. At first blush, it can be stated simply that literate thought comprises two complex constructs—*literate* and *thought*. Upon further reflection, it might be surmised that literate thought also incorporates aspects from other concepts such as *language*, *literacy*, *cognition*, and *comprehension*.

Traditionally, the term *literate* has been used to describe individuals who possess erudition and can access and interpret printed or written scholarly texts or materials (Olson, 1994; Paul, 2009; Paul & Wang, 2006a). These assertions can be inferred from the above passage by Rubin

(1995), who highlights the thought and memory aid associated with writing. As is discussed later, the process of writing serves several functions, one of which is to facilitate our external representations of reality. Indeed, writing is only one form of an external representation of reality.

It is possible to develop literate thought, or to become literate, in the *through-the-air* or *face-to-face* mode using spoken or sign communication or, specifically, the primary forms of verbal languages. This is implied, in part, in the second passage above by Paul and Wang (2006a). The through-the-air mode is the *real engine* for thought and communication and upon which secondary representations such as print or written language, Braille, and so on, are based (Paul, 2009; Pinker, 1994)—a point that is reiterated throughout this book.

This should not be construed as an *either–or* dichotomy; it is important to develop high levels of thought in both through-the-air and secondary (or captured) modes. In fact, it is doubtful that individuals can reach a competent level of literate thought in the secondary mode without also having competence in the primary or through-the-air mode (Cain & Oakhill, 2007; Nation, 2005; Perfetti, Landi, & Oakhill, 2005). With respect to linguistic and cognitive demands, there are similarities and differences between these two broad modes, as discussed later. Nevertheless, we argue that, in general, literate thought is mode-independent (i.e., not dependent on a specific mode).

In this chapter, we begin our response to at least two broad questions:

1. What does it mean to be literate?

2. What is literate thought?

To address these questions, it is necessary initially to discuss perspectives on writing (as part of literacy), particularly those views related to or implied by the two passages at the beginning of the chapter. The intention is to examine a few basic tenets of external representations and internal representations—the latter of which entails historical background on oral literacy or the oral tradition.

Subsequently, this chapter proceeds to a rendition of the concept of literate or, in this case, a literate mind. Finally, we describe the major requisites and relate literate thought to other areas that include New and Multiple Literacies, psychological and disciplinary models, and critico-creative thinking. These key concepts provide the background and insights into the remainder of this book, including discussions of specific populations of students such as those with language/learning, sensory, and cognitive/developmental disabilities, and those who are English language learners (ELLs).

PERSPECTIVES ON WRITING

Rubin (1995)

Rubin (1995) asserted that, without the benefits associated with writing, it would be extremely labor-intensive to learn, acquire, use, or develop information from complex subjects such as physics, mathematics, and philosophy. Considering the sheer amount of available data in these disciplines, it is difficult to imagine how individuals could solve problems or develop theories if they had to depend on their personal memories without the aid of written language. Reasoning further, it has to be wondered whether religion with its sacred texts, and literature (based on spoken language), in particular, are even possible without writing.

Writing seems to be a tool that assists in the external representations of reality or meaning. External representations can be manifested as outlines, semantic or word maps, advance or graphic organizers, summarizations, syntheses, briefs, reports, and so on. The nature of internal representations (defined as being inside the head, cognitive representations) is often affected by the use and organization of external representations via the use of external aids or apparatus (e.g., pen and paper, computer, etc.). In fact, Rubin (1995) argued that it is doubtful that one can represent information internally (i.e., cognitively) without exposure to an external representation or external activity (e.g., observation of an event, etc.). After the initial exposure or experience, individuals can use their metacognitive (defined as thinking about thinking) skills to develop further their internal representations.

Ong (1982) and others (e.g., Luria, 1976) argued strongly that it is the specific phenomenon of writing (or written language) that made it possible for the complexity and development of thought present in societies that have print and technology. Thus, there would be no serious complex ideas or disciplines if it had not been possible to capture information via the use of typography (print) or chirography (handwriting). Ong expressed the value and influence of writing emphatically:

> Oral cultures indeed produce powerful and beautiful verbal performances of high artistic and human worth, which are no longer even possible once writing has taken possession of the psyche. Nevertheless, without writing, human consciousness cannot achieve its fuller potentials, cannot produce other beautiful and powerful creations. In this sense, orality needs to produce and is destined to produce writing. Literacy, as will be seen, is absolutely necessary for the development not only of science but also of history, philosophy, explicative understanding of literature and of any art, and indeed for the explanation of language (including oral speech) itself. (p. 15)

If we consider carefully the remarks of Ong (1982), we can ask an interesting array of questions. For example, is writing per se responsible for the development of complex disciplines such as science or mathematics? Is writing related to a certain type of complex thought found in societies that have written language or literacy? Does writing affect the further development of spoken (or sign) language? Finally, with respect to one major goal of this book: Is writing (and reading) absolutely indispensable for the development of literate thought?

Before leaving the first passage, it should be highlighted that several scholars, notably, Luria, Ong, and others, have commented on the assertion that writing produces global effects on thinking and memory (e.g., see Olson, 1994; Rubin, 1995). It is now clear—albeit still debatable—that, if there are effects of writing, then these must be considered along with the effects of schooling, which often confound the issue due to the required tasks associated with literacy practices in the classrooms (e.g., answering levels of questions, providing levels of interpretations, and so on; see additional discussions in Scribner & Cole, 1981; Street, 1984). In any case, it might be that writing actually produces specific effects on thinking associated with a specific task such as working on a mathematics problem, composing poetry, or solving language puzzles, rather than global effects on thinking in general.

Paul and Wang (2006a)

Paul and Wang (2006a) offer another position on writing, namely, that it is only one external form of captured information, which can aid the process of thinking during the representation and understanding of reality. This focus is on the product of writing (i.e., what is captured on paper or electronically) and not the process, which these researchers do acknowledge is equally as important. Essentially, this means that there are other external forms of captured information that are equivalent to or can provide similar benefits as does writing (Paul, 2009; Paul & Wang, 2006b; Wang, 2005). Given the range of difficulties that students, particularly students with disabilities, have with print (i.e., reading and writing), which can impede their growth in the development of complex cognition and through-the-air verbal language skills, Paul and Wang (2006a, 2006b) argued for the use of other external forms of captured information, in addition to print, in schools for instructional purposes (see also Chapters 3 and 6 to 9).

A similar analogy has also been made by Walmsley and Allington (1995), who suggested that part of the difference between good and poor or struggling readers and writers can be explained by instructional tasks reflective of weak content and impoverished information. Good readers and writers continue to improve intellectually because they can access challenging texts and are required to perform complex cognitive or metacognitive tasks in both the written and through-the-air modes. On the other hand, poor or struggling readers and writers are exposed to high interest, low vocabulary, easy-reading books and are also engaged in less rigorous, more literal, less-demanding cognitive and linguistic activities in the through-the-air mode.

From another standpoint, using inaccessible print or written language materials predominantly or solely can induce cognitive impoverishment or cognitive deprivation. This assertion has been compared to that of the *Matthew Effects* in reading as described by Stanovich (1986). Stanovich argued that good readers tend to become even better readers and can read to learn mainly via the process of reading voraciously. He labeled this situation as *the rich get richer*. On the other hand, *the poor actually become poorer* in the case of struggling or poor readers.

Poor readers do not read widely or frequently and tend to lag further and further behind their better-reading counterparts. As implied by Warmsley and Allington (1995) as well as Paul and Wang (2006a, 2006b), these readers (and writers) are not provided with opportunities to continue their acquisition of knowledge via the increasing development of their cognitive and metacognitive skills relative to their chronological age levels.

In Paul and Wang's (2006a, 2006b; see also, Wang, 2005) view, print literacy (reading and writing) is not the only road to the development of literate thought. Specifically, writing is not a general, global change agent; rather, writing is one form of captured information which influences the way individuals think and use their memory processes. There are other forms of captured information that do not involve print, such as the use of audiobooks (on CDs or DVDs) or videobooks (i.e., signing books on DVDs). Whether these *alternative* forms of captured information are equivalent to writing (process- and product-wise) is an open debate (see also, the discussion in Chapters 2 and 3). If so, then they can also serve, at the least, as external aids for thought and memory, and this would have pervasive educational or instructional implications for children and adolescents, particularly the ones who struggle immensely with information presented in print or written language venues.

Writing and External Representation

To recap, there are two broad types of representation—external and internal—and both are comprised of or influenced by cognitive and social processes, practices, strategies, and so on. As mentioned previously, external representations refer to processes and products outside the head whereas internal representations refer to actions inside the head.

We have argued that writing is one tool for producing and representing information externally. It aids in the development of memory and thinking and reduces the demands on memory to permit reflection and refinement. A complex process notwithstanding, writing can be viewed as one external form of captured information.

To minimize confusion, it is important to emphasize that we have labeled writing as one type of captured information. As discussed further in this book (see Chapters 2 and 3), writing is a reflection—albeit roughly—of the sounds of speech and even influences how one thinks about one's spoken language. Through writing, individuals can learn and develop a better and deeper understanding of intricacies related to phonology and other language components. Writing is also a form of communication and is driven by the activities of one's spoken language and cognition. Individuals write to convey what they know and to figure out (or construct) what it is that they think they know. Thus, writing is a mechanism for constructing meaning and reality—albeit it is not the only mechanism for this purpose.

Table 1-1 provides a summary of the broad views of writing.

Table 1-1. Highlights of Views of Writing

One View of Writing
- Without the benefits (i.e., as an aid for thought and memory) associated with writing, it would be extremely difficult to learn, acquire, use, or develop information from complex subjects such as physics, mathematics, and philosophy.
- If there are effects of writing, then these must be considered along with the effects of schooling, which often confounds the issue due to the required tasks associated with literacy in the classrooms.
- Writing produces specific effects on thinking associated with a specific task such as working on a mathematics problem, writing a poem, or solving a logic problem, rather than global effects on thinking in general.

A Second View of Writing
- The use of print literacy predominantly or solely with poor or struggling readers/writers can induce cognitive impoverishment or cognitive deprivation.
- Writing is only one form of captured information, which can and does influence the way individuals think and use their memory processes. There are other forms of captured information, not involving print, such as the use of audiobooks (on CDs or DVDs) or the use of videobooks (i.e., signing books on DVDs).

Additional Remarks on Writing
- Writing is a representation—albeit roughly—of the sounds of speech or of the spoken language and even influences how one thinks about one's spoken language.
- Via writing, individuals can learn and develop a better and deeper understanding of the intricacies of their spoken language (e.g., its phonology, morphology, syntax, and its use to express ideas and so on).
- Writing is a form of communication and is driven by the activities of one's spoken language and cognition. Individuals write to convey what they know and write to figure out (or construct) what it is that they think they know.

ORALITY AND INTERNAL REPRESENTATION

As mentioned previously, literate thought can be developed in the spoken (or sign) language mode as well—that is, via the processes and products associated with the use of face-to-face or through-the-air communicative interactions, which may not be captured or represented externally (e.g., by external aids such as paper and pencil, etc.). Although this type of literate thought is or can be complex, it is different from the type of thought that is aided by writing or any other external aid. This becomes evident in a discussion on orality or the oral tradition (Denny, 1991; Feldman, 1991; Olson, 1989, 1991; Rubin, 1995).

In describing orality, it should be possible to begin to conceptualize what it means to be literate—in the broad sense—that is, in a sense that transcends traditional literacy skills (e.g., reading and writing). The emphasis here is on the construction of internal representations of reality or meaning. There are constraints associated with the use of this mode (i.e., the limitations of human memory and cognitive processes).

To understand the issues of orality and constraints, let us start with Bruner (1986), who argued that there are basically two processes of thought or cognitive functioning that can be used to construct a model of reality or of meaning about events. One can be labeled the *narrative* and the other is the *logical argument*. Although both processes are complementary, each cannot be reduced to the other because they are radically different. Specifically, they are different with respect to their criteria for quality, creativity, and coherence.

In general, *logical argument* is most useful for the development of theories, laws, and other abstract entities, and requires external representational aids to be most effective. In contrast, the *narrative* functioning deals mostly with concrete ideas and events and is dependent on human memory and thinking within an internal mode of representation (i.e., inside the head). In other words, meaning is typically conveyed through the use of concrete, observable actions set in the realm of the narrative; there is no penchant for the deep, layered abstract representations of truths (Olson, 1994; Ong, 1982; Rubin, 1995).

As a consequence, the narrative is the predominant or sole form of cognitive functioning in the oral tradition or orality (particularly in nonliterate or nonprint cultures). How does the use of orality work? How do individuals construct meaning or reality via remembering situations, events, and dialogues in the oral mode? There have been attempts to analyze the oral tradition within the structure of psychological models such as schemas, scripts, story grammars, and other various comprehension models (Olson, 1994; Rubin, 1995; see also the discussions of several reading and comprehension models in Israel & Duffy, 2009; Paul, 2001, 2009).

In short, the oral traditions rely on themes presented in a narrative that emphasizes the use of words, which are rhythmic or cohere in some fashion (e.g., ballads, songs, mnemonic or visual imagery) to aid in the internal representation of meaning or reality. Although the recall of the message is serial, the message itself is constrained by the organization of meaning, imagery, and even by the patterns of sounds (Olson, 1994; Ong, 1982; Rubin, 1995). With respect to the constraints of rhythm, for example, Rubin remarked that:

> . . . rhythm functions like other constraints or forms of organization to limit word choice, in this case to words with the correct number of syllables or stress patterns. In addition, the rhythm provides a global organization, allowing singers to select, substitute, and add or delete whole rhythmic units (e.g., verses) and still continue. Rhythm also emphasizes certain locations within lines, which facilitates other constraints, such as the placing of rhyme and alliteration on stressed syllables. (pp. 11-12)

There is little question that the use of the oral mode establishes constraints on thinking and memory because it does not employ the use of external representations. However, this does not mean that orality is not as complex as literacy (i.e., writing) or does not involve the use of genres (e.g., fiction, nonfiction). Although it has been argued that writing has led to the separation of text and the interpretation of the message associated with the text, this is also the case in the use of orality (Denny, 1991; Feldman, 1991; Olson, 1989, 1994). Thus, it is possible to develop literate thought in the oral mode, especially if individuals can access the message and reflect on it to provide interpretations by constructing a range or layers of meanings. Such endeavors are affected by the quality of one's cognition, particularly one's ability to remember, store, organize, and retrieve information, ranging from the simple to the complex.

Consider the following scenario as support for the above assertions. Prior to and even after the invention of the printing press, a substantial number of individuals still depended on others to convey information through the use of the oral mode (Olson, 1989). Individuals, designated as *readers*, would present the latest news, rulings, or nuanced information by reading the script to a specific community in a specific location. These readers did not participate in the discussion or debate—this was reserved for the group of listeners. The tasks of the reader (or, possibly someone else) were to read the document, reread it if necessary, and to record the major points or reactions offered by the community of listeners. The listeners had to use their memories to debate the main points or to pass on important information to others.

The learning of trades was conducted primarily through oral discussions and apprenticeships. To develop the skills of a cobbler, for example, an individual would shadow the activities of an actual cobbler, first observing and listening intently to the wisdom of the master and then taking on and accomplishing increasingly difficult tasks until full mastery. Observation and apprenticeship are considered to be applicable even for modern occupations (e.g., teachers, doctors, etc.), albeit these vocations are usually accompanied by printed works.

In essence, anthropological data demonstrate that—similar to writing—oral genres also represent a separation of text and interpretation, which permits reflection and abstraction (Feldman, 1991; Olson, 1989, 1994). The separation of the content from the interpretation of the text is critical for the development of literate thought (or any other type of reflective or critical thinking). This separation is often said to represent the compelling power and influence of writing (see Chapter 3).

The quality of literate thought associated with orality can be quite different from that which entails the use of external representations such as writing. This is due to the limitations and constraints of internal representations versus those of external representations. It has been demonstrated that oral cultures that exist within a larger mainstream culture with print literacy are quite different from oral cultures within a larger society that is virtually nonliterate or does not possess print literacy (Olson, 1994; Rubin, 1995). Individuals are affected by the conditions of literacy (i.e., writing), and this shapes their thinking about and use of information in the oral traditional mode within the larger literate (i.e., print-based) society. This influence can be seen in the organization and presentation of the information in the traditional oral mode; that is, individuals have developed a complex, nuanced use of spoken language, resulting in a rather sophisticated organization and presentation of their thoughts (e.g., larger vocabulary, longer sentences, more complicated, difficult ideas, etc.). In the rest of the book, we examine further the concept of representation, both internally and externally.

Table 1-2 provides a summary of major points for the oral tradition or orality.

Table 1-2.   Highlights of the Oral Tradition or Orality

Orality and Internal Representation

- The narrative is the predominant or sole form of cognitive functioning in the oral tradition or orality (particularly in nonliterate or nonprint cultures).
- The narrative deals mostly with concrete ideas and events and is dependent on human memory and thinking within an internal mode of representation, that is, inside the head. In other words, meaning is conveyed through the use of concrete, observable actions set in the realm of the narrative; there is no penchant for the abstract representations of truths.
- The oral traditions rely on themes presented in a narrative that emphasizes the use of words that are rhythmic or cohere in some fashion (e.g., ballads, songs, mnemonic or visual imagery) to aid in the internal representation of meaning or reality.
- There is little question that the use of the oral mode establishes constraints on thinking and memory, especially because it does not employ the use of external representations.
- Orality is as complex as literacy (i.e., writing) and also involves the separation of text and the interpretation of the message.

LITERATE MIND

We have reached the point where we can provide an initial response to one of our two questions presented at the beginning of the chapter: What does it mean to be *literate*? Or, to put it metaphorically, what does it mean to possess a literate mind? The concept literate should be compared to that of *illiterate*. Similar to other ill-structured, slippery, complex notions, it is difficult to define or even describe these terms adequately.

Let us start by stating that literate, or having a literate mind, refers to an individual's ability to access (e.g., perceive visually or auditorally) and interpret (comprehend, apply, etc.) learned (e.g., serious, scholarly, academic, nuanced) information either through-the-air or in captured modes. This is a rather simple description, but it broadens the traditional concept of being literate as well as that of illiterate, especially if the focus is on captured forms of information.

Historically, literate and illiterate have been associated with only print literacy. Traditionally, if a person was considered literate, then this meant that s/he could access and interpret information captured in the print or written mode. Conversely, if a person was labeled illiterate, then s/he could not access and interpret information captured in the print mode at a certain literacy level in society (e.g., functional literacy).

These traditional descriptions present problems when considering historical figures such as Socrates and Homer. Socrates did not read or write anything; his philosophy was recorded (i.e., written) by one of his most famous pupils, Plato (e.g., see discussion in Copleston, 1985). Homer, the exemplar for the oral tradition or orality, was blind; as one account goes, he dictated his most famous stories [poems] (e.g., *The Illiad*, *The Odessey*) to his listeners with one or more persons recording (writing down) what he said.

There are several controversies regarding the historical Homer as well as the manner involving the composition of his poems. In any case, given the constraints of human memory, Homer is purported to have begun each new episode by synthesizing or summarizing the events of the previous one. This is distracting to most individuals who read, for example, *The Illiad*. Nevertheless, it is hypothesized that Homer employed this technique to ensure that he remembered where he left off by asking if his listeners concurred with his summary (Homer, 1898).

It would be shortsighted or, perhaps, erroneous to label either Socrates or Homer as illiterate. For that matter, it would be narrow to label individuals who are blind or severely dyslexic as illiterate if they have been able to access print information in alternative formats such as audiobooks or videobooks (Braille literacy is a special condition, which is discussed in Chapter 7). The above situations require a reconceptualization of the notions of literate and illiterate in light of what is required to develop literate thought, especially in a captured mode.

An individual who possesses a literate mind or is literate is able to engage in reflective or literate thinking (i.e., reasoning, etc.) on a range of learned information in any type of mode. Within this framework, a person is illiterate if s/he cannot access and interpret learned information in any mode—not just via the print mode. Thus, let us suppose that a person can access and interpret *Moby-Dick* via an audiobook mode but not via the print mode. This person is still considered literate, in our view.

At the least, we should describe the modes, through-the-air or captured, in which an individual is considered literate or illiterate, rather than simply label someone as being literate or illiterate in general. This leads to our second question posed at the beginning of the chapter: What is literate thought?

LITERATE THOUGHT

In previous publications (Paul, 1998, 2001, 2006, 2009; Paul & Wang, 2006a, 2006b; Wang, 2005), literate thought has been described as the ability to think creatively, critically, logically, rationally, and reflectively on information presented in either a through-the-air mode or captured or preserved as in print, CD, or DVD. Admittedly, this is a rather vague description, given the slippery or ill-structured concepts contained in the description, namely, *creativity, criticism, logic, rationality,* and *reflectivity.* However, it will become clear that literate thought involves—but is more than—what Bruner (1986) has termed *logical argument* and what others have labeled *metacognition* (Baker & Brown, 1984) or *critico-creative thinking* (Norris, 1992).

At the least, literate thought incorporates three types of thinking—*critical, imaginative,* and *wild*—often used to create new ideas or to solve problems in diverse areas such as science, art, and philosophy (see discussion in Beveridge, 1980). There is no doubt that *thinking* is difficult to define or describe as it is also slippery or can be labeled as an ill-structured or ill-defined concept. Thinking can be random or organized; it can be creative, critical, logical, rational, and reflective—similar to the description of literate thought provided earlier.

It seems that thinking is too ambiguous and that it might be unproductive to inquire about thinking in general. For example, it has been argued that the focus of the development of critical thinking—or any other type of structured, deliberate, reflective thinking—should be within a specific discipline or content area, albeit some attention can be given to the development of general thinking skills (Kuhn, 2005; Norris, 1992; see also, Chapter 5). Consider this example: Chess players are good with a certain type of thinking related to the game such as planning ahead, visualizing moves, examining board positions quickly, and so on. This does not mean that chess players can use the same skills effectively in other domains that require similar areas of expertise. In fact, there seems to be evidence that chess players cannot perform as well beyond the constraints of the game of chess (Rubin, 1995; see also, Tulving & Craik, 2000).

The concept of thinking has interested scholars and philosophers for centuries. Dewey (1933) expounded on the various types of thinking, especially a type of thinking that is most effective for and should be the main goal of education—reflective thinking or reflective thought. Dewey's description is probably most applicable to the emphasis of this book—albeit he seemed to highlight critical thinking skills and the use of a scientific approach in his rendition of reflective thought:

> Active, persistent, and careful consideration of any belief or supposed form of knowledge in the light of the grounds that support it and the further conclusions to which it tends constitutes *reflective thought.* (p. 9)

One perspective on a few components, activities, and processes associated with literate thought has been captured somewhat by the description of *creative cognition* by Smith (1995, p. 33):

> Creative cognition involves many complex mental activities, such as formulating and reconceptualizing problems, generating divergent ideas, transcending mental blocks, visualizing, exploring ideas, discovering interesting combinations of ideas, using and adapting one's expert knowledge, discovering insight, and refining ideas. Examples of basic cognitive processes that underlie these activities include encoding, storage and retrieval of information, attention, mental imaging, conceptualization, analogical reasoning and rule-based thinking, and metacognition.

If a coherent, adequate understanding of literate thought is to be developed, then it is necessary to construct a model or a narrative compilation of strategies or skills that incorporates findings from several domains that have been researched such as language, literacy, cognition, and comprehension—domains mentioned at the beginning of this chapter (Israel & Duffy, 2009; Kintsch, 1998; Kintsch & Rawson, 2005). Literate thought, similar to the construct of comprehension, needs to be understood from a multiple-perspective, multifaceted view. The focus in this chapter is on describing briefly three broad requisites and on highlighting the issue of decontextualized literate language.

Requisites of Literate Thought

There are three broad requisites of literate thought (Paul, 2001, 2009; Paul & Wang, 2006a, 2006b; Wang, 2005):

1. Adequate proficiency in a bona fide language;

2. Understanding and application of a metalanguage or specialized vocabulary associated with a specific discipline or area and with general society or culture; and,

3. Ability to access and interpret decontextualized literate language.

Other factors to consider include overall cognitive ability, experience, the affective domain, and so on. Nevertheless, the above three broad requisites are of importance and relevance here.

Literate thought is not an all-or-nothing phenomenon. The development of or proficiency in the three major areas above is not an all-or-nothing phenomenon either. This is instructive to remember when working with children with disabilities or those who are English language learners (ELLs), who exhibit a wide range of experiences as well as varying levels of proficiency in the use of English, both in the spoken and written modes.

Bona Fide Language

To describe briefly what it means to possess a bona fide language is a challenging task, given the myriad of theories and models that exist, involving either cognitive, social, or environmental/behavioral factors and their computations or combinations (Lund, 2003; Paul, 2001, 2009; Pence & Justice, 2008). A simplified view is offered here: Possessing a bona fide language should mean that an individual has developed a level of proficiency in the integrative use of the major language components such as phonology, morphology, syntax, semantics, and pragmatics (for a detailed description of these components and language development, see Crystal, 1995, 1997, 2006; Pence & Justice). Most children develop an adequate language level by the time they start formal schooling—at about age 5 or 6—with the more difficult aspects of phonology accomplished by age 8 or so.

There is little argument that an adequate level of proficiency in a language—however this is defined or described—is critical for the subsequent development of print literacy skills (reading and writing), for an understanding of disciplines such as mathematics and science, and for continued growth in cognition and metacognition (McGuinness, 2004, 2005). Nevertheless, there is more to reading, writing, and content knowledge than just possessing language skills. In a similar vein, possessing a bona fide language is necessary, but not sufficient, for literate thought.

Metalanguage

The second major requisite for the development of literate thought is the acquisition and use of a metalanguage. The term *metalanguage*—as used here—refers to the specialized (or *rare*) vocabulary or terminology, often associated with a particular discipline, content area, or topic. For example, to develop a deep understanding of the game of baseball, individuals need a working knowledge or familiarity of terms such as *balk, bean ball, bunt, double play, fielder's choice, forced play, hit, hit-and-run, home run, pitch out, run-batted-in, spit ball, steal, suicide bunt,* and so on. It also helps to be knowledgeable about the rules of the game of baseball.

It is critical to understand these terms as they are applicable to events in a baseball game. For example, in everyday colloquial usage, the word *theory* has a more general meaning than that which occurs in scientific disciplines. These colloquial usages can cause problems for individuals when they encounter the manner in which such terminology is used in specialized disciplines or content areas (for related discussions, see Baker & Brown, 1984; Israel & Duffy, 2009; Pearson & Fielding, 1991; Pearson & Stephens, 1994).

Another perspective on metalanguage can be gleaned from the controversial work of Hirsch and his colleagues (Hirsch, 1987; Hirsch, Kett, & Trefil, 2002). Hirsch has argued that the development of reading, particularly critical reading in general and in specific content areas such as physics, mathematics, and so on, is dependent on a working knowledge or familiarity of terminology or concepts in the wider culture of society. This has been coined *cultural literacy* (Hirsch; Hirsch, Kett, & Trefil).

Returning to our game of baseball, consider the following statement:

> *Both the trajectory and spin of the knuckleball are most effective if the velocity of the pitch does not exceed 100 kilometers per hour. Otherwise, the movement is not sufficiently erratic or fluttery, making it somewhat easier for the batter to hit the ball.*

To comprehend the above statement, an individual needs an understanding of basic terms in mathematics and physics as well as basic terms in the topic of baseball. In fact, the use of vocabulary and concepts from other fields or disciplines tends to deepen and broaden the understanding of a particular topic. This use is common in school settings and even in academic texts or materials (Hirsch, 1987; Hirsch, Kett, & Trefil, 2002). In sum, both a specialized and broad metalanguage is important for the development of literate thought.

Decontextualized Literate Language

The third major requisite for literate thought is proficiency in handling decontextualized literate language. Typically, decontextualization should be contrasted with contextualization. In both situations, however, one can use literate language, albeit contextualization provides more support to aid with understanding or comprehension.

Let us consider contextualization. Spoken (or signed) communicative exchanges can occur in through-the-air or face-to-face contexts. Such exchanges are considered natural (i.e., typical manner for receiving and expressing information) and redundant (i.e., the use of overlapping cues—verbal and nonverbal—to minimize misunderstandings). For example, if there is a breakdown in communication, individuals might repeat the statement, gesture or pantomime, rephrase the statement by using different words or paraphrase, or use concrete examples, demonstrations, or explanations with visual supports (e.g., pictures, objects, graphic designs, etc.).

Contextualized language is grounded in the immediate context—the here-and-now, the concrete and visible. It is presumed that the sender (speaker, signer) and receiver (listener, watcher) share basic background experiences or knowledge and a common language related to the topic of conversation.

Up until the preschool years, the language and interactions of children and parents is predominantly contextual with a minimal use of literate or even abstract expressions. Consider the following example.

Parent: *This is an elephant (showing a picture). Tomorrow, we will go to the zoo and see lots of animals. The elephant is one animal that we will see. Let's look at the elephant. Here's the elephant's nose (pointing to the trunk of the elephant). It is also called a trunk. Now you point to the elephant's nose.*

Child: *[Points to the elephant's trunk].*

Parent: *The elephant has four legs. Can you point to the legs?*

Child: *[Points to each of the four legs]. That's a tail! [Pointing to the tail of the elephant].*

Parent: *Yes, that is the elephant's tail. The tail is long [uses finger to trace the length of the tail].*

Decontextualization refers to situations that have been removed from context (i.e., not live or current) and that have been captured such as in print, audio, or video. Thus, materials in print such as textbooks, children's literature, or audiobooks, and videobooks are examples of decontextualization. If we capture the above exchange between the parent and child in print or on a DVD with audio (and no print), this would become a decontextualized event with the use of contextualized language. Even though the event is captured, it should be fairly easy for children (or anyone else) to understand.

On the other hand, most of the information in school or learned situations presented in either the face-to-face mode (e.g., lectures, discussions, debates, etc.) or in the captured mode (e.g., in print texts or videos) contains decontextualized *literate language*. This type of language relies heavily on the use and understanding of language itself, in order for individuals to construct meaning of the topics of conversations or the meaning of texts (i.e., captured information). Consider the following example of literate language use, which can be presented in context (i.e., live or current) or captured and decontextualized in print (as it is here) or on videotape.

Teacher: *Today, we are going to discuss the American Civil War. You have been reading about the Civil War for the past week. Yesterday, someone said that the Civil War was similar to another event in American history. Does anyone remember what was discussed?*

Student: *Yes, Jane said that the American Revolution should actually be considered a civil war. Because America was still part of Great Britain, this revolution was actually a civil war.*

Teacher: *Very good! Now let's discuss the causes of the Civil War. Then, for fun, we can compare the causes of the Civil War with the causes of the American Revolution. Despite the similarity between these two conflicts, they do have different causes or maybe not.*

Much of the academic learning and success in schools requires the development and use of decontextualized literate language (Bailey, 2007;

Shanahan, 2009). And, much of this information is presented via written materials or print. In academic settings, the interactions involve participants (e.g., students, readers) who have read, listened to, or viewed a text and are requested to perform specific tasks such as taking a test, retelling a story, answering questions, or relating, sharing, or discussing/debating the information.

Table 1-3 provides a few principles related to the use of decontextualized and contextualized language.

Table 1-3. Characteristics of Decontextualized and Contextualized Language

---

Decontextualized Language
- The construction of meaning involves the use of literate language with the dialogue and other elements being independent of the communicative context or situation.
- Comprehension is dependent on proficiency in the language utilized, including the structures.
- Much of the language used in classroom situations and in academic texts is reflective of decontextualized language.
- In general, the nature of shared knowledge and experiences is not explicit; thus, there are cognitive and experiential demands placed on the reader or listener.
- Comprehension or understanding is facilitated by knowledge of the metalanguage of specific topics and, sometimes, by knowledge of the general metalanguage associated with general societal usage (as in cultural literacy).

Contextualized Language
- Comprehension of the message is supported by redundancies and other cues associated with interpersonal communications or interactions (e.g., repetitions, paraphrasing, non-verbal cues, etc.).
- The construction of meaning or understanding is a process of negotiation between the speaker/signer and the listener/watcher.
- This type of language is reflective of everyday, nonacademic conversations or dialogues and is often used predominantly with young children or those for whom English is not a first language (in the initial stages).
- Nonlinguistic and situational or context cues are critical and present in this type of language use.
- Shared background knowledge and experiences and shared language are present.
- Focus is on the *here-and-now*, the concrete.

LITERATE THOUGHT AND OTHER DOMAINS

To render a more complete description of literate thought, it is indispensable to become familiar with basic information from other related domains. For example, in the subsequent chapters of this book, we synthesize a few salient theoretical and research findings from ill-structured, seemingly diverse areas such as the New and Multiple Literacies (Chapter 3), cognitive and disciplinary models (Chapter 4), and critico-creative thinking (Chapter 5). Taken together, we assert that the goal of education is to develop literate and critical thinking skills (see also, Kuhn, 2005). Brief introductory descriptions of these areas are presented below.

New and Multiple Literacies

There has been a proliferation of *literacy* terms emulating from the concept of the New and Multiple Literacies (Bloome & Paul, 2006; Paul, 2006). For sure, the meaning of the word *literacy* is now broader than possessing the ability to read or write (see Chapter 3). Influenced by the New and Multiple Literacies (defined as digital media literacy, for example, e-books, hand-held devices such as wireless phones, Blackberries, iPad and other microcomputers) and sociocultural models of literacy (e.g., Israel & Duffy, 2009), we have a growing scholarly field called *Literacy Studies*.

Literacy Studies is not concerned with the development of specific skills in literacy, that is, reading and writing. Rather, the focus is on the social contacts of individuals with the various forms of literacy. Theorists and researchers are interested in the roles that literacy (the broad view) plays in the lives of individuals within social institutions such as schools, places of worship, and other locations (e.g., restaurants, etc.) in communities. Knowledge of literacy practices, contexts, and other aspects of language use (speaking, signing, etc.) results from the social construction of reality—the main epistemology of this field (see Noddings, 1995; Phillips & Soltis, 2004; Pring, 2004; Ritzer, 2001, for accessible descriptions of social constructivism).

Tyner (1998) provided one framework for categorizing the multitude of literacy-related terms that have emerged from the New and Multiple Literacies. She has categorized two groups of literacies: tool literacies and literacies of representation (see also, Chapter 3). *Tool literacies* refer to those entities that are used to manipulate information such as computer literacy and technological literacy (e.g., text messaging, etc.). *Literacies of representation* entail specific domains of information or knowledge such as mathematics literacy, medical literacy, and legal literacy as well as the traditional print or script literacy. Other examples of literacies of representation are discussed later in this text.

In Chapter 3, the impact and contribution of the New and Multiple Literacies are explored with respect to understanding literate thought. These new types of literacies seem to challenge our current assumptions of knowledge—especially knowledge generated by behavioral or cognitive frameworks. The effects or implications of the New and Multiple Literacies on the development of literate thought in children with disabilities or those who are English language learners are examined more extensively in Chapters 6 to 9.

Cognitive and Disciplinary Structures

There is no doubt that literate thought has been influenced predominantly by cognitive models of language and knowledge, albeit contributions from social and cultural viewpoints are acknowledged in this book. In Chapter 4, the emphasis is on two broad domains: cognitive models and disciplinary structures (see also Phillips & Soltis, 2004). There are clearly other viable cognitive domains, which are mentioned in this text; however, the above two domains offer critical insights pertinent to our interests.

Cognitive models are concerned with the manner in which individuals construct or develop their understanding of topics and ideas in their environment (Phillips & Soltis, 2004). The influence of the childhood development models of Piaget and Vygotsky, and other theories on cognitive information-processing and cognitive flexibility are also discussed. From one standpoint, the *name* of the cognitive model might not be critical given that there are a preponderant number of positions ranging from predominantly cognitive to cognitive social (Lund, 2003; Pence & Justice, 2008; Phillips & Soltis, 2004). Rather, what needs to be explicated is the fact that individuals are actively involved in the cognitive *construction* of meaning or reality (Israel & Duffy, 2009). Such construction is influenced pervasively by a number of factors, including the relationship between language and thought.

The construct of disciplinary structures poses epistemological challenges for theorists, researchers, and practitioners (Donovan & Bransford,

2005; Israel & Duffy, 2009; Phillips & Soltis, 2004). It can be debated whether a discipline such as mathematics or science has a structure (often called knowledge structure). It seems clear that, for example, some mathematical concepts are easier than others and are often acquired or learned early. Intuitively—and there is some supportive research—any particular discipline seems to have a structure with concepts on varying difficulty levels. Thus, an individual may need to understand a piece of information at one stage before proceeding to learning information in the next stage. With respect to mathematics, one needs to understand addition prior to engaging in multiplication.

The work of Rand Spiro on cognitive flexibility (e.g., Spiro, Collins, & Ramchandran, 2007; Spiro, Vispoel, Schmitz, Samarapungavan, & Boerger, 1987; see also, Cartwright, 2009) provides a different, perhaps differentiating, perspective on this issue. Spiro and his colleagues argue that a distinction needs to be made between well-structured disciplines such as science and mathematics and ill-structured ones such as history and philosophy. Inadvertently, this seems to be a distinction between the so-called *hard* sciences and the *soft* disciplines.

In our view, there is a range of structures from well-organized to loosely-organized within all disciplines. It seems that disciplines such as physics and chemistry contain more well-structured concepts that can be arranged hierarchically with respect to levels of difficulty. On the other hand, sociology and education possess mostly ill-structured concepts, which certainly have coherence but not strict levels of difficulty. The overall type of structure associated with a discipline may be reflective of its status as a *science*, with regard to the accumulation of knowledge or the rendition of logical arguments (Noddings, 1995; Pring, 2004; Ritzer, 2001). In any case, the notion of disciplinary structure does impact the nature and development of literate thought.

To develop high levels of literate thought, we argue that there needs to be a match between the *level* of cognitive development of the individual and the *difficulty* of the required tasks associated with the structure of the discipline. Most breakdowns in learning in school and clinical settings are due to mismatches between these two broad entities. Thus, a certain degree of understanding seems to be necessary for fostering effective instructional or clinical practices (Fenstermacher & Soltis, 2004; Phillips & Soltis, 2004). Specifically, there are formidable challenges for educators and clinicians in considering this issue for children with disabilities or for children who are English language learners.

Critico-Creative Thinking

Another aspect of literate thought is the ability to engage in critical or critico-creative thinking. By now, it should not be a surprise that it is difficult to define or describe critico-creative thinking because it is also an ill-structured domain (Norris, 1992). To borrow Spiro's rendition of a Wittgenstein phrase, critico-creative thinking requires crisscrossing-the-landscape strategies (Spiro et al., 2007; Spiro et al., 1987; see also, Cartwright, 2009). This means that it is critical to access multiple cognitive features (strategies, perspectives, skills) for addressing and resolving problems from multiple perspectives.

In Chapter 5, we examine whether it is possible to develop general critical thinking skills or whether these skills need to be related to a specific discipline such as mathematics, science, social studies, psychology, and so on. It might be that skills in one domain do not apply indiscriminately to working on problems in another domain. On the other hand, it has been argued that there are general guidelines for developing thinking skills with the most robust example being the application of the concept of metacognition from reading to all other content areas, especially mathematics and science (Baker & Beall, 2009; Donovan & Bransford, 2005; Paris & Stahl, 2005).

One of the most challenging topics is the evaluation of critico-creative thinking. What does it mean to be an effective critico-creative thinker? Who makes this determination and how? It seems that—at the least—individuals need a deep understanding of a specific topic or content area in order to develop skills associated with being a critical thinker in that topic or content area.

Possessing a deep understanding is necessary, but not sufficient for critico-creative thinking. Individuals also need to examine critically all prominent views—including contradictory ones—on a particular position or topic in a particular domain. After much dialogue and reflection, one can state his or her current position, which should always be tentative (see, e.g., reflective thinking or thought in Dewey, 1933). This is considered the strong version of critico-creative thinking (Applegate, Quin, & Applegate, 2008; Brown & Keeley, 2007; Flage, 2004; Halpern, 1997; Kuhn, 2005). The strong version leads or should lead to a refinement or further development of one's thinking.

There is also a weak version of critico-creative thinking in which the objective is simply to defend one's view against the attacks of others. In essence, one's view does not or might not actually change or evolve in this situation (Applegate, Quin, & Applegate, 2008; Brown & Keeley, 2007; Flage, 2004; Halpern, 1997; Kuhn, 2005). This can lead to what has been labeled paradigm inflexibility or paradigm incommensurability (Kuhn, 1996; Nickles, 2003), resulting in substantial ongoing conflicts within disciplines or between individuals holding different worldviews (Noddings, 1995; Phillips & Soltis, 2004; Pring, 2004; Ritzer, 2001).

Obviously, labeling critico-creative thinking as strong, weak, or some other descriptor is open to interpretation. Critico-creative thinking seems to involve reasoning, problem solving, deductive or inductive thinking, hypothesis testing, and other skills. Regardless of the type of critico-creative thinking and despite the difficulties in defining and evaluating it, many educators seem to believe that this is an important skill to develop, especially in the content areas. Ironically, critico-creative thinking may be related to one's conception of the structure of a discipline, including its methodology and research approaches.

EDUCATION FOR THINKING AND THE FUTURE

There have been numerous debates on the grand aim of formal education or schooling (Fenstermacher & Soltis, 2004; Noddings, 1995; Pring, 2004; Rippa, 1997). These debates have been influenced by the status of education and educational research within the university and the academic community. The following question has been debated vociferously: Is education a science, an art, or something else (Pring, 2004)? Whatever education is, there has been a wide proliferation of goals, ranging from the basic development of the three Rs (reading, writing, and arithmetic) to the lofty goal of assisting individuals to be meaningfully engaged in a participatory democracy (Fenstermacher & Soltis; Noddings; Pring; Rippa).

Kuhn (2005) reiterates some of these goals in her book, but settles on the goal of developing critical thinking skills, particularly inquiry and argument skills, as the most important aim of education. We concur with her main points; nevertheless, in our view, the goal of education should be to develop literate thought, and this is reiterated in Chapter 10.

Literate thought has cognitive, social, and affective dimensions; nevertheless, literate thinking—indeed all forms of reflective thinking—is predominantly an individual activity. Students—including those with disabilities and those who are ELLs—need to be encouraged to develop higher levels of literate thinking with respect to any particular topic, discipline, or area of interest in school and social settings. All students can develop and improve in the area of literate thought. A number of students require a tremendous amount of assistance, opportunities, and encouragement, especially if one corollary is to help students become independent thinkers.

What does the future look like? What will be the nature of an effective literate-thinking person? Much of the focus has been on methods such as employing the scientific approach and reflecting on or understanding an empirical reality. However, this view may be shortsighted. With the proliferation of ideas about virtual realities, multiple realities, and possible realities, educators and clinicians need to extend their strategies so that students can handle these different types of realities.

In one sense, as discussed in Chapter 10, we might need a new dose of the *humanities* within all of the content areas or disciplines. Indeed, the approaches and attitudes associated with the humanities seem to be important not only for critical or reflective thinking but also for a type of thinking labeled as *wild* (or *imaginative*), mentioned previously (Beveridge, 1980). In any case, the focus should be on the development of imagination, intuition, creativity, and, of course, literate thought. In fact, all of these skills might be mandatory for survival in a *brave new world*.

SUMMARY

The intent of this chapter is to introduce the reader to the concepts of literate thought and related issues. We provide a few underpinnings of literate thought and connect this construct to others such as the New and Multiple Literacies, cognitive and disciplinary models, and critico-creative thinking.

A few major points are:

- The capacity to think and the manner of thinking have been influenced by the invention of writing. As an external aid to thought and memory, writing facilitates thinking and permits reflection and interpretation of texts.

- Writing produces specific effects on thinking associated with a specific task such as working on a mathematics problem, writing a poem, or solving a logic problem, rather than global effects on thinking in general.
- Other external forms of captured information are, might be equivalent to, or can provide similar benefits as does writing. Examples include audio books and videobooks (without the accompaniment of print).
- Given the range of difficulties that students, particularly students with disabilities, have with print (i.e., reading and writing), which can impede their growth in the development of complex cognition (or thinking skills), it is critical to use other external forms of captured information, in addition to print, in schools for instructional purposes.
- The oral traditions rely on themes presented in a narrative type of cognitive functioning that emphasizes the use of words that are rhythmic or cohere in some fashion (e.g., ballads, songs, mnemonic or visual imagery) to aid in the internal representation of meaning or reality.
- It is possible to develop literate thought in the oral mode, especially if individuals can access the message and reflect on this message to provide interpretations or, in other words, to construct a range of meanings.
- A literate mind refers to an individual's ability to access and interpret learned (e.g., serious, scholarly, academic) information.
- Literate thought has been described as the ability to think creatively, critically, logically, rationally, and reflectively on information presented in either a through-the-air mode or captured or preserved as in print, CD, or DVD.
- The three broad requisites of literate thought are:
  1. Adequate proficiency in a bona fide language;
  2. Understanding and application of a metalanguage or specialized vocabulary associated with a specific discipline or area and with general society or culture; and,
  3. Ability to access and interpret decontextualized literate language.
- The multifaceted concept of literate thought is related to and influenced by other ill-structured, seemingly diverse, domains such as the

New and Multiple Literacies, cognitive and disciplinary models, and critico-creative thinking skills.

QUESTIONS FOR REFLECTION AND DISCUSSION

1. What are a few broad views or perspectives of writing?

2. Discuss a few points regarding the nature of internal and external representations of reality.

3. According to the authors, what does it mean to be literate or illiterate?

4. What is literate thought? List and briefly describe the three broad requisites.

5. List and describe the major domains that have influenced the model of literate thought.

REFERENCES

Applegate, M., Quin, K., & Applegate, A. (2008). *The critical reading inventory: Assessing students' reading and thinking.* Upper Saddle River, N.J.: Pearson/Merrill/ Prentice Hall.

Bailey, A. (Ed.). (2007). *The language demands of school: Putting academic English to the test.* New Haven, CT: Yale University Press.

Baker, L., & Beall, L. (2009). Metacognitive processes and reading comprehension. In S. Israel & G. Duffy (Eds.), *Handbook of research on reading comprehension* (pp. 373-388). New York: Routledge.

Baker, L., & Brown, A. (1984). Metacognition skills and reading. In P. D. Pearson, R. Barr, M. Kamil, & P. Mosenthal (Eds.), *Handbook of reading research* (pp. 353-394). White Plains, NY: Longman.

Beveridge, W. (1980). *Seeds of discovery.* New York, NY: W.W. Norton & Company.

Bloome, D., & Paul, P. (Guest Editors). (2006). *Theory into Practice: Literacies of and for a diverse society, 45*(4).

Brown, M. N., & Keeley, S. (2007). *Asking the right questions: a guide to critical thinking.* Upper Saddle River, N.J.: Pearson/Prentice Hall.

Bruner, J. (1986). *Actual minds, possible worlds.* Cambridge, MA: Harvard University Press.

Cain, K., & Oakhill, J. (Eds.). (2007). *Children's comprehension problems in oral and written language.* New York: Guilford Press.

Cartwright, K. (2009). The role of cognitive flexibility in reading comprehension: Past, present, and future. In S. Israel & G. Duffy (Eds.), *Handbook of research on reading comprehension* (pp. 115-139). New York: Routledge.

Copleston, F. (1985). *A history of philosophy: Book 1.* New York: Doubleday.

Crystal, D. (1995). *The Cambridge encyclopedia of the English language.* New York: Cambridge University Press.

Crystal, D. (1997). *The Cambridge encyclopedia of language* (2nd ed). New York: Cambridge University Press.

Crystal, D. (2006). *How language works.* London, England: Penguin Books.

Denny, J. P. (1991). Rational thought in oral culture and literate decontextualization. In D. Olson & N. Torrance (Eds.), *Literacy and orality* (pp. 66-89). New York, NY: Cambridge University Press.

Dewey, J. (1933). *How we think: A restatement of the relation of reflective thinking to the educative process.* New York: D. C. Heath & Company.

Donovan, M., & Bransford, J. (Eds.). (2005). *How students learn: History, mathematics, and science in the classroom.* Washington, DC: The National Academies Press.

Feldman, C. (1991). Oral metalanguage. In D. Olson & N. Torrance (Eds.), *Literacy and orality* (pp. 47-65). New York, NY: Cambridge University Press.

Fenstermacher, G., & Soltis, J. (2004). *Approaches to teaching.* New York: Teachers College, Columbia University.

Flage, D. (2004). *The art of questioning: An introduction to critical thinking.* Upper Saddle River, NJ: Pearson/Prentice Hall.

Halpern, D. (1997). *Critical thinking across the curriculum: A brief edition of thought and knowledge.* Mahwah, N.J.: Erlbaum.

Hirsch, E.D. (1987). *Cultural literacy: What every American needs to know.* Boston, MA: Houghton Mifflin.

Hirsch, E.D., Kett, J., & Trefil, J. (Eds.). (2002). *The new dictionary of cultural literacy* (3rd ed.). Boston, MA: Houghton Mifflin Company.

Homer. (1898). *The Illiad.* [Translated by Samuel Butler]. Retrieved December 27, 2010, from http://www.sacred-texts.com/cla/homer/ili/index.htm.

Israel, S., & Duffy, G. (Eds.). (2009). *Handbook of research on reading comprehension.* New York: Routledge.

Kintsch, W. (1998). *Comprehension: A paradigm for cognition.* Cambridge: Cambridge University Press.

Kintsch, W., & Rawson, K. (2005). Comprehension. In M. Snowling & C. Hulme (Eds.), *The science of reading: A handbook* (pp. 209-226). Malden, MA: Blackwell.

Kuhn, D. (2005). *Education for thinking.* Cambridge, MA: Harvard University Press.

Kuhn, T. (1996). *The structure of scientific revolutions* (3rd ed.). Chicago: University of Chicago Press.

Lund, N. (2003). *Language and thought.* New York: Routledge.

Luria, A. (1976). *Cognitive development: Its cultural and social foundations.* Cambridge, MA: Harvard University Press.

McGuinness, D. (2004). *Early reading instruction: What science really tells us about how to teach reading.* Cambridge, MA: The MIT Press.

McGuinness, D. (2005). *Language development and learning to read: The scientific study of how language development affects reading skill.* Cambridge, MA: The MIT Press.

Nation, K. (2005). Connections between language and reading in children with poor reading comprehension. In H. Catts & A. Kamhi (Eds.), *The connections between language and reading disabilities* (pp. 41-54). Mahwah, NJ: Erlbaum.

Nickles, T. (Ed.). (2003). *Thomas Kuhn.* New York: Cambridge University Press.

Noddings, N. (1995). *Philosophy of education.* Boulder, CO: Westview Press.

Norris, S. (Ed.). (1992). *The generalizability of critical thinking: Multiple perspectives on an educational ideal.* New York: Teachers College Press, Columbia University.

Olson, D. (1989). Literate thought. In C. K. Leong & B. Randhawa (Eds.), *Understanding literacy and cognition* (pp. 3-15). New York: Plenum Press.

Olson, D. (1991). Literacy and objectivity: The rise of modern science. In D. Olson & N. Torrance (Eds.), *Literacy and orality* (pp. 149-164). New York: Cambridge University Press.

Olson, D. (1994). *The world on paper.* Cambridge: Cambridge University Press.

Ong, W. (1982). *Orality and literacy: The technologizing of the word.* London: Methuen.

Paris, S., & Stahl, S. (Eds.). (2005). *Children's reading comprehension and assessment.* Mahwah, NJ: Erlbaum.

Paul, P. (1998). *Literacy and deafness: The development of reading, writing, and literate thought.* Needham Heights, MA: Allyn & Bacon.

Paul, P. (2001). *Language and deafness* (3rd ed.). San Diego, CA: Singular/Thomson Learning.

Paul, P. (2006). New literacies, multiple literacies, unlimited literacies: What now, what next, where to? A response to "Blue listerine, parochialism & ASL literacy." *Journal of Deaf Studies and Deaf Education, 11*(3), 382-387.

Paul, P. (2009). *Language and deafness* (4th ed.). Sudbury, MA: Jones & Bartlett.

Paul, P., & Wang, Y. (2006a). Multiliteracies and literate thought. *Theory into Practice, 45*(4), 304-310.

Paul, P., & Wang, Y. (2006b). Literate thought and deafness: A call for a new perspective and line of research on literacy. *Punjab University Journal of Special Education* (Pakistan), *2*(1), 28-37.

Pearson, P. D., & Fielding, L. (1991). Comprehension instruction. In R. Barr, M. Kamil, P. Mosenthal, & P. D. Pearson (Eds.), *Handbook of reading research* (2nd ed.) (pp. 815-860). New York: Longman.

Pearson, P. D., & Stephens, D. (1994). Learning about literacy: A 30-year journey. In R. Ruddell, M. Ruddell, & H. Singer (Eds.), *Theoretical models and processes of reading* (4th ed.) (pp. 22-42). Newark, DE: International Reading Association.

Pence, K., & Justice, L. (2008). *Language development from theory to practice.* Upper Saddle River, NJ: Pearson/Merrill/Prentice Hall.

Perfetti, C., Landi, N., & Oakhill, J. (2005). The acquisition of reading comprehension skill. In M. Snowling & C. Hulme (Eds.), *The science of reading: A handbook* (pp. 227-247). Malden, MA: Blackwell.

Phillips, D., & Soltis, J. (2004). *Perspectives on learning.* New York: Teachers College Press.

Pinker, S. (1994). *The language instinct: How the mind creates language.* New York: William Morrow & Company.

Pring, R. (2004). *Philosophy of educational research* (2nd ed.). New York: Continuum.

Rippa, S. A. (1997). *Education in a free society: An American history* (8th ed.). White Plains, NY: Longman.

Ritzer, G. (2001). *Explorations in social theory: From metatheorizing to rationalization.* Thousand Oaks, CA: Sage Publication.

Rubin, D. (1995). *Memory in oral traditions: The cognitive psychology of epic, ballads, and counting-out rhymes.* New York: Oxford University Press.

Scribner, S., & Cole, M. (1981). *The psychology of literacy.* Cambridge, MA: Harvard University Press.

Shanahan, C. (2009). Disciplinary comprehension. In S. Israel & G. Duffy (Eds.), *Handbook of research on reading comprehension* (pp. 240-260). New York: Routledge.

Smith, S. (1995). Creative cognition: Demystifying creativity. In C. Hedley, P. Antonacci, & M. Rabinowitz (Eds.), *Thinking and literacy: The mind at work* (pp. 31-46). Hillsdale, NJ: Erlbaum.

Spiro, R., Collins, B., & Ramchandran, A. (2007). Reflections on a post-Gutenberg epistemology for video use in ill-structured domains: Things you can do with video to foster complex learning and cognitive flexibility. In R. Goldman, R. D. Pea, B. Barron, & S. Derry (Eds.), *Video research in the learning sciences.* Mahwah, NJ: Lawrence Erlbaum Associates.

Spiro, R., Vispoel, W., Schmitz, J., Samarapungavan, A., & Boerger, A. (1987). Knowledge acquisition for application: Cognitive flexibility and transfer in complex content domains. In B. Britton & S. Glynn (Eds.), *Executive control processes in reading* (pp. 177-199). Hillsdale, NJ: Erlbaum.

Stanovich, K. (1986). Matthew effects in reading: Some consequences of individual differences in the acquisition of literacy. *Reading Research Quarterly, 21,* 360-407.

Street, B. (1984). *Literacy in theory and practice.* Cambridge: Cambridge University Press.

Tulving, E., & Craik, F. (Eds.). (2000). *The Oxford handbook of memory.* New York: Oxford University Press.

Tyner, K. (1998). *Literacy in a digital world: teaching and learning in the age of information.* Mahwah, NJ: Lawrence Erlbaum Associates.

Walmsley, S., & Allington, R. (1995). Redefining and reforming instructional support programs for at-risk students. In R. Allington & S. Walmsley (Eds.), *No quick fix: Rethinkinq literacy programs in America's elementary schools* (pp. 19-44). New York: Teachers College Press.

Wang, Y. (2005). *Literate thought: Metatheorizing in literacy and deafness.* Unpublished doctoral dissertation, Ohio State University, Columbus.

FURTHER READING

Blackburn, S. (1999). *Think: A compelling introduction to philosophy.* New York: Oxford University Press.

Ellsworth, N., Hedley, C., & Baratta, A. (Eds.). (1994). *Literacy: A redefinition.* Hillsdale, NJ: Erlbaum.

Heidegger, M. (1968). *What is called thinking?* New York: Harper & Row. [Translated by J. G. Gray].

Korner, S. (1970). *Categorical frameworks.* Oxford: Oxford University Press.

Olson, D., & Torrance, N. (Eds.). (1996). *Modes of thought: Explorations in culture and cognition.* New York: Cambridge University Press.

CHAPTER 2

Comprehension and Literate Thought

The study of thinking has been characterized by a multitude of different approaches, first in philosophy and the arts, later in science. Many scientific disciplines today are concerned in one way or another with the study of thinking, or higher-level cognition, the somewhat fuzzy term currently preferred in cognitive science and cognitive psychology. . . .

Comprehension may be another paradigm for cognition, providing us with a fairly general though perhaps not all-encompassing framework within which cognitive phenomena can be explained.

Kintsch, 1998, pp. 1-2

There are many definitions of comprehension, but little consensus, perhaps because the boundaries of the topic are so broad and so poorly marked. Reading comprehension is only a subset of an ill-defined larger set of knowledge that reflects the communicative interactions among the intentions of the author/speaker, the content of the text/message, the abilities and purposes of the reader/listener, and the context/situation of the interaction. Early definitions of reading comprehension focused on thinking and reasoning about text . . . whereas recent national reports have emphasized constructive and interactive processes of reading comprehension.

Paris & Hamilton, 2009, p. 32

In this chapter, we provide more details on the multifaceted concept of literate thought. In our model, *literate thought* is defined as the use of goal-directed, conscious, deliberate, organized thinking in a creative, logical, and reflective manner. This type of thinking is most applicable for the resolution of problems or for any other similar desired outcome.

We include the two passages above on the concept of comprehension because this construct is a major component of or perhaps a paradigm for literate thought. Whether viewed as a problem-solving activity or a paradigm for cognition (Kintsch, 1998), clearly comprehension is an ill-structured, ill-defined, complex phenomenon (e.g., see Fox & Alexander, 2009). The second passage (Paris & Hamilton, 2009) attests to the difficulty of describing comprehension and traces its trajectory from thinking/reasoning to constructive/interactive processes. Although both passages address reading or print comprehension specifically, the second one reminds us that comprehension is part of a larger *communicative interactive* process involving authors/speakers and readers/listeners.

With a focus on comprehension, we portray literate thought as reflective of two broad processes—access and interpretation—to be presented later in more detail. Basically, one must have access to the message before one can construct/interpret an understanding (or model) that might have several levels, layers, or applications. In relation to the concept of communicative interaction, we focus mostly on captured forms of information involving the use of through-the-air language such as speech and sign as well as a representation of the language form in print or the written form—in this case, English. The concepts of sign literacy (i.e., captured signed information) and caption literacy (e.g., subtitles or captions used in the media such as movies and television) are mentioned briefly here, and caption literacy is discussed in further detail in the chapter on sensory disabilities (Chapter 7).

It is important also to highlight the relationship between print (script) literacy and spoken language comprehension. Specifically, this is the relationship between the concept of *reading* comprehension and that of *listening* comprehension. This is pertinent for the development of literate thought via the various means of captured information, for example, using audiobooks (compact disks [CDs]) or videobooks (digital video disks [DVDs]), which do not utilize the medium of print (e.g., an alphabetic writing system such as English). In particular, this exposition refers to external forms of captured information other than the use of print as discussed in Chapters 1 and 3.

We have mentioned several key concepts thus far that are the focus of this chapter: comprehension, access/interpretation, captured forms of verbal information, and the relationship between print comprehension and listening comprehension. Another key concept that needs to be addressed—and one that is an eye-opener—are the myths associated with print literacy. The presence of print literacy or the condition of a substantial number of individuals with the ability to read and write at a mature literate level is often associated with societal characteristics such as civilization, participatory democracy, technological advances, and cognitive development.

On the other hand, illiteracy (with respect to print) is often associated with anarchy, crime, and third-world conditions such as little medical or technological advancements (Olson, 1994). One major assumption of this view is that literate thought is only possible or predominantly possible via the comprehension and use of print literacy (discussed in Chapter 1 as well). In other words, the most prestigious or beneficial captured form of information is in print, the written language of society. Our goal in this book is to debunk these myths and argue that literate thought is mode-independent, that is, independent of the nature of a specific mode of captured information. This argument is further developed using Vygotsky's model (1962, 1978) in Chapter 3.

Before proceeding, let us consider the following example. Suppose that one group of students was requested to *read* the ensuing passage whereas a second equivalent group had to *listen* to it:

> There are real standards. We must fight soggy nihilism, skepticism, and cynicism. We must not believe that anything goes. We must not believe that all opinion is ideology, that reason is only power, that there is no truth to prevail. Without defenses against postmodernism irony and cynicism, multiculturalism and relativism, we will all go to hell in a handbasket.

> The sides in this conflict have various names: absolutists versus relativists, traditionalists versus postmodernists, realists versus idealists, objectivists versus subjectivists, rationalists versus social constructivists, universalists versus contextualists, Platonists versus pragmatists. These do not all mean the same, and some people who stand on one side or the other would be choosy about allowing them to apply to themselves. So for the moment they simply act as pointers. (Blackburn, 2005, p. xiii)

Putting aside the various contributions of prior or background knowledge, the use of metacognitive abilities, and other access/interpretation issues, we can ask several questions focusing on the anticipated findings of this small thought experiment:

- With respect to the concept of literate thought, does it matter whether one can comprehend the passage via reading or listening (or viewing/watching as in sign)?
- Is a particular type of comprehension—print or listening or viewing—constrained by text variables such as specific vocabulary and complex syntactic structures?
- Are the skills for print comprehension different from or similar to those for listening or viewing comprehension? Do these groups of skills vary across specific groups of individuals (e.g., across age level, experiences, type of disability, etc.) and different situations and contexts?
- What is the relationship, if any, between listening/viewing comprehension and print comprehension? Does this relationship reveal insights into the mode of captured information (e.g., print versus non-print CD or DVD)?

We address these questions and more in this chapter and in the rest of this book. To remove the suspense immediately, our goal is to demonstrate (actually reiterate) that literate thought is independent of the captured form of verbal information as long as there is equivalency across the various captured forms. What equivalency means, in our view, also needs to be demonstrated in an empirical (or fact independent or objective) manner. To explicate these issues, we begin with a brief discussion of comprehension.

COMPREHENSION

There is no widely accepted definition or theory on reading comprehension or even listening comprehension (Fox & Alexander, 2009; Paris & Hamilton, 2009). Research on comprehension has been influenced by long-standing debates regarding the location of meaning (Bartine, 1989, 1992). Specifically, it has been argued that meaning is situated predominantly in the text or in the reader's head; alternatively it is the result of an interaction or transaction between the reader and text. These debates engendered the tenor of the various theories or models, which entail the use of processes such as extracting and assembling information, constructing and integrating meaning, and connecting layers of meanings and information (Israel & Duffy, 2009; Ruddell & Unrau, 2004).

Despite the variety of models, there seems to be a consensus that comprehension is an ill-structured, ill-defined, broad concept that is affected by several groups of factors such as text (e.g., language structure, genre), reader (e.g., age, language and cognitive abilities, prior knowledge, metacognitive skills, motivation, and interest), context (e.g., classroom literacy practices, teacher–student interactions), and task (e.g., test-taking, pleasure reading, retelling, sharing, scanning, etc.). On the other hand, there is no consensus on the most effective way to assess comprehension, even if some agreement can be reached on selected aspects of its definition or description within the purview of the groups of factors mentioned above.

For our purposes, it is important to describe various levels of comprehension within a text (intratextual or textual) and across texts (intertextual). The genre of a text—that is, narrative (e.g., novels) or expository (e.g., academic texts)—also needs to be considered in any description. Although our focus is on accessing and understanding forms of captured information, we recognize the contributions to comprehension of exposure and discussion of information in the face-to-face or through-the-air discourses. In fact, developing through-the-air general comprehension skills contributes or may contribute to the acquisition of print comprehension capabilities or, in our case, to the acquisition of comprehension skills associated with any form of captured information.

Intratextual and Intertextual Comprehension

If we observe a sample of classroom literacy practices, it would be safe to conclude that much of what passes for comprehension, including comprehension instruction and assessment, focuses on—rightly or wrongly—the use of single texts or passages (Israel & Duffy, 2009; see also, Paris & Stahl, 2005). We can label this type of comprehension as *intratextual comprehension*, which is also known as *text* or *textual comprehension* (National Reading Panel, 2000; see also, Fox & Alexander, 2009).

Within a printed text, for example, a reader needs to comprehend at various levels that range from a word to sentence to longer discourse, and include the entire text or passage. As aptly stated by Cain and Oakhill (2007):

> At the word level, the reader must decode the individual words on the page . . . At the sentence level, the comprehender needs to work out the syntactic structure and sense of each sentence. Simply deriving the meanings of individual words and sentences is insufficient: In order to construct a mental model of the text, the comprehender needs to integrate information from different sentences to establish coherence and to incorporate background knowledge and ideas (retrieved from long-term memory) to make sense of details that are only implicitly mentioned . . . (p. xii)

Let us see how this operates with the following example.

> *Katherine was traveling at 40 miles per hour in her local neighborhood. She was in a hurry because she did not want to be late for her daughter's recital. It was not long before Katherine heard a siren. With a frustrated, exasperated look on her face, Katherine noticed a red-and-blue light on top of a police car turning rapidly. The ticket cost her $150 dollars and a demerit mark on her license with the Transportation Bureau. After checking the time on her cell phone, it became apparent that Katherine's daughter was going to be extremely disappointed.*

Setting aside the issues associated with the use of short passages for assessing comprehension (e.g., see Paris & Stahl, 2005), we can demonstrate the various layers of comprehension that are necessary to build a mental model of the meaning of this passage. For example, the reader needs to know the meanings of words and phrases such as *traveling*, *in a hurry*, and *recital*. The reader can surmise that Katherine was driving a vehicle, albeit it is not clear what kind of car, truck, and so on. Using inferential skills, the reader understands why and from whom Katherine received a ticket, even though such information is not explicit in the passage. In addition, the reader can surmise that Katherine exceeded the speed limit (i.e., traveled faster than what was allowable) and that was the reason for receiving a ticket (actually called a *speeding* ticket). The reason for breaking the speed limit or traveling too fast was because Katherine was afraid of being late to her daughter's recital. The last line, referring to the daughter's impending disappointment, should cause the reader to assume that Katherine was indeed late to the recital.

Young readers may have had the experience of their parents driving fast to arrive at some function on time. Older readers, especially those who drive, can relate to the embarrassment and frustration of Katherine and even to the reasons why individuals put themselves in such situations. These affective aspects are also part of the comprehension model developed by readers.

In essence, reading comprehension involves access to letters and words that readers need to identify rapidly and automatically. Rapid, automatic word identification skills facilitate and actually activate the comprehension processes and vice versa. Comprehension thus entails several layers moving from letters and words to longer discourses and even beyond the words on the page. Basically, this is what is involved in textual or intratextual comprehension.

With *intertextual comprehension*, one perspective is that readers construct a mental model of the topic under consideration by integrating information across the various texts or passages involved (Israel & Duffy, 2009). For example, suppose that readers encounter several passages on the topic of bats. After completing one passage, readers construct a mental model and then construct additional mental models after reading more passages on the same topic. Simplistically, readers eventually need to integrate (actually, connect) the information and end up with a tentative mental model of their understanding of bats. Typically this involves a process of critical reading, based on the application of critical thinking skills (discussed in Chapter 5).

Another perspective on intertextual reading involves repeated readings of the same passage. Individuals may have had additional experiences (via reflective thinking or dialogues) on the topic of bats. These experiences may have resulted in new information or enhanced or deepened understanding. When individuals read the initial passage again, they thus enhance or broaden their previously-constructed mental model of the passage. This enhancement is similar to the effect that individuals may have upon rereading a classic story or book of which they only had a limited or impoverished understanding years earlier. Our view of enhancement is similar to Langer's notion of *envisionment building* (Langer, 1989, 2004).

Much of the discussion of intertextual comprehension entails the emerging world of the New and Multiple Literacies, which involves not only multiple modes of information (e.g., print, graphics, illustrations) but also multiple texts that are both static and dynamic (e.g., hypermedia) (Fox & Alexander, 2009; Paul & Wang, 2006a, 2006b; Tyner, 1998). Fox and Alexander stated that these new emerging literacies compel us to broaden our concept of text comprehension to include issues such as (p. 232):

- Non-traditional forms of text, including oral discussions and graphic representations
- Text features only possible or only emphasized in electronic environments, such as use of color, interactivity, animations, and iconic cues indicating links
- Readers' capability to modify, enhance, program, link, collapse, and collaborate when using forms of electronic text
- Explicitness or directness of connections and the degree of congruence among multiple texts

This is just a thumbnail sketch of the complex process of comprehension, particularly print comprehension, at the intratextual (or textual) and intertextual levels. It is clear that intertextual comprehension issues will engender new and more complex models of comprehension that proceed beyond the use of terminology such as extraction, construction, integration, and connection. In addition, it should be emphasized that intratextual or intertextual comprehension applies to any mode of captured information, not only to print or script. To enhance our understanding of literate thought, we need to proceed to the notion of listening comprehension and relate this to the development of reading (or print) comprehension as well as to other modes of captured information.

Listening and Reading Comprehension

At first glance, there might be biased conceptions associated with the phrase, *listening comprehension*, which would render it not as high-level or complicated as reading comprehension or even underestimates the influences of listening comprehension on reading achievement. In fact, the impetus for much of the biased information might be due to views on the notion of *listening* (see also, related discussions on orality in Chapter 1).

The foregoing discussion has been epitomized aptly by the classic work of Sticht and James (1984), particularly in the introduction to their chapter:

D. P. Brown, a blind educator, completed his doctoral dissertation 30 years ago at Stanford University. In it, he analyzed relationships among oral and written language skills . . . He argued that listening to and comprehending spoken language is different from listening to nonlanguage sounds, which is something the prelanguage infant can do. He argued that, just as reading is not called looking, though it certainly involves looking while processing language symbols, listening while processing language signals should not be called merely listening. Listening, so he argued, is a parallel term to looking, and it causes confusion to have the term also serve as the oral language counterpart to reading. So he coined the term auding to refer to the process of listening to language and processing it for comprehension. (p. 293)

It thus can be stated that listening comprehension refers to general oral language comprehension skills such as speaking and listening (i.e., *auding*). The value and contributions of general language comprehension skills to the development of print comprehension have been investigated by a number of scholars (e.g., Nation, 2005, and the various discussions and reviews in Cain & Oakhill, 2007; Catts & Kamhi, 2005a, 2005b; Hoffman, 2009; Sticht, Beck, Hauke, Kleiman, & James, 1974; Sticht & James, 1984). McGuinness (2004, 2005) argued that general overall language problems (e.g., lack of proficiency in phonology, morphology, syntax, and semantics) contribute immensely to reading difficulties beyond the issue of decoding or even phonemic awareness. Cain and Oakhill maintained that there might not be one language profile that fits all children with reading/language difficulties, albeit there are common general language comprehension difficulties (e.g., synthesis, inferencing, etc.) across all readers. These general language comprehension difficulties lead to problems of inferences and other print comprehension areas at various levels of the passage, that is, at the word, phrase, sentence, and passage levels.

Simple View of Comprehension? Reading Comprehension

There seems to be a general consensus—albeit contentious—that listening comprehension (i.e., general language comprehension) and decoding skills contribute to reading (print) comprehension development (e.g., Cain & Oakhill, 2007; Hoffman, 2009). While this may provide substantial support for what has been called the *Simple View of Reading* (Hoover & Gough, 1990) as argued by Cain and Oakhill, the exact contributions and manner of influence involving both decoding and listening comprehension to overall reading comprehension have been contested (Hoffman). Reading comprehension is a complex entity involving more than just decoding and listening comprehension skills. For example, the

Simple View of Reading does not consider, in an in-depth manner, overall cognitive skills and knowledge such as prior knowledge, metacognition, and inferencing or synthesis.

Clearly, the relationship between listening comprehension and reading comprehension is in need of further research, particularly the findings expounded nearly four decades ago by Sticht et al. (1974; see also, the discussions in Cain & Oakhill, 2007; Hoffman, 2009; and Sticht & James, 1984):

1. Performance on measures of ability to comprehend language by auding will surpass performance on measures of ability to comprehend language by reading during the early years of schooling until reading skill is learned, at which time ability to comprehend by auding and reading will become equal.

2. Performance on measures of ability to comprehend language by auding will be predictive of performance of measures of ability to comprehend language by reading after the decoding skills of reading have been measured.

3. Performance on measures of rate of auding and rate of reading will show comparable maximal rates of languaging and conceptualizing for both processes, assuming fully developed reading decoding skills.

4. Training in comprehending by auding of a particular genre (e.g., "listening for the main idea") will transfer to reading when that skill is acquired. Conversely, once reading skill is acquired, new cognitive content learned by reading will be accessible by auding. Again, this reflects the model's position that reading and auding simply represent alternative in-roads to shared language competencies and cognitive content. Thus, additions to this content become equally accessible by auding and reading, once the latter is acquired (p. 2).

Although Sticht et al. (1974; see also Sticht & James, 1984) offered evidence for the first three statements above, only limited evidence was proffered for number 4. Nevertheless, there is research demonstrating that progress in reading comprehension is impeded if there are general auding or language comprehension problems (see reviews in Cain & Oakhill,

2007; Catts & Kamhi, 2005a, 2005b). This implies that progress in reading comprehension cannot proceed without a parallel or comparable level of progress in listening or language comprehension.

It is also possible that, at the highest level (e.g., beyond high school reading materials), reading print is easier to comprehend, initially, than listening to print, mainly due to the complex and condense language and cognitive variables associated with this level of print materials. Reaching this level of print comprehension might be difficult without an adequate development level of listening comprehension. As argued by Hoffman (2009), it is also possible that reading comprehension requires much more than just decoding plus listening comprehension skills.

Simple View of Comprehension? Non-Print Modes

With respect to literate thought, there should be theoretical discussions and research endeavors on similar relationships within the various modes of captured information discussed in this chapter and elsewhere. For example, would the findings of Sticht et al. (1974) apply analogously for the following relations?

- Listening comprehension and comprehension of audiobooks
- Viewing comprehension (similar to listening) and comprehension of videobooks (involving signing only or signing plus a video)
- Listening/viewing comprehension and videobooks (involving any combinations or permutations of speech, sign, and either static or dynamic video)
- Listening/viewing comprehension and comprehension of multi-media

We have no doubt that comprehension involves more than just *listening or viewing* general language skills in the above examples. In essence, we hypothesize that much of the challenge comes with addressing the nuances associated with the captured form of information (i.e., decontextualized literate language, etc.) as well as other general comprehension skills (e.g., use of prior knowledge, metacognition). Still, it has to be wondered: If someone has good listening or language comprehension skills, will this make it somewhat easier to understand a story or passage in the performance literacy mode (e.g., book on tape) than in the print literacy mode, especially if this person has difficulty with print? In the absence of strong research evidence, we argue that it would be easier, but performance literacy comprehension, in our example, requires more than just good listening or language comprehension skills. We return to these issues later in this book.

Comprehension and Literate Thought

As mentioned previously, Kintsch (1998; see also, 2004) has remarked that comprehension might be considered a model for cognition or some aspects of cognition. Given the overlap of components and processes between theories of comprehension (Israel & Duffy, 2009) and our simple model of literate thought, we can also assert that literate thought is a model for some aspects of general cognitive processing. As such, literate thought is pervasively influenced by cognitive models of processing, whether in general, or specifically, as in the case of reading or literacy development (e.g., see discussion of cognitive-processing models in Ruddell & Unrau, 2004).

This predominant dependence on cognition does not preclude the influences of social and cultural factors such as 1) the effects of the home environment, 2) the quality of interactions between peers and between teachers and students, 3) the use of specific teaching strategies or literacy practices in social interactive situations, and so on. We acknowledge the influences of social forces, including the notion that mental or cognitive process might be social or historical in origin (Luria, 1976; Vygotsky, 1978; see also, Chapter 3). There is little doubt that social factors influence and enhance the development of cognition (and language).

Nevertheless, our focus here is to discuss the components and processes of literate thought mostly from a cognitive perspective. We do not maintain that literate thought is an inside-the-head model only. However, even the best teaching–learning situations or the most enriching literacy environments or practices will not contribute immensely to the development of literate thought (or any other cognitive activity) if individuals do not possess the ability to access and interpret these realms of experiences via the use of their cognitive processes such as summarizing, synthesizing, and so on.

We are aware of the new wave of social and cultural foci, especially on the development of literacy (see Gee, 2004; Halliday, 2004). However, we do not believe that this means that cognition is *out* and socioculturalism is *in*. Hayes (2004) makes this point eloquently, and we quote his passage at length, with respect to the study of writing:

> There are two reasonable arguments that might lead to abandoning cognitive studies of writing. First, one might argue that all there is to know has already been learned about the relation of writing to topic knowledge, to language structure, to working memory capacity, and so on, and therefore, no further investigations are necessary. However this argument would not be easy to defend. Second, one might argue that all the issues that can be investigated through cognitive measures such as working memory capacity or reading level are better or more conveniently studied through social factors such as race, class, or gender. The validity of this position certainly has not been demonstrated nor is it likely to be.
>
> . . . Just as we would think a carpenter foolish who said, "Now that I have discovered the hammer, I am never going to use my saw again" so we should regard a literacy researcher who says, "Now that I have discovered social methods, I am never going to use cognitive ones again." Our research problems are difficult. We need all available tools, both social and cognitive. Let's not hobble ourselves by following a misguided fad. (p. 1411)

In our view, it would be misguided to abandon a discussion of cognitive processes and components in order to develop higher levels of literate thought, of course, with some attention to social factors. As discussed later in this book in the chapters on children and adolescents with disabilities, a number of cognitive factors account for their reading difficulties, for example, short-term memory, phonological strategies, and inference or coherence skills. We argue that the bulk of problems with literate thought development for many children and adolescents may also be due to specific or similar cognitive factors.

Our discussion of access and interpretation issues in the next section thus is markedly influenced by cognitive-processing models of reading and literacy (Israel & Duffy, 2009; Ruddell & Unrau, 2004). The primary reason for this influence is that we are interested in accessing and interpreting forms of captured information, of which print literacy (i.e., reading) is one type (Paul & Wang, 2006a, 2006b). As discussed in Chapter 1, the cognitive skills and processes needed for accessing and interpreting forms of captured information are quite different from—and may be more demanding than—those needed for through-the-air, uncaptured information.

Table 2-1 presents a summary of the major points on comprehension and its influence on our model of literate thought.

ACCESS/INTERPRETATION

In our comprehension model of literate thought, it is critical to highlight the processes of access and interpretation. In this chapter, the access/interpretation processes are related to two forms (or modes) of captured information: print (or script) and performance (oral or sign). Caption and other modes are discussed later in this book (Chapters 3 and 6–8). Similar to models associated with reading (or print) comprehension, there is a reciprocal relationship between access and interpretation. This is analogous to the relationship between decoding and comprehension (McGuinness, 2004, 2005; Ruddell & Unrau, 2004; Snowling & Hume, 2005).

There is no broad consensus on the meanings of access and interpretation. In general, to have access to stimuli means that one possesses a code or mechanism to sense, perceive, or process the information. Any attempt to describe the construct of access and even interpretation entails the use of a particular *memory* model. We shall leave it to others to debate the construct of memory (Foster & Jelicic, 1999; Tulving & Craik, 2000).

To access verbal information in a captured form, individuals need to possess the capacity to receive or perceive such information related to the structure of the stimuli. For example, it is often stated that individuals need to *decode* stimuli (letters, words) on the printed page in order to be able to comprehend or build a model of what the text means (see Israel & Duffy, 2009; Ruddell & Unrau, 2004). The meaning of the construct of decoding is shrouded with controversy, yielding a number of models on early reading and literacy. Despite the range of models, it can be asserted that if individuals cannot decode, they are not likely to comprehend the printed message. It is possible to think of comprehension as a form of encoding, actually the flip side of decoding (McGuinness, 2004, 2005).

This same decoding–encoding framework can be applied to any form of captured information. Despite the script literacy bias of the terms, we can say that individuals need to decode the spoken (or signed) message that has been captured in order to comprehend (or begin to comprehend) it, similar to the discussion of listening comprehension and its relation to print comprehension, earlier in this chapter (Cain & Oakhill, 2007; Catts

Table 2-1.   A Few Factors Associated with Comprehension and Relationship to Literate Thought

Remarks on Comprehension
- There is no widely accepted definition or theory on reading comprehension or even listening comprehension.
- Research on comprehension has been influenced by longstanding debates regarding the location of meaning.
- Comprehension is an ill-structured, ill-defined, broad concept, affected by several groups of factors such as text (e.g., language structure, genre), reader (e.g., age, language and cognitive abilities, prior knowledge, metacognitive skills, motivation and interest), context (e.g., classroom literacy practices, teacher-student interactions), and task (e.g., test-taking, pleasure reading, retelling, sharing, scanning, etc.).
- Comprehension can be discussed at the intratextual or textual level (i.e., within the text) or at the intertextual level (i.e., involving several or multiple texts).

Listening/Viewing Comprehension and Reading Comprehension
- Listening comprehension refers to general oral language comprehension skills such as speaking and listening (i.e., auding).
- General language comprehension difficulties lead to problems of inferences and other print comprehension skills at various levels of the passage, that is, at the word, phrase, sentence, and passage levels.
- There seems to be a general consensus—albeit contentious—that listening comprehension (i.e., general language comprehension) and decoding skills contribute to reading (print) comprehension development.
- With respect to literate thought, there should be theoretical discussions and research endeavors on similar relationships within the various modes of captured information.

Comprehension and Literate Thought
- Given the overlap of components and processes between theories of comprehension and the simple model of literate thought, it can also be asserted that literate thought is a model for some aspects of general cognitive processing.
- Literate thought is not an inside-the-head model only. Even the best teaching–learning situations or the most enriching literacy environments or practices, however, will not contribute immensely to the development of literate thought (or any other cognitive activity) if individuals do not possess the ability to access and interpret these realms of experiences via the use of their cognitive processes such as summarizing, synthesizing, and so on.
- The cognitive skills and processes needed for accessing and interpreting forms of captured information are quite different from—and may be more demanding than—those needed for through-the-air, uncaptured information.

& Kamhi, 2005a, 2005b; Sticht & James, 1984). There is little doubt that listening (or watching) comprehension for audio or video books has attention, memory, visual, and auditory components, but we have argued that listening is the oral language counterpart of reading (Cain & Oakhill; Catts & Kamhi, 2005a, 2005b; Sticht & James). As is discussed later in this book, this becomes even more complicated with caption literacy, which involves, at the least, both listening and reading comprehension as well as viewing a video component.

Similar to comprehension, the concept of interpretation has several layers (e.g., word, phrase, sentence, connected discourse, and passage or passages) and involves the use of critical thinking skills (see Chapter 5). The process of interpretation is influenced by factors that also influence comprehension such as prior knowledge, metacognition, and other text and reader factors (e.g., sociocultural influences and so on). In Chapter 1, we discussed the importance of possessing a metalanguage (e.g., specialized vocabulary) as part of the prior knowledge of an individual in developing literate thought. In essence, this highlights the need for possessing prior knowledge of the information (and other aspects such as language structures, etc.) in the passage as well as of a wider knowledge of the culture in which one resides, which can illuminate and enhance one's understanding of a particular passage (e.g., the cultural literacy concept of Hirsch, 1987; Hirsch, Kett, & Trefil, 2002).

From another perspective, it is possible to access the language of print but not be able to use the information (i.e., understanding and applying information). Basically, this means that the individual does not possess higher-level comprehension skills (use of prior knowledge, metacognition, inference, etc.). The main point here is that the use of the word, *access*, is not synonymous with the interpretation or the meaning associated with a passage or even with the application of that interpretation or meaning. Of course, access to the language of a captured mode helps the individual in this process, especially if s/he is required to perform tasks in this particular mode only.

As mentioned previously, there is or should be a relationship between access and interpretation. This is analogous to the relationship between decoding and comprehension for reading and even between that of oral language and print comprehension (Cain & Oakhill, 2007; Catts & Kamhi, 2005a, 2005b; Israel & Duffy, 2009). Two big constructs often are used to describe this relationship: *threshold* and *reciprocity*.

In order for this relationship to become operationalized, there needs to be a level of competence or proficiency in both areas of access and interpretation. This level of competence can be labeled as a threshold. When an individual reaches a threshold in a specific area, this means that s/he can use that area to develop or enhance the other one. In addition, an individual does not necessarily have to achieve the highest threshold level before being able to use a particular domain (through access or interpretation) to obtain a deeper understanding of it.

As an example, many reading theorists (e.g., Adams, 1990; Chall, 1996; Rumelhart, 2004) have maintained that children need to proceed beyond the learning to read stage—namely, possessing a threshold in, for example, decoding and comprehension—in order to read to learn, which is an independent entity. In reading to learn, children learn more about their language as well as about the reading process. In second language learning, Cummins (1984, 1988, 1989; see also, Chapter 9) has proposed a threshold hypothesis, which basically states that an individual needs a certain working level of proficiency in one language before that language can be used in acquiring a second language.

In our literate thought model, we argue that individuals need to develop a reasonable level of threshold in both access and interpretation and to develop further in each domain separately in order for one domain to facilitate and enhance the other. When a threshold has been reached, there can be reciprocity. The particular mode of captured information (e.g., print, audio, video of verbal language) is not critical. Nevertheless, access skills in one mode (e.g., print) do not necessarily transfer to access skills in another different mode (e.g., sign). This becomes a critical issue for some d/Deaf or hard of hearing students, whose first language is American Sign Language (discussed in Chapter 7). There is a distinction between being deaf and being Deaf. The former refers to the audiometric definition of deafness, whereas the latter refers to identifying with the Deaf culture, which has its own set of values, social structure, forms of artistic expression, and, most importantly, its own language, American Sign Language (ASL) (Wang, Kretschmer, & Hartman, 2008).

Regardless of the mode of captured verbal information—print, audiobook, or videobook—individuals need to have specific access skills. If too much energy or time is spent accessing information, then there will be breakdowns with interpretation. To paraphrase Stanovich (1991, 1992), we hypothesize that it is possible for individuals to have adequate access skills but poor interpretation skills. However, the opposite is not true, especially if we are within the same mode of captured information: It is impossible for an individual to have adequate interpretation skills without a working level of access skills. No access, no interpretation.

With this understanding of access and interpretation and the concomitant constructs of threshold and reciprocity, we can proceed to the specific forms of captured verbal information in the next section.

FORMS OF CAPTURED VERBAL INFORMATION

Paul and Wang (2006a, 2006b) asserted that the term *literacy* should be reconceptualized as a form of captured verbal information (see also, the discussion in Chapter 3). Verbal information is information rendered via the use of a verbal language (speech, sign, Braille, writing), symbols (e.g., mathematics, chemistry), and visuals (e.g., graphics, illustrations, pictures, artwork, etc.). It should be clarified that there are not always sharp distinctions between these categories. For example, computer communication devices may use visuals plus voice plus symbols to assist individuals with limited speaking or communication skills in expressing needs. Chinese characters are certainly a type of written language or script literacy whereas a case can be made that Braille employs both verbal language (a representation, for example, of the alphabetic system) and symbols (e.g., for contractions, numerals, or even for letters). Finally, it is obvious that script (print) literacy may also contain symbols and visuals.

The point to be made here is that the above information has been captured (saved, preserved, etc.) in a certain form. The form of the captured information indicates the name of the literacy, albeit we might need to compromise or focus on a predominant category. Simplistically, the written language of English, French, or Chinese is labeled *script literacy* (also known as *written* or *print literacy*). In fact, any form of written language can be labeled script literacy. Braille can be labeled Braille literacy, but this can also be a type of script or mathematical literacy (e.g., consider the Nemeth Braille system).

This concept of captured information becomes even more complex when one considers the use of subtitles or captions (at the bottom of a television program or movie). In this book, we have labeled this caption literacy; however, this type of literacy entails the use of script, voice or sign, and a video (i.e., moving pictures). The access and interpretation skills needed for caption literacy are different from those required for script or print literacy, albeit there are some overlaps.

Given the ubiquitous nature and prestige of script literacy, the ensuing section focuses on the rendering of that literacy into a captured through-the-air form such as speech or sign, which is labeled *performance literacy*. The previous information on listening comprehension can be applied to our discussion of performance literacy. There are other types of performance literacy, which proceeds beyond the use and transliteration of script literacy. Other types of verbal language literacy (Braille, caption, communication boards, etc.) are covered in the ensuing chapters of this book, particularly in the chapters on children with disabilities (e.g., Chapters 6–8).

Script (Print) Literacy

Much of the information disseminated in learning institutions such as schools, colleges, and universities is rendered via the use of print, which refers to the traditional view of the term literacy. Our concept of script literacy refers to this traditional view of literacy, namely, writing or written language as embodied in typographic (type or print) or chirographic (handwritten) venues. This *World on Paper* (Olson, 1994) not only refers to information captured on paper but also electronically in print via a written language system, such as the alphabet or the Mandarin (Chinese characters) system.

Individuals can read script literacy information or express their thoughts in writing. There are access and interpretation skills for both reading and writing. Writing involves reading and much more (e.g., see Hayes, 2004). Despite the purported overlapping underpinnings between reading and writing, most of the theorizing and modeling has been on print or script comprehension, that is, reading (Ruddell & Unrau, 2004). Within this purview, the access skills for script literacy are print-related skills (e.g., word identification, knowledge of the language of print) whereas interpretation skills are those that are used to perform tasks such as answering questions, making inferences, and offering generalizations. Access is similar to word identification or decoding skills and interpretation is similar to comprehension skills.

It is no surprise that there are numerous models of the reading process with some overlaps (Israel & Duffy, 2009; McCarthey & Raphael, 1992; Mitchell, 1982; Ruddell & Unrau, 2004). Using the framework of

Ruddell and Unrau, there are cognitive-processing models and others such as dual coding, transactional, aptitude-influences, and sociocognitive. To simplify (and it is not simple), reading is a constructive, multiple-contextualized entity involving an array of processes such as linguistics, cognitive, social, and political. Paul (2003, 2009; Trezek, Wang, & Paul, 2011) has argued that these processes can be grouped into areas such as text (e.g., orthography, grammar, genres), reader (e.g., prior knowledge, metacognition, affective behaviors), task (e.g., purpose of reading, type of assessment used), context (e.g., cultural or political influences, school effects), and the interactions or combinations of these areas (**Table 2-2**; additional elaboration on print factors can be found in Chapter 6).

With respect to Table 2-2, we can surmise that any model of reading needs to incorporate aspects of all four areas (text, reader, task, and context), delineate major components within the areas, discuss internal processes, and demonstrate relationships between and among the compo-

---

Table 2-2.   A Few Factors Associated with the Reading Process

Text
Print knowledge
Letter knowledge
Letter–sound correspondences
Orthography
Word meanings
Syntax
Other discourse structures
Literary genres
Reader
Prior knowledge
Metacognition (strategies)
Inferential ability
Motivation/interest
Task
Purposes of reading/writing
Setting or time issues
Evaluation issues
Context
Social and cultural areas
Classroom culture
Home environment

Source: Paul (2009).

nents. This conceptual framework can also be applied to any mode of captured information, especially those modes that embody verbal language (e.g., performance literacy, caption literacy).

McGuinness (2005) asserts that reading can be stated as a decoding–encoding entity, which she believes are two sides of the same coin. *Decoding* refers to word identification or access, and *encoding* can refer, broadly, to the output such as writing, spelling, or overall comprehension or interpretation (mentioned previously in this chapter). In her work, McGuinness (2004, 2005) argued that this decoding–encoding entity is more difficult for opaque languages, such as English, for which one letter may have several sounds or one sound can be translated into different letters. This assertion has also been corroborated in a research review of the acquisition of literacy by d/Deaf and hard of hearing children and adolescents in three countries: United States, China, and South Korea (Wang, Lee, & Paul, 2010).

McGuinness (2005) criticized several of the fundamentals of current reading models. Her main contention is that these models do not incorporate many of the findings conducted by language researchers on, for example, the acquisition of English. In our view, knowledge of the language of print is critical for reading development; nevertheless, reading is much more than the knowledge and use of a language. In fact, this is true for access and comprehension in any other mode of captured verbal information.

Despite the proliferation of models, it has been difficult to paint a coherent picture of the reading acquisition or reading comprehension process (Israel & Duffy, 2009; Ruddell & Unrau, 2004). This presents a challenge in proffering suggestions and implications for literacy instruction. Nevertheless, the focus on factors in the four areas mentioned above (text, reader, task, context) is based on a synthesis of major findings discussed in sources such as Adams (1990), Anderson, Hiebert, Scott, and Wilkinson (1985), Snow, Burns, and Griffin (1998), and even the recommendations of the National Reading Panel (2000). Important areas for literacy instruction, particularly reading, need to include aspects such as phonemic awareness, phonics, vocabulary, fluency, and comprehension.

In the ensuing chapters of this text, we discuss the language and literacy development of children and adolescents with specific disabilities and those who are English language learners (ELLs). These populations not only provide similarities with respect to development and problems with script literacy, but also enhance our thesis that literate thought should be facilitated and developed in modes of captured information in addition to print.

Merits of Print Literacy

Prior to discussing our construct of performance literacy, it is important to debunk a few assumptions associated with script literacy (Olson, 1994; Paul, 2009; Paul & Wang, 2006a, 2006b). Olson (1994) provides the best treatment of this concept. This researcher lists six beliefs associated with writing (pp. 3–7):

1. Writing is the transcription of speech.

2. The superiority of writing to speech.

3. The technological superiority of the alphabetic writing system.

4. Literacy as the organ of social progress.

5. Literacy as an instrument of cultural and scientific development.

6. Literacy as an instrument of cognitive development.

Each belief above could take an entire chapter to provide background and contrary evidence. By no means is the case closed; however, these assumptions have been challenged both empirically and theoretically (see also, Olson, 1994; Rubin, 1995; and Chapter 1 of this book). With respect to literate thought, the focus here is on items 1, 2, and 6. Chapter 3 of this book provides additional details on the purported merits of script literacy within a historical framework and the context of the New and Multiple Literacies.

Current research on reading and writing (e.g., see discussions in Israel & Duffy, 2009; Ruddell & Unrau, 2004) should put to rest the assumption that writing is simply speech written down (#1). Although speech or, more precisely, the conversational or through-the-air form of the language is the real engine of the use of language (Pinker, 1994), writing is hardly a transcription of this entity. We have discussed additional views on writing in Chapter 1. It can be averred also that writing requires more than just the skill of reading and general language comprehension skills.

It is tempting to view writing as superior to speech, given all of the false starts, memory lapses, and so on associated with speech. Considering writing as a technological device notwithstanding, this view is actually related to myth number 1 and, indeed, may be a contradiction. In short, it is best to view writing as being dependent on speech (or through-the-air manifestations such as signing), which represents the major deliverance of thoughts in the mind. As noted by Olson (1994), "writing, though important, is always secondary" (p. 8).

Given the concept of literate thought, from a different perspective it can be argued that performance literacy (discussed later) can be as rigorous and organized as script literacy (or written language). Via the use of technology, individuals can edit and refine their spoken or signed thoughts and present them in a manner analogous to writing. In fact, it is often forgotten that the process of writing, especially in an organized, coherent fashion, requires the art of revision and editing. Granted, performance literacy is still different from the act of performance (i.e., uncaptured through-the-air speech or sign); nevertheless, similar to writing, it is dependent on the performance form (i.e., speech or sign).

It should be clear that assumption number 6 should be refuted by the contents (empirical and theoretical findings) of this book. The contributions of script literacy, particularly writing, to the development of cognition are certainly acknowledged. However, we agree strongly with Olson (1994), who asserted that "it is simply a mistake . . . to identify the means of communication with the knowledge that is communicated. Knowledge can be communicated in a number of ways—by speech, writing, graphs, diagrams, audio tapes, video" (p. 12).

In short, writing, similar to other *products*, is a manifestation of cognition. There is a reciprocal relationship between writing and cognition and, in fact, this relationship is influenced by social and cultural factors as well. What is really needed is a theory or model that explicates the interrelationships among language, literacy, mind, and culture.

Performance Literacy

In this book and elsewhere (Paul, 2001, 2006, 2009; Paul & Wang, 2006a, 2006b; Wang, 2005), the construct, *performance*, simply refers to the through-the-air presentations or communicative interactions in the conversational or primary form of a language. The most common form is speech. Other forms include sign (for d/Deaf individuals) or communicative devices. Here we restrict the use of the construct performance to the use of speech or sign for full-blown languages (e.g., English, French,

American Sign Language, Chinese Sign Language, etc.). Communication devices typically have symbol systems (symbols, pictures, icons, etc.), and this represents a form of captured information even though such devices are primarily used for communicative interactions (see Chapter 8). Assisted speaking devices, such as those used by individuals who have had a laryngectomy, can still be considered as being within the purview of performance.

So if literacy is a form of captured information, then performance literacy refers to information presented in the oral or conversational form of the language (i.e., nonscript-based form) that has been captured on CDs and DVDs. Information in the performance literacy mode can range from dinner conversations to classroom lectures to the reading/signing of information in books and other print materials. Performance literacy does not contain print. Common examples are the audio book (e.g., Kindle, Nook, etc.) and book-on-tape (cassette recordings) often used by individuals who are blind or visually impaired.

The concept of performance is related to that of *orality*. The notion of performance thus has been influenced by research on *orality* and the *oral tradition*, discussed in Chapter 1 (Denny, 1991; Feldman, 1991; Olson, 1991). With respect to the use of speech, insights from the previous discussion of listening comprehension can be applied here, particularly if we are referring to listening to a passage or story from print. If the captured information is in sign—either American Sign Language or some form of sign English—then there needs to be a discussion of watching or viewing comprehension, which is analogous to listening or oral language comprehension, especially for passages or stories that have been transliterated (sign English) or translated (American Sign Language) from printed English. The complicated concept of watching or viewing comprehension is discussed further in Chapter 7.

The capture of script literacy information in a performance literacy mode does not render such information as being easier to comprehend. The previous discussion on factors that impact comprehension is also applicable here. The content of information in the performance literacy mode thus can be as complex and as difficult as information presented in the written mode.

In other words, performance literacy materials can contain decontextualized or literate academic language, which is reflective of the vocabulary and grammar of script literacy (see also, the discussion in Chapter 1).

Consider, again, the examples of talking or signing books. Theoretically, it is possible to capture in the performance literacy mode all information electronically from newspapers or other printed materials such as legal documents and textbooks.

Similar to the discussion for script literacy, performance literacy also has access and interpretation issues. For captured audio materials, individuals need adequate listening skills to access the captured information. For video materials with *sound*, individuals must have not only viewing and listening skills, but also the ability do both in some simultaneous fashion. The issue becomes even more complicated if an interpreter (e.g., interpreter's bubble) is used along with the video and with speaking narrator/characters. Regardless of the condition for performance literacy, the skills needed for interpretation or comprehension are similar to those for script literacy.

Comparison of Script and Performance Literacy

We have argued thus far that the major differences between the modes of script and performance literacy concern the type of access skills needed by individuals. We do not deny that there may be differentiating effects of these modes on the use of memory and other cognitive domains; however, this is an area of future research (as is mentioned later). It can be argued theoretically that the interpretation skills (e.g., use of literate language, prior knowledge, metacognitive skills, etc.) needed for understanding a story or passage in the performance literacy mode, for example, are roughly similar to those for understanding the same story or passage in the print (script) mode.

Nevertheless, there are a few attributes uniquely attributed to each mode that might cast a few doubts on the equivalency factor. For example, the performance literacy mode can involve the use of speakers and/or signers, who present information (e.g., reading or telling a story) and are affected by speaker or signer characteristics. These characteristics include the author's or user's voice, presentation or speaking style, and rate and emphasis of speaking and signing, all of which can affect an individual listener's or viewer's interpretation of the story.

Another major difference between script and performance literacy is that of control. For example, the viewer has little or no control over the presentation in the performance literacy mode, and this is different from the control evident in his or her reading of print (e.g., proceeding at one's own pace). In addition, the notion of *lookback* (defined as reading the print again) is different from that of *viewback* (or *listenback*), which is limited to the amount of information that remains on screen as well as the length of time that the video frames are present. That is, given the current state of technology, it might be easier and more convenient to lookback with print than to viewback (or listenback) with video (or audio).

Finally, the perceptual field of print is broader than that associated with the presentations of verbal information in video and/or audio texts. Specifically, even with repeated viewings or listenings, the viewer/listener may not see or hear more than one frame at a time or can only hear one sentence at a time sequentially, whereas a print user can work with a whole page, containing much more information. The effects of the perceptual fields on comprehension for these modes need to be investigated further.

A few highlights on access/interpretation and script and performance literacy are presented in **Table 2-3**.

IMPLICATIONS FOR RESEARCH

There is little doubt in our minds that there will be ongoing research on the effects of print literacy, particularly the use of literacy in multimedia environments. This research is bound to yield new and more complex models of comprehension, which should also affect our understanding of the development of literate thought. Individuals need to access and interpret print to be successful at reaping the benefits of our current technologically driven societies.

Our hope is that scholars see the need for research on captured through-the-air modes such as performance literacy. Through-the-air modes can further our understanding of the concept of listening comprehension or general language comprehension skills. This line of research should not be accomplished in lieu of or supplant the research on script literacy in either traditional or multimedia modes.

In our view, performance literacy should not be used in place of script literacy. It simply is another avenue for students to work with decontextualized information that is roughly similar to the decontextualized information in print. It is not yet clear if performance literacy can facilitate access to the complex language structures often used in script literacy.

Table 2-3. Major Highlights of Access/Interpretation and Script and Performance Literacy

---

Access and Interpretation/Comprehension
- Access can have at least two broad components: access to the language of the captured information and access to the content/meaning of the information. These two components can be separated for discussion purposes.
- It is possible to access (i.e., via decoding skills) the language of print but not be able to use the information (i.e., understanding and applying information). It is equally possible to access and use information through the performance-based mode (speech and/or signs) of your native language, but not understand the language of English print that contains the same information.
- The main point here is that the use of the word *access* is not synonymous with the interpretation or the meaning associated with a passage or even with the application of that interpretation or meaning. Access to the language of a captured mode helps the individual in this process, especially if s/he is required to perform tasks in this particular mode only.

Script Literacy
- Refers to information captured on paper or electronically via the use of a written language system (e.g., letters, characters).
- The access skills for script literacy are print related skills (e.g., word identification, knowledge of the language of print) whereas interpretation skills are those that are used to perform tasks such as answering questions, making inferences, and offering generalizations.
- Many merits of script literacy have been challenged and are currently undergoing intensive investigations.
- With script literacy, the reader has control, that is, he or she can move his or her eyes at a comfortable speed across the print. The reader can reread or read ahead, if desirable.

Performance Literacy
- Combines aspects of both script (e.g., the language used in print venues) and caption media/literacy (e.g., video, the language of monologues and dialogues).
- Performance refers to information presented in the oral or conversational form of the language (i.e., nonscript-based form), ranging from dinner conversations to classroom lectures to the reading/signing of information in books and other print materials.
- Performance literacy materials may contain decontextualized or literate language, which closely resembles the vocabulary and grammar of script literacy.
- Performance literacy should not be used in lieu of script literacy. It is just another avenue for students to work with decontextualized information that is roughly similar to the decontextualized information in print.

Source: Based on discussions in Paul (2009); Paul & Wang (2006a, 2006b); and Wang (2005).

However, it can expose students to these structures and to the nature of information at various difficulty levels. There is a need for research focusing on the decontextualized nature of performance literacy information and on the development of skills for working with this type of information.

Paul and Wang (2006b, p. 35) have suggested that future researchers should explore the following questions:

1. What are the contributions of performance literacy to the development of literate thought and as a possible instrument for cognitive development, in general?

2. What are some possible ways for enhancing and developing performance literacy skills in children and adolescents? Will these methods improve access to script literacy, particularly the language of print? Will they improve students' understanding of script literacy information?

3. What are the implications and effects of using the performance literacy mode in bilingual-bicultural situations?

In addition to the above questions, researchers should explore differences between script literacy and performance literacy with respect to:

- The complex structures of the language/information
- Influences of the reader or interpreter on comprehension for audio books and video books
- The ability of individuals to access and interpret print information that has been converted into audio or video texts
- Ease of lookback techniques for print versus those that might be needed (e.g., listenback or watchback) for video or audio text
- The effects of the perceptual fields of both modes
- The contributions of general listening/viewing or language comprehension skills to the various modes of captured information (print, audio, video)

As we reiterate throughout this book, the goal is not to select one mode of presenting information over another or to show the manner in which one mode is more beneficial than the other. In short, the goal is to develop literate thought. The mode of information should be immaterial, except with reference to the preferences and needs of the individual/

receiver. Whether all modes of captured information are equal is an open researchable question.

SUMMARY

The intent of this chapter is to introduce the concept of comprehension as it relates to the discussion of literate thought and modes of captured forms of information. We discuss listening comprehension and its relationship to print comprehension and provide insights into types of literacy such as print and performance. More research must be done on the non-print forms of captured information and the manner in which these forms are affected by skills associated with general listening or viewing language comprehension.

Major highlights of this chapter are as follows:

- Literate thought is the use of goal-directed, conscious, deliberate, organized thinking in a creative, logical, and reflective manner. This type of thinking is most feasible or applicable for the resolution of problems or for any other similar desired outcome.
- Whether comprehension is viewed as a problem-solving activity or a paradigm for cognition, it is an ill-structured, ill-defined, complex phenomenon, affected by several groups of factors such as text, reader, context, and task.
- Comprehension is part of a larger *communicative interactive* process involving authors/speakers and readers/listeners.
- Listening comprehension refers to general oral language comprehension skills such as speaking and listening (i.e., auding). There seems to be a general consensus—albeit contentious—that listening comprehension (i.e., general language comprehension) and decoding skills contribute to reading (print) comprehension development.
- Literate thought is not an inside-the-head model only. However, even the best teaching–learning situations or the most enriching literacy environments or practices will not contribute immensely to the development of literate thought (or any other cognitive activity) if individuals do not possess the ability to access and interpret these realms of experiences via the use of their cognitive processes such as summarizing, synthesizing, and so on.

- Within a comprehension model, literate thought is reflective of two broad processes, access and interpretation.
- In general, to have access to stimuli means that one possesses a code or mechanism to sense, perceive, or process the information.
- Similar to comprehension, the concept of interpretation has several layers (e.g., word, phrase, sentence, connected discourse, passage, or passages) and involves the use of critical thinking skills.
- There is or should be a relationship between access and interpretation. This is analogous to the relationship between decoding and comprehension for reading and even between that of oral language comprehension and print comprehension.
- *Literacy* should be reconceptualized as a form of captured verbal information. Verbal information is information rendered via the use of a verbal language (speech, sign, Braille, writing), symbols (e.g., mathematics, chemistry), and visuals (e.g., graphics, illustrations, pictures, artwork, etc.). There are not always sharp distinctions between these categories.
- The concept of script literacy refers to the traditional view of literacy, namely, writing or written language as embodied in typographic (type or print) or chirographic (handwritten) venues.
- The construct, *performance*, simply refers to the through-the-air presentations or communicative interactions in the conversational or primary form of a language. Performance literacy refers to information presented in the oral or conversational form of the language (i.e., nonscript-based form) that has been captured on CDs and DVDs.
- The goal is to develop literate thought; the mode of information should be immaterial, except with reference to the preferences and needs of the individual/receiver. Whether all modes of captured information are equal is an open researchable question.

These first two chapters provide a foundation for the concept of literate thought and related areas. In the next chapter, we discuss a few tenets of one related area, the New and Multiple Literacies, which offer interesting and challenging implications for the development of literate thought. With the emphasis on cultural and social models, it might be that these new forms of literacies, in conjunction with new comprehension models, will shake loose the predominant cognitive framework of literate thought. Or, as a few scholars believe (see reviews in Gaffney & Anderson, 2000; Paul, 2009), these new areas might be an elaborated extension of the paradigm for cognition.

QUESTIONS FOR REFLECTION AND DISCUSSION

1. Why is literate thought independent of the specific mode or form of captured information?

2. Define the concept of comprehension.

3. With respect to literate thought, what insights can be gained by a better understanding of the traditional term, *listening comprehension*?

4. Describe the concepts of *access* and *interpretation* as they relate to print (script) literacy and performance literacy.

5. Compare and contrast script literacy and performance literacy.

REFERENCES

Adams, M. (1990). *Beginning to read: Thinking and learning about print*. Cambridge, MA: The MIT Press.

Anderson, R., Hiebert, E., Scott, J., & Wilkinson, I. (1985). *Becoming a nation of readers: The report of the commission on reading*. Washington, DC: The National Institute of Education and The Center for the Study of Reading.

Bartine, D. (1989). *Early English reading theory: Origins of current debates*. Columbia, SC: University of South Carolina Press.

Bartine, D. (1992). *Reading, criticism, and culture: Theory and teaching in the United States and England, 1820-1950*. Columbia, SC: University of South Carolina Press.

Blackburn, S. (2005). *Truth: A guide*. New York: Oxford University Press.

Cain, K., & Oakhill, J. (Eds.). (2007). *Children's comprehension problems in oral and written language*. New York: Guilford Press.

Catts H., & Kamhi, A. (Eds.). (2005a). *The connections between language and reading disabilities*. Mahwah, NJ: Erlbaum.

Catts, H., & Kamhi, A. (2005b). *Language and reading disabilities* (2nd ed.). Boston, MA: Pearson/Allyn & Bacon.

Chall, J. S. (1996). *Stages of reading development.* (2nd ed.). New York: McGraw-Hill.

Cummins, J. (1984). *Bilingualism and special education: Issues in assessment and pedagogy.* San Diego, CA: College-Hill Press.

Cummins, J. (1988). Second language acquisition within bilingual education programs. In L. Beebe (Ed.), *Issues in second language acquisition: Multiple perspectives* (pp. 145-166). New York, NY: Newbury House.

Cummins, J. (1989). A theoretical framework for bilingual special education. *Exceptional Children, 56*, 111-119.

Denny, J. P. (1991). Rational thought in oral culture and literate decontextualization. In D. Olson & N. Torrance (Eds.), *Literacy and orality* (pp. 66-89). New York, NY: Cambridge University Press.

Feldman, C. (1991). Oral metalanguage. In D. Olson & N. Torrance (Eds.), *Literacy and orality* (pp. 47-65). New York, NY: Cambridge University Press.

Foster, J., & Jelicic, M. (Eds.). (1999). *Memory: Systems, process, or function?* New York: Oxford University Press.

Fox, E., & Alexander, P. (2009). Text comprehension: A retrospective, perspective, and prospective. In S. Israel & G. Duffy (Eds.), *Handbook of research on reading comprehension* (pp. 227-239). New York: Routledge/Taylor & Francis Group.

Gaffney, J., & Anderson, R. (2000). Trends in reading research in the United States: Changing intellectual currents over three decades. In M. Kamil, P. Mosenthal, P. D. Pearson, & R. Barr (Eds.), *Handbook of reading research* (Vol. III) (pp. 53-74). Mahwah, NJ: Erlbaum.

Gee, J. (2004). Reading as situated language: A sociocognitive perspective. In R. Ruddell & N. Unrau (Eds.), *Theoretical models and processes of reading* (5th ed.) (pp. 116-132). Newark, DE: International Reading Association.

Halliday, M. A. K. (2004). The place of dialogue in children's construction of meaning. In R. Ruddell & N. Unrau (Eds.), *Theoretical models and processes of reading* (5th ed.) (pp. 133-145). Newark, DE: International Reading Association.

Hayes, J. (2004). A new framework for understanding cognition and affect in writing. In R. Ruddell & N. Unrau (Eds.), *Theoretical models and processes of reading* (5th ed.) (pp. 1399-1430). Newark, DE: International Reading Association.

Hirsch, E. D. (1987). *Cultural literacy: What every American needs to know.* Boston, MA: Houghton Mifflin.

Hirsch, E. D., Kett, J., & Trefil, J. (Eds.). (2002). *The new dictionary of cultural literacy* (3rd ed.). Boston, MA: Houghton Mifflin.

Hoffman, J. (2009). In search of the "Simple View" of reading comprehension. In S. Israel & G. Duffy (Eds.), *Handbook of research on reading comprehension* (pp. 54-66). New York: Routledge/Taylor & Francis Group.

Hoover, W., & Gough, P. (1990). The simple view of reading. *Reading and Writing, 2*, 127-160.

Israel, S., & Duffy, G. (Eds.). (2009). *Handbook of research on reading comprehension.* New York: Routledge.

Kintsch, W. (1998). *Comprehension: A paradigm for cognition.* Cambridge: Cambridge University Press.

Kintsch, W. (2004). The construction-integration model of text comprehension and its implications for instruction. In R. Ruddell & N. Unrau (Eds.), *Theoretical models and processes of reading* (5th ed.) (pp. 1270-1328). Newark, DE: International Reading Association.

Langer, J. (1989). *The process of understanding literature* (Center for Learning & Teaching of Literature: Research Monograph, 2.1). Albany, NY: SUNY Albany.

Langer, J. (2004, May). *Developing the literate mind.* Paper presented at the meeting of the International Reading Association, San Diego, CA.

Luria, A. R. (1976). *Cognitive development: Its cultural and social foundations* (M. Lopez-Morillas & L. Solotaroff, trans). Cambridge, MA: Harvard University Press.

McCarthey, S., & Raphael, T. (1992). Alternative research perspectives. In J. Irwin & M. Doyle (Eds.), *Reading/writing connections: Learning from research* (pp. 2-30). Newark, DE: International Reading Association.

McGuinness, D. (2004). *Early reading instruction: What science really tells us about how to teach reading.* Cambridge, MA: The MIT Press.

McGuinness, D. (2005). *Language development and learning to read: The scientific study of how language development affects reading skill.* Cambridge, MA: The MIT Press.

Mitchell, D. (1982). *The process of reading: A cognitive analysis of fluent reading and learning to read.* New York, NY: Wiley.

Nation, K. (2005). Connections between language and reading in children with poor reading comprehension. In H. Catts & A. Kamhi (Eds.), *The connections between language and reading disabilities* (pp. 41-54). Mahwah, NJ: Erlbaum.

National Reading Panel. (2000). *Report of the National Reading Panel: Teaching children to read – An evidence-based assessment of the scientific research literature on reading and its implications for reading instruction.* Jessup, MD: National Institute for Literacy at EDPubs.

Olson, D. (1991). Literacy and objectivity: The rise of modern science. In D. Olson, & N. Torrance (Eds.), *Literacy and orality* (pp. 149-164). New York, NY: Cambridge University Press.

Olson, D. (1994). *The world on paper.* Cambridge: Cambridge University Press.

Paris, S., & Hamilton, E. (2009). The development of children's reading comprehension. In S. Israel & G. Duffy (Eds.), *Handbook of research on reading comprehension* (pp. 32-53). New York: Routledge/Taylor & Francis Group.

Paris, S., & Stahl, S. (Eds.). (2005*). Children's reading comprehension and assessment.* Mahwah, NJ: Erlbaum.

Paul, P. (2001). *Language and deafness* (3rd ed.). San Diego, CA: Singular/Thomson Learning.

Paul, P. (2003). Processes and components of reading. In M. Marschark & P. Spencer (Eds.), *Handbook of deaf studies, language, and education* (pp. 97-109). New York: Oxford University Press.

Paul, P. (2006). New literacies, multiple literacies, unlimited literacies: What now, what next, where to? A response to "Blue listerine, parochialism & ASL literacy." *Journal of Deaf Studies and Deaf Education, 11*(3), 382-387.

Paul, P. (2009). *Language and deafness* (4th ed.). Sudbury, MA: Jones & Bartlett Learning.

Paul, P., & Wang, Y. (2006a). Multiliteracies and literate thought. *Theory into Practice, 45*(4), 304-310.

Paul, P., & Wang, Y. (2006b). Literate thought and deafness: A call for a new perspective and line of research on literacy. *Punjab University Journal of Special Education* (Pakistan), *2*(1), 28-37.

Pinker, S. (1994). *The language instinct: How the mind creates language.* New York, NY: William Morrow & Company.

Rubin, D. (1995). *Memory in oral traditions: The cognitive psychology of epic, ballads, and counting-out rhymes.* New York: Oxford University Press.

Ruddell, R., & Unrau, N. (Eds.). (2004). *Theoretical models and processes of reading* (5th ed.). Newark, DE: International Reading Association.

Rumelhart, D. (2004). Toward an interactive model of reading. In R. Ruddell & N. Unrau (Eds.), *Theoretical models and processes of reading* (5th ed.) (pp. 1149-1179). Newark, DE: International Reading Association.

Snow, C., Burns, S., & Griffin, P. (Eds.). (1998). *Preventing Reading Difficulties in Young Children.* Washington, DC: National Academy Press.

Snowling, M., & Hulme, C. (Eds.). (2005). *The science of reading: A handbook.* Malden, MA: Blackwell.

Stanovich, K. (1991). Word recognition: Changing perspectives. In R. Barr, M. Kamil, P. Mosenthal, & P. D. Pearson (Eds.), *Handbook of reading research* (2nd ed.) (pp. 418-452). White Plains, NY: Longman.

Stanovich, K. (1992). Speculations on the causes and consequences of individual differences in early reading acquisition. In P. Gough, L. Ehri, & R. Treiman (Eds.), *Reading acquisition* (pp. 307-342). Hillsdale, NJ: Erlbaum.

Sticht, T., Beck, L., Hauke, R., Kleiman, G., & James, J. (1974). *Auding and reading: A developmental model.* Alexandria, VA: Human Resources Research Organization (HumPRO).

Sticht, T., & James, J. (1984). Listening and reading. In P. D. Pearson, R. Barr, M. Kamil, & P. Mosenthal (Eds.), *Handbook of reading research* (pp. 293-317). New York: Longman.

Trezek, B., Wang, Y., & Paul, P. (2011). Processes and components of reading. In M. Marschark & P. Spencer (Eds.), *Handbook of deaf studies, language, and education* (Vol. 1, Part 2) (pp. 99-114). New York: Oxford University Press.

Tulving, E., & Craik, F. (Eds.). (2000). *The Oxford handbook of memory.* New York: Oxford University Press.

Tyner, K. (1998). *Literacy in a digital world: teaching and learning in the age of information.* Mahwah, NJ: Lawrence Erlbaum Associates.

Vygotsky, L. (1962). *Thought and language.* Cambridge, MA: The MIT Press.

Vygotsky, L. (1978). *Mind in society: The development of higher psychological processes.* Cambridge, MA: Harvard University Press.

Wang, Y. (2005). *Literate thought: Metatheorizing in literacy and deafness.* Unpublished doctoral dissertation, Ohio State University, Columbus.

Wang, Y., Kretschmer, R., & Hartman, M. (2008). Reading and students who are d/Deaf or hard of hearing. *Journal of Balanced Reading Instruction, 15*(2), 53-68.

Wang, Y., Lee, C., & Paul, P. (2010). An understanding of the literacy levels of students who are deaf/hard-of-hearing in the United States, China, and South Korea. *L1-Educational Studies in Language and Literature, 10*(1), 87-98.

FURTHER READING

Brown, D. (1954). *Auding as the primary language ability.* Unpublished doctoral dissertation, Stanford University, California.

Carroll, J. B. (1964). *Language and thought.* Englewood Cliffs, NJ: Prentice-Hall.

Huey, E. (1908/1968). *The psychology and pedagogy of reading.* Cambridge, MA: The MIT Press.

Yuill, N., & Oakhill, J. (1991). *Children's problems in text comprehension: An experimental investigation.* Cambridge: Cambridge University Press.

CHAPTER 3

New and Multiple Literacies

Historically, literacy has been viewed as the ability to decode print-based texts, and this definition still pervades in many education circles today. Such a view was limited even before the development of new digital technology, in that typographic literacy extends far beyond decoding and encompasses meaning making, functional use of texts, and critical analysis . . . In a rapidly growing digital world, however, such a narrow perspective is even more limiting. We view literacies as plural, consisting of multiple competencies and practices, each shaped by different contexts, purposes, and uses . . . This perspective recognizes the emergence of new digital literacies that focus not only on foundational skills and practices of reading and writing, but also on the skills, knowledge, and attitudes that enable complex ways of getting and making meanings from multiple textual and symbolic sources.

Warschauer & Ware, 2009, p. 215

In the not too distant past, the primary foci of education were on the acquisition of skills: simple reading, writing, and calculating. Furthermore, as suggested by the passage above, the definition of literacy was limited to reading and writing print-based texts (i.e., script literacy as discussed in Chapters 1 and 2). At present, with advanced and powerful technology, information and knowledge are growing at an unprecedentedly rapid rate in media much broader than print-based texts.

To negotiate the complexities of contemporary plural society, individuals are expected to develop the required intellectual tools and learning strategies to acquire knowledge in multimedia that enables them to use goal-directed, conscious, deliberate, organized thinking in a creative, logical, and reflective manner about social phenomena, science and technology, mathematics, history, and the arts. In short, individuals are now educated to become self-sustaining, lifelong learners who can develop literate thought to access and interpret information in multiple modes (see the discussion of literate thought in Chapter 2). The emergence of this transformed goal for education has launched a new line of research on literacy and will have a pervasive influence on individuals, particularly those labeled as struggling readers and writers.

This chapter starts with a discussion on the definition of literacy. Then, we explore the New and Multiple Literacies through different lenses and paradigms. In essence, we investigate and provide our perspectives on the following questions, which serve as themes for the chapter: How do the New and Multiple Literacies impact our understanding of literate thought? Do these new types of literacies challenge our assumptions about knowledge? What are the effects for children with disabilities or those who have traditional language or literacy problems?

DEFINITION OF LITERACY

What is literacy? What is the value of being literate? What additional parameters does technology bring to the concept of literacy? The answers to these questions are increasingly complicated by influences from multi-disciplinary research endeavors such as literacy education, educational technology, cognitive psychology, sociology, cultural anthropology, film/video studies, art, media theory, game studies, literary criticism, social theory, critical pedagogy, cultural studies, and so on. As discussed in earlier chapters, the answers to these questions are influenced by whether one holds a narrow or broad perspective on the concepts of literacy, who is defined as literate, and even illiteracy.

Traditional Literacy

The historical origin of the term *literacy* can be traced to *literature* (Williams, 1983), which once combined the adjectival meaning of being discerning and knowledgeable with the noun that describes a body of writing on generally acknowledged aesthetic merit. The contemporary meaning of *literature* only includes the latter with its own adjective, *literary*, whereas from the end of the nineteenth century, literacy became a new word to describe the general and necessary skills to read and write typographic (type or print) and chirographic (handwritten) materials.

There has been a common naïve belief in the magical transformative power of simply learning to read and write, which is also conventionally considered as an instrument of precision and power.

Clanchy's (1993) historical study, *From Memory to Written Record: England 1066-1307*, reported that handwritten records introduced in medieval English were used mainly as legal and business records to measure ownership, business transactions, census, and so on. Eventually, complex systems were developed to serve as a mechanism of social control at that time. The rise of the notion of literacy for the general populace in later centuries typically was connected with the invention of the printing press and subsequent availability of written documents, and a democratic and rational society as well as economic growth and industrial development. Any deterioration in literacy has posed problems for a democratic and progressive society. This superficial perception of literacy leads to the notion that illiteracy is a social problem analogous with poverty, malnutrition, and disease, and people who cannot read are pathetic and disadvantaged (Olson, 1994).

As discussed in Chapters 1 and 2, the traditional perception of literacy mistakenly identifies the means of communication with the knowledge that is communicated. In other words, it confounds the *means* of literacy education with the *ends* of literacy education. Olson (1994) believes that the emphasis on the means detracts from the importance of the content being communicated, and he maintains:

> Literacy in Western cultures is not just learning the abc's; it is learning to use the resources of writing for a culturally defined set of tasks and procedures. . . . Literacy is not just a basic set of mental skills isolated from everything else. It is the evolution of those resources in conjunction with the knowledge and skill to exploit those resources for particular purposes that makes up literacy. That is why literacy and literate competence can have a history. . . . We require a much more diversified notion of literacy. (p. 43)

Freire's (1970, 1973, 1985) work on critical literacy also challenged the idea of defining literacy with respect to the framework of a competitive marketplace. According to Freire, the brutal competition in capitalist societies means that some individuals have to lose in order for others to win and the social inequity would exist forever. He believed that the dominant culture defines literacy and the reading and writing skills that are accepted by the mainstream society as tools to reinforce social status. Minority groups have to passively accept the dominance of mainstream culture by learning their literacy in order to survive in the competition.

Freire and Macedo (1987) criticized the current practice of using print literacy to separate literates from illiterates in the schools of the United States. They wrote, "this large number of people who do not read and write and who are expelled from school do not represent a failure of the schooling class; their expulsion reveals the triumph of the schooling class. In fact, this misreading of responsibility reflects the schools' hidden curriculum" (p. 121).

Along the cultural/power parameter of literacy, Kaestle (1991) suggested the existence of a *cultural price* tagged to literacy:

> The uses of literacy are various. As a technology, it gives its possessors potential power; as a stock of cultural knowledge within a given tradition, literacy can constrain or liberate, instruct or entertain, discipline or disaffect people. Princeton historian Lawrence Stone once remarked that if you teach a man to read the Bible, he may also read pornography or seditious literature; put another way, if a man teaches a woman to read so that she may know her place, she may learn that she deserves his. (p. 27)

New and Multiple Literacies

Although the social control feature of written records still exists today, the emergence of new media, such as newspapers, radio, videos, televisions, computers, and so on, complicates the situation. In Tyner's (1998) *Literacy in a Digital World*, the concept of literacy is refined to accommodate the information age:

> In this book, I investigate a third way to use literacy as a source of social power and that is the ability to decode information in a variety of forms, analogous to the reading of print, but also applicable to audio, graphics, and the moving image, a process that Paolo Friere and Donaldo Macedo (1987) call 'reading the world.' If citizens can also manipulate and understand the processes to create messages and distribute them, that is, 'writing the world,' then literacy practices accrue maximum benefit to the individual. It would be false to say that this vision of literacy would automatically translate into an equal distribution of social power. It is obvious that those who control both the channels of distribution and the skillful production of compatible content have access to the most favorable opportunities to influence social policy through sustained creative effort. Nonetheless, a sophisticated and powerful vision of literacy shows potential to enable each person to at least join the debate by skillfully negotiating within the exist-

ing power structure, as well as outside it. And this is why it is urgent that everyone has access to literacy in its most powerful forms. (p. 4)

We (Paul, 1998, 2001, 2006, 2009; Paul & Wang, 2006a, 2006b; Wang, 2005) agree that, instead of narrowly defined as mechanic skills (i.e., reading and writing) involving typographic and chirographic materials, *literacy* should be defined broadly as forms of captured information, including *script literacy, performance literacy, caption literacy* (see also Chapter 2), *computer literacy, Internet literacy, digital literacy, information communication technology (ICT) literacy, scientific literacy, literacies of technology, visual literacy, mathematical literacy,* and so on. To benefit maximally from literacy, individuals in the information age thus need to access information (i.e., decode information in various forms) and know how to interpret the information (i.e., manipulate and understand the processes to create messages and distribute them). Such a broadly defined literacy includes not only print literacy but also the New and Multiple Literacies, which also can be defined as *media literacy* (with more emphasis on understanding), *information literacy* (with more emphasis on access), *new media literacies,* and *multiliteracies.*

Accordingly, the purposes of the New and Multiple Literacies expand from social control to: 1) support democracy, self-expression, participation, and socially active citizenship (Kellner, 2000); 2) offer knowledge economy, competitiveness, and choice; and 3) sustain lifelong learning, cultural expression, and personal fulfillment (Livingstone, Van Couvering & Thumim, 2009).

The potential danger in the field is the tendency to promote one form of literacy over another. The competition is the same as arguing which tool is better: a hammer, screw driver, or knife (see also the discussion in Chapter 2). Although the printed word changed and incorporated oral traditions, print culture did not wipe out oral tradition. Similarly, radio, television, and computers overlap with other literacy technologies because these electronic communication technologies incorporate both oral and print conventions. In fact, book sales are at the all-time historical high in today's information age. There is no magic about any particular literacy. The pen, book, and computer are only literacy artifacts that are used as technologies to record information, which is the end product (Clanchy, 1993).

In his landmark book, *The Labyrinths of Literacy*, Graff (1995) provided some powerful conclusions about literacy:

1. Literacy is historically founded and grounded; that is, literacy cannot be completely understood without knowing the sociohistorical forces of its time.

2. Literacy is fundamentally complex; therefore, *strong* theories of literacy fail.

3. No mode or means of learning and communicating is neutral, and literacy is not an exception.

4. Alphabetic literacy (i.e., reading and writing) is an exceptionally valuable set of competencies among other literacies.

5. No set of literacies is superior to others.

6. Reading and writing are not easy to learn, so blaming individual learners for their failure to learn and advance is irresponsible of schools or society.

7. The presence and significance of multiple paths of learning literacy should not be lost in the triumph of one correct path.

8. The practices that equated literacy learning (here meaning reading and writing) with elementary education have restricted and stratified both literacy and education.

9. There is no one route to near-universal literacy and associated modern concomitants, and, similarly, there is no one route in terms of literacy to economic development, industrialization, democraticization, and the like.

PARADIGMS OF THE NEW AND MULTIPLE LITERACIES

We adopt the technology and literacy model proposed by Warschauer and Ware (2009) to categorize paradigms of the New and Multiple Literacies as learning, change, and power. Instead of promoting one particular paradigm, we believe that the co-existing paradigms of the New and Multiple Literacies should work collaboratively for paradigmatic commensurability.

Table 3-1 provides a summary of the three paradigms.

Learning Paradigm

The *learning paradigm* concerns the use of the New and Multiple Literacies to enhance students' literacy learning in general, which is measured by their performance on standardized reading and writing assessments. The popularity of this view has increased since the No Child Left Behind Act of 2002, which favors evidence-based, mainly quantitative, research. The representative studies within the learning paradigm include various software-based programs to engage students in multimedia literacy activities such as drill-and-practice, individualized reading instruction, extensive reading management, automated writing evaluation, and so on (see the review in Warschauer & Ware, 2009). The emphasis is on multiple ways of improving reading and writing skills, rather than

Table 3-1.   Paradigms of the New and Multiple Literacies

Factor	Details
Learning	
Fields of inquiry	Educational technology, educational administration, educational policy
Goal	Raise test scores and improve student learning
Research interests	Technology's impact on learning and literacy outcomes
Change	
Fields of inquiry	New literacy studies, cultural and media studies, game studies, computers and writing
Goal	Make schooling relevant by valuing new literacies
Research interests	Relationship between home and school literacy practices
Power	
Fields of inquiry	Sociology, economics, development studies, critical pedagogy
Goal	Empower youth through knowledge, access, and skill with socially relevant tools
Research interests	Relationship of access and use to educational and social equity

Source: Adapted from Warschauer & Ware (2009).

enhancing broader literacy skills such as multimedia and hypertext development or Internet-related skills of locating, storing, evaluating, and critiquing information. The New and Multiple Literacies are considered means to meet the end of developing print literacy skills.

Change Paradigm

The *change paradigm* considers the technologies used in the New and Multiple Literacies as revolutionary transformations in production, distribution, and acquisition of information similar to the invention of the printing press in the fifteenth century. Considering school as a conservative institution, supporters of the change paradigm advocate a fundamental educational reform to replace current modes of literacy instruction with those more representative of the technologies used outside of school, for example, television, computer, video gaming, and so on (Warschauer & Ware, 2009). The primary objective of the change paradigm is to build an effective pedagogical bridge between school-based and home-based literacies. Technology, literacy, culture, and society are considered intimately intertwined.

Power Paradigm

Advocates of the power paradigm consider the New and Multiple Literacies as being closely related to social, economic, and educational power. They propose transformative pedagogical approaches such as project-based technology-mediated literacy learning that moves away from the prescribed and scripted print literacy practices that are currently in vogue in schools (Warschauer & Ware, 2009). Advocates of the power paradigm are most likely to argue that the use of print literacy, particularly school texts, is limited and restrictive and does not prepare students for the diversity of the twenty-first century (e.g., see various articles in Bloome & Paul, 2006).

MEDIA OF THE NEW AND MULTIPLE LITERACIES

Few people question that we are currently in a state of disequilibrium as we attempt to integrate our knowledge of reading comprehension based on print literacy with our emerging knowledge or view of comprehension in the New and Multiple Literacies (Dalton & Proctor, 2009). In general, print literacy is linear, static, temporally and physically bounded, and often with an explicit purpose, authorship, and authority. The New and Multiple Literacies are nonlinear, multimodal, interactive, heavily visually oriented, unbounded in time and space, and often with ambiguous delivery of authorship and authority. Some print literacy skills such as decoding and fluent reading might still be required in certain New and Multiple Literacies activities such as reading a Web-based text, but many do not involve these basic print literacy skills. An example is watching a YouTube.com video demonstration on how to change the oil in a car. Other New and Multiple Literacies activities require additional literacy skills that are irrelevant to print literacy skills, for example, the ability to identify the most effective key words in a Web-based search that will provide the specific information desired.

Table 3-2 summarizes factors influencing literacy development in the New and Multiple Literacies compared with those of print literacy (a detailed discussion of a few prominent factors for print literacy can be found in Chapters 2 and 6).

Many media of the New and Multiple Literacies are intertwined. In the ensuing sections, we highlight only two of the most popular media: Internet and video gaming.

Internet

A momentous global milestone was reached in 2005 when the one-billionth individual began reading, viewing, writing, and communicating online. Furthermore, with the exponential growth rate, approximately half of the world's population will be online by 2012 and Internet access will be virtually omnipresent sometime thereafter (Coiro, Knobel, Lankshear, & Leu, 2009a). In the United States, 94% of students aged 12 to 17 years have home access to the Internet (Lawless & Schrader, 2009). As noted by Coiro, Knobel, Lankshear, and Leu, (2009b):

> The Internet is the largest single repository of information to have been compiled in the history of our civilization. Moreover, as each person contributes to it, the amount of online information grows at a ferocious rate. This poses an interesting paradox: the more information that appears online, the more challenging it is to turn this information into knowledge. (p. 209)

Table 3-2. Summary of Factors Influencing Literacy Development in the New and Multiple Literacies Compared with Print Literacy

Reader Factors	Print Literacy	New and Multiple Literacies
Word recognition and fluency	Key factors in determining reading level and text choice.	Speech- or sign-based digital text diminishes the impact of word recognition and fluency; instead, listening or signing comprehension becomes a better indicator of reading level and text choice.
Vocabulary	One of the strongest predictors of comprehension; support via context, glossary or bold font words.	Influence of vocabulary knowledge may be reduced by more extensive just-in-time supports, such as: glossary hyperlinks, multimedia representations, access to online tools (e.g., dictionary, thesaurus, encyclopedia, and language translation), and access to social network of experts and peers.
Metalinguistic awareness	Syntactic awareness is important for monitoring comprehension for word recognition errors that produce ungrammatical and/or meaningless sentences. Pragmatic awareness is essential for comprehending and keeping track of the ideas exchanged during a dialogue and for understanding the goals and purposes of the dialogue. Limited support is offered in print text, for example, the different usage of punctuation marks for various purposes of communication.	Speech- or sign-based digital text can help the reader to utilize awareness of conventions in using spoken or sign language to understand different types of meanings conveyed in the dialogue signaled in speech by intonation, pause and intensity, or in signing by facial expression, pause and signing space.
Passage-specific prior knowledge	Prior knowledge of text structure helps the reader to organize information in the text in ways that facilitate comprehension. Supplementary aids include:	Influence of passage-specific prior knowledge may be mediated by broader array of just-in-time supports, such as: layers of information via hyperlinks within and

	graphics, graphic organizers, informational callouts, literacy analysis notes, etc.	across hypertexts, multimedia representations, tools for really simple syndication (RSS) feeds and indexing, and access to social network of experts and peers.
Topic-specific prior knowledge	World knowledge and domain-specific knowledge assist the reader's comprehension by helping him/her to draw inferences on the concepts encountered in texts that are related to knowledge they have already acquired. Supplementary aids include: graphics, graphic organizers, informational callouts, etc.	Similarly, influence of topic-specific prior knowledge may be mediated by a broader array of just-in-time supports, such as: layers of information via hyperlinks within and across hypertexts, multimedia representations, online encyclopedia or language translation, content Web sites, tools for RSS feeds and indexing, and access to social network of experts and peers.
Cognitive and metacognitive strategies	In development of comprehension, it is indispensable to have general cognitive strategies such as critical analysis, inference, and reasoning as well as problem solving, and metacognitive strategies that are employed to think about and maintain control over reading. However, limited support is provided by print text, for example, graphic organizers, reflection questions, main idea statements, summaries, and so on.	The reader is able to flexibly use resources and tools described above to locate information, evaluate information, synthesize across multiple sources, and conduct collaborative learning.
Engagement and motivation	It is not enough to simply possess knowledge and skills in reading, the reader must have the willingness or motivation to actually use the various strategies and skills. Affect factors in print include: genre, author, quality of illustrations and aesthetics, writing quality, perceived relevance, text choice, purpose for reading, etc.	In addition to the affect factors in print, the reader's interest is also mediated by options for multimedia, hyperlinked content, interactivity, social interaction, and choice of supports.

Source: Adapted from Dalton & Proctor (2009).

Historically, print and audiovisual texts were produced in scarcity with only a few people having access to the production and distribution system, which "maintained a strong distinction between producers and consumers, with key filters operating to select material to be distributed in accordance with criteria of cultural quality, editorial values, professional production conventions, and political or market pressures" (Livingstone et al., 2009, p. 112). Compared with the authoritative and carefully selected texts available in a library, the Internet provides individuals with a variety of primary sources, which might be overwhelming for many underprepared users. In particular, new waves of social practices and new types of communities (e.g., Facebook, Twitter, wiki, Flickr, blogging, etc.) have mushroomed across cyberspace.

Meanwhile, writing on the Internet and other word processors is considered to be more of a social process with more collaborations, sharing, and revisions than in the pencil-and-paper venue (see the reviews in Bangert-Drowns, 1993; Cochran-Smith, 1991). Furthermore, in a meta-analysis comparing writing with computers to pencil-and-paper writing in grades kindergarten through 12 (K-12), Goldberg, Russell, and Cook (2003) found that writing with a word processor resulted in a greater length and higher quality of text, although there was no evidence that learners were more engaged and motivated.

As a special feature of the Internet, hypertext has received substantial attention. Reading hypertext is not simply point-and-click but a complicated point-read-think-and-click process (Tapscott, 1988). It places high demands on critical-reading skills because Web readers need to constantly ask themselves why they are reading a particular Web text and always assess the reliability of the texts (Kuiper & Volman, 2009). As critical consumers of the Internet, readers need to deconstruct the information, identify bias, and ask whose voice is represented, whose is not, and why (Dalton & Proctor, 2009).

Another unique characteristic of the Internet is the nonverbal visual component, which requires Web readers to read visual information and judge it on its functionality, meaning, and relationship to the text (Kuiper & Volman, 2009). The visual information can be an animated graphic, photo slide show, diagrams, equations, symbols, artifacts, gestures, audio/video clip, or image with little accompanying verbal information. Based on Paivio's (1986) dual-coding theory and Mayer's (1997, 2001) multimedia learning theory, visual/pictorial and auditory/verbal information are processed via separate channels. Meaningful multimedia learning occurs when the visual/pictorial and auditory/verbal representations are connected to form an integrated knowledge model. Due to limited cognitive capacity, multimedia learning should minimize the learners' extraneous processing, manage their essential processing, and foster their generative processing (see the details of each principle in Mayer, 2009).

Collectively, while promoting democracy and freedom, the Internet also demands access and navigation skills that are not necessary in print literacy, for example, successful Web-search strategies mentioned earlier. In addition, a more refined critical evaluation skill is required for Internet users to negotiate conflicting information presented online. Other than locating and critiquing sources, Internet-based literacy skills also include storing sources, communicating and sharing perspectives with each other through e-mail correspondence, instant messaging, file sharing and so on, establishing online discourse communities, and judging the friendliness or usability of digital tools to work effectively and efficiently, all of which go beyond traditional vocabulary and text comprehension in print literacy (Kulikowich, 2009). Internet literacy requires an integrated sum of numerous sub-skills.

Table 3-3 provides a summary of the special features and required unique literacy skills of the Internet compared with those of print literacy.

Video Gaming

Landmark studies conducted by Gee (2003, 2007) identified video gaming as a new literacy because, consistent with gaming conventions, players access and interpret images, actions, words, sounds, and movements to encode and decode the meanings in the game. Players participate in the game as a form of social practice. Gee (2003) suggested that advantages of video gaming might include situated learning, reducing the consequences of failure, the benefits of affinity groups, and the power of information given on-demand or just-in-time instead of just-in-case.

One of the most popular educational gaming software programs is *JumpStart World* (http://www.jumpstart.com; Knowledge Adventure, Torrance, CA), which creates an adventure-based three-dimensional (3D) virtual world that is personalized for each player to learn math, reading, and critical thinking skills. For example, if a child is reading below grade level, the game can dispense more reading-related activities. Specifically, it can be easily used as a zone of proximal development (Vygotsky, 1962,

Table 3-3. Summary of Special Features and Required Unique Literacy Skills of the Internet

Special Features	Required Unique Literacy Skills
Hypertext	Access, locate, and navigate information
	Critically evaluate why reading a particular Web text
	Assess the reliability of the Web texts
	Construct knowledge from various sources
Web search	Aware of successful Web-search strategies, such as how to choose appropriate and effective keywords
Visual information	Read visual information
	Judge visual information on its functionality, meaning, and relationship to the text
Capability to save information	Know how and where to store information in multiple hardware
Various communicating and sharing tools	Know how and where to communicate and share perspectives with each other through e-mail correspondence, instant messaging, file sharing, etc.
Online discourse communities	Know how and where to establish or join online discourse communities
Other digital tools	Judge the friendliness or usability of digital tools to work effectively and efficiently

1978) that "scaffolds" players because the next dispensed game is based on the performance of the previous game. For example, if the player is struggling with the difference between a long vowel /ā/ and the short vowel /ă/ in a game, then a range of different games working on this concept will follow until the player demonstrates proficiency. The player can create his/her own character and, after a few activities, even their own pets.

The JumpStart World is an interactive game where the player's character can explore several different areas (e.g., StoryLand, ScienceLand, FutureLand, AdventureLand, etc.) to earn medals to go to the next world. It has various JumpStart characters with different personalities with whom the player's character will interact. These friendly characters will not only talk about the importance of eating a healthy breakfast daily but also how having friends means sharing your things, and then ask the player character to do that in the game. JumpStart World also includes a massively multiplayer online (MMO) game where children can race against each other to earn points on educational exercises.

IMPACT OF THE NEW AND MULTIPLE LITERACIES ON LITERATE THOUGHT AND ASSUMPTIONS ABOUT KNOWLEDGE

More than two millennia ago, Plato claimed that using the technology of literacy was a relatively minor problem compared to what people did with the information that literacy made available to them (Tyner, 1998). That is, the technology of literacy (e.g., reading and writing) is not as important as the purpose of literacy. We propose to connect the purpose of being literate with the concept of literate thought, which refers to the ability to access and interpret captured information (Paul, 1998, 2001, 2006, 2009; Paul & Wang, 2006a, 2006b; Wang, 2005; see also, Chapter 1).

Literacy involves management of the language and thought in which we are engaged. In other words, literacy involves accessing and interpreting information via communicative interactions and cognitive activity (e.g., metacognition). *Accessing information* means to be able to decode the message or to obtain the content/meaning, which refers to the semantic content of the information. *Interpreting information* means to reflect on the information to solve problems or to develop other higher-level critical thinking skills. There is no doubt that different literacies have different modes of communication. The question is whether these different modes of communication result in different ways to access and interpret information during communicative interactions and during an individual's thinking endeavors.

Modes of Literacy and Accessing Information

One major difference between script literacy and performance (i.e., speaking or signing) is that, during communication, script literacy is relatively permanent whereas performance is transient, meaning that it progresses with time (Ong, 1977; see also, the discussion on performance and performance literacy in Chapter 2). More specifically, script literacy provides us with "a concrete, thing-like appearance" (Saljo, 1988, p. 3), whereas performance is more elusive. It thus is easier to register authority in script than in performance, which might explain to some degree the reason for the heavy reliance on script in assessment and in viewing script literacy as a prerequisite for civilization today.

Ong (1967) agrees that, because of the motionlessness of writing, it is possible to return and correct it, which is an impossible task for speech or the performance mode. In essence, reading and writing as communicative practices have been a part of Western culture long enough to have become obviously perceived as a natural and neutral way of conveying a message. In a sense, script literacy has been considered as "an essential ingredient of implicit Western ethnocentrism" (Saljo, 1988, p. 1).

It therefore is not surprising that print literacy has been considered the legitimate literacy in Western schools. Olson (1974) believes that dramatically challenging print literacy's crucial role in schooling is impossible; it is an essential part in the formation and communication of information on science and philosophy. In addition, it is accessible to both producers and receivers. Nevertheless, Saljo (1988) argues that such a schooled literacy is a specific mode of literacy geared towards the needs of a special social institution, which considers reading and writing as ends in themselves rather than as means to accomplish other tasks. In other words, the fixation on reading and writing has been a crucial mistake in our education system, which has led to misunderstanding the richness of literate thought in other modes.

Although it is too radical to deny the contribution of print literacy to communication and civilization, we need to devote more attention to the previous marginalized literacy (e.g., New and Multiple Literacies) and recognize that literacy assists communicative interactions and makes us better thinkers not only by print, but also by other modes. It is well accepted that literacy assists us to view the multiplicity of the world and expands our vision; it also helps us to respect our interconnectedness with other people and the intrinsic pluralism of meaning (Langer, 1995).

It might be difficult for some people to admit that, at the same time, literacy itself is a multimode entity. There is no way to quantitatively measure the different modes of literacies, but it is suggested that they are equal to each other as well as independent of each other. There is research on individuals contributing to the discussions of printed texts, which were offered orally (Olson, 1989; see also, Chapter 1). Furthermore, we have valued the civilized world long before the invention of printing and still treasure the role of oral (performance) literacy today.

We need to recognize that modern technology makes an enormous contribution to the development of oral (performance) literacy. For example, print literacy is a form of decontextualized information (see Chapter 1) that separates textual information from the reader's interpretation. Some scholars argue that print literacy is an essential foundation for language and communication because it concentrates on the problem of human intersubjectivity and joint communication concern in social interaction by transferring decontextualized pieces of information from sender to recipient (Saljo, 1988). In contrast, as previously mentioned, performance typically is delivered in face-to-face, live, contextualized circumstances, which might put it in a disadvantageous position in communication.

With the development of technology, information presented in speech or signing can be captured in audio or video electronic media (e.g., audio books, audio taped lectures, audio CDs, DVDs, etc.) and be viewed as performance literacy (see also, Chapter 2). Or, in the video materials, the same information can be signed together with a print component to make it caption literacy. The information is separated from the initial speaker or signer and can be decontextualized. Print literacy therefore has no privilege over performance literacy for being decontextualized information.

Literacy can be considered as the combination of the captured information itself and the mode of the information or, in other words, the content (namely, meaning) of the information and the vehicle of the information. Different literacies might have different vehicles—because information is exchanged by speech, signing, or print—but at the same time have roughly the same content. For example, the same lecture can be signed by the interpreter or documented as a print record. The vehicles of information can be understood as nonessential as long as there is roughly the same meaning communicated.

Modes of Literacy and Interpreting/Utilizing Information

If it is accepted that different modes of literacy are equivalent and self-sufficient for accessing information, what are their roles in utilizing information, for example, in creative, critical, and reasonable thinking?

Vygotsky (1962, 1978) believes that cognitive development depends on the internalization of psychological tools, which can be defined as outside sign-stimuli influencing human behavior. Each sign has a specific meaning. We can understand signs as nonessential carriers of meaning, so signs retreat to the edge and semantics come to the center of internalization. If substituting one semiotic system for another while retaining its semantics is possible, the internalization processes can be similar, which indicates that the development processes are similar as well. For example, students who are d/Deaf or hard of hearing can use alternative symbolic systems (i.e., signing or speech) to gain the similar semantics. Their literate thought development process thus could be similar to that of students with normal or typical hearing.

The core of Vygotsky's theoretical framework is that mental processes cannot be understood without understanding the tools and signs that mediate them (Wertsch, 1985). *Mediation*, an essential concept in psychological tools, means "the use of certain signs or symbols in mental processing. It involves using something else to represent behavior or objects in the environment. The signs or symbols can be universal or specific to a small group, such as a family or classroom, or they can be specific to a particular person" (Bodrova & Leong, 1996, p. 21). Although Vygotsky never restricted the notion of mental tools to language, he argued that language played a preeminent role in mediation. Furthermore, he claimed that semiotic functions, such as the generalizing or abstracting function, would be difficult, if not impossible, to carry out in the absence of a bona fide language (Vygotsky, 1962, 1978).

Bodrova and Leong (1996) reiterated the role of language as a mental tool, an actual mechanism for thinking:

> Language makes thinking more abstract, flexible, and independent from the immediate stimuli. Through language, memories and anticipations of

the future are brought to bear on the new situation, thus influencing its outcome. When children use symbols and concepts to think, they no longer need to have the object present in order to think about it. Language allows the child to imagine, manipulate, create new ideas, and share those ideas with others. It is one of the ways we exchange social information with each other. Thus, language has two roles; it is instrumental in the development of cognition and is also itself part of cognitive processing. (p. 13)

The basic element of language is the word. A word can be utilized to refer to objects and to identify properties, actions, and relationships. Words organize things into systems. That is to say, words codify our experience.

The basic function of a word is its referential function or, using Vygotskian terminology (Vygotsky, 1962), *object reference*. In the absence of words, human beings would have to deal only with things that could be perceived and manipulated directly. With the help of language, however, humans can deal with things that we have not perceived even indirectly and with things that were part of the experience of earlier generations. Words thus add another dimension to our world; we humans have a double world (Luria, 1982). We humans can not only regulate our perceptions, we can also regulate our memories by utilizing images because we can contrive these images at will even in the absence of the objects. We can control our actions, which means that words give rise not only to a bilateral world but also to voluntary action, which could not exist without language. Furthermore, human beings can carry out trial-and-error thinking and other cognitive actions in the absence of real objects. In other words, we can act internally. Internalization occurs when external behaviors *grow into the mind* while maintaining the same structure, focus, and function as their external manifestation (Vygotsky & Luria, 1993).

A word not only substitutes for or represents an object but also analyzes it by isolating and generalizing the properties of the object or, in other words, by incorporating it into a system of complex associations and relationships. When we use a word to refer to some object, we automatically include it in a peculiar category. Such an abstracting and generalizing function is known as its *meaning*. Luria claimed that because the powers of abstraction and generalization are the most important functions of thinking, a word is a *unit of thought*. He further argued that by abstracting and generalizing the property of an object, a word becomes an instrument of thought and a means of communication (Luria, 1982).

In brief, a word not only duplicates the world, it also serves as a powerful instrument for analyzing the world (and even for imagining future worlds!). Luria concluded: "language is a system of codes adequate for independently analyzing an object and expressing any of its features, properties, and relationships. The word is the foundation of the system of codes which ensures the transition from the sensory to the rational world" (Luria, 1982, p. 39). The word—not reading and writing skills—therefore becomes the main instrument of human conscious activity or, in our view, the mental tools of literate thought. Such an understanding of literate thought does not limit the mode of the word to print and suggests that literate thought could be mode-independent.

Conclusion

It is hard to imagine written language as a mother tongue because it is a strenuous process involving enormous learning efforts. Compared to written language, speech is easy because sounds are spontaneously produced and speech progresses through simple play with sounds (Ong, 1967; Saljo, 1988). "Oral speech evolves naturally in the process of social interaction between children and adults," whereas "written speech emerges as the result of special learning" (Luria, 1982, p. 165). Olson also argued: "Writing is dependent in a fundamental way on speech. One's oral language, it is now recognized, is the fundamental possession and tool of mind; writing, though important, is always secondary" (Olson, 1994, p. 8).

Olson further claimed:

> We don't want to say that we think in writing. Rather, writing offers us a set of options for cognition, options we choose among when we write. There is no magic about writing. It is not merely transcription, but neither is it a medium that operates independently of speech and thought. Writing, as Gombrich said of art, offers us a formulary into which we insert information. If there is no space on the formulary for a certain kind of information, it is just too bad for that information. Scholars have become increasingly attentive to what our formulary, our writing, leads us to overlook, but we also continue to believe that what it allows us to capture more than compensates for what is lost. Hence, we look forward to a long literate tradition and with it increased interest in understanding just what all literacy involves. (p. 292)

That is, the development of literate thought is not dependent on a particular mode of captured information, and the New and Multiple

Literacies are justified and equally respected as vehicles for the development of literate thought. This reconceptualized description of literacy does not discard or replace traditional print literacy. On the contrary, it is a more complex reformulated framework that incorporates and integrates more than one mode of literacy, allowing individuals more choices to accomplish the goal of literacy education.

It is hypothesized that literacy development in an alternative mode might contribute to the development of print literacy as well. Such an understanding of literacy will provide significant contributions to the field, especially for the traditionally marginalized populations who cannot benefit sufficiently from the traditional reading world, for example, children with disabilities or those who have traditional language/literacy problems such as many English language learners (ELLs).

CHILDREN WITH DISABILITIES AND ELLs

By adding the additional dimension of technology, the reconceptualized literacy connects the concept of literate thought with the goal of literacy, which significantly broadens the choices for children with disabilities and those who have traditional language/literacy problems (e.g., ELLs) to access and interpret captured information. Meanwhile, the pervasive reliance on pencil-and-paper standardized tests as a means of assessment might be viewed as oppression for many struggling readers, who encounter great difficulties in accessing information in the print mode and cannot keep up with the *standard*. The linear understanding of what constitutes academic success thus has left these children behind. Using the New and Multiple Literacies with alternative assessments should promote equity and social justice in learning and, hopefully, bridge the achievement gap in schools as well.

Such an understanding of literacy might change the way we view the literacy performance of children with disabilities or those who have traditional language/literacy problems (see the reviews in Chapters 6–9). It might be possible that children with disabilities or those who have traditional language/literacy problems have not received full credit for their literacy skills—that is, literacy in the broad sense. It might be impossible for them to reach the same level as their peers on print tests for school information that is conventionally offered in print. On the other hand, it might be possible that they can gain skills and utilize the same school information in alternative modes, and use alternative assessments for their academic achievement. Let's take science education as an example.

New and Multiple Literacies in Science Education

Many students with disabilities or ELLs have difficulty accessing academic content information such as science that traditionally has been presented in print. For example, in traditional text-based science instruction, much of the information that reflects school knowledge is obtained through printed texts. Heavily reliant on textbooks as the major tool, conventional science instruction and assessment present a problem for struggling readers who cannot successfully access and utilize the information in print. Studies show that the pattern of low performance was similar across the literature on traditional science assessments for students with disabilities and ELLs where the tests require students to read and write in print and their performance is evaluated mainly on the written product (Cawley & Parmar, 2001; Donohoe & Zigmond, 1988; Harnisch & Wilkinson, 1989).

Facing such a challenge, some researchers have tried to teach and improve reading and writing skills of students with disabilities (e.g., Barman & Stockton, 2002; Borron, 1978; Cawley & Parmar, 2001) within the context of science. But the question is: do students need to read to be taught or to be assessed for science knowledge and skills?

It is necessary to reconceptualize and broaden our current notion of literacy in the classroom. Students with disabilities, including those who are struggling readers, and ELLs might need opportunities to gain and think about complex information through a captured (i.e., preserved, saved, or documented) mode other than print—that is, in a speaking and/or signing literacy mode or other modes in the New and Multiple Literacies. Oral or sign literacy (i.e., performance literacy) (Paul, 1998, 2001, 2006, 2009; Paul & Wang, 2006a, 2006b; Wang, 2005) might be another legitimate route for developing scientific conceptual knowledge for these students.

Students with disabilities and ELLs need to be able to access and utilize information that has been typically presented in print literacy materials. Information presented in print (books, journals) can be transliterated and captured in oral (e.g., talking books) or sign (e.g., video books) forms. Furthermore, children can be taught skills and/or have numerous opportunities for working with such captured information (e.g., studying, remembering, synthesizing, etc.).

In traditional text-based science classrooms, the majority of instruction focuses on the acquisition of factual knowledge. However, inquiry-based science instruction emphasizes conceptual knowledge that is more likely to be generalized than factual information. The conceptual approach only considers scientific knowledge that helps students make sense of their surroundings as meaningful. Within such a conceptual approach, students act as involved performers instead of detached observers and their comprehension of the subject matter is contextually contingent and grounded in experience (Cawley & Parmar, 2001; Stoddart, Pinal, Latzke, & Canaday, 2002; see also, the discussion in Chapter 4).

In essence, through the contextualized use of the New and Multiple Literacies in scientific inquiry, students with disabilities and ELLs can develop and practice metacognitive thinking skills while simultaneously enhancing their scientific conceptual understanding. The curricular integration of inquiry-based science instruction and the New and Multiple Literacies is a promising practice for them to access a general education curriculum. Such a universal design perspective has received increasing attention in the field of education.

Universal Design

The dynamic flexibility of the New and Multiple Literacies offers new opportunities to meet the individual needs of a wide spectrum of learners. As an instructional design framework, *Universal Design for Learning (UDL)* has become popular in education.

> Universal Design for Learning (UDL) is based on the application of universal design in architecture and industrial design, where it is standard practice to design physical spaces, structures, and tools so that access is ensured for the full spectrum of individuals, including those with physical or sensory disabilities. For example, sidewalk curb cuts and closed captioning on TV are two examples of universal design. A key premise of universal design is that society benefits as a whole from innovation that originally targets a specific user group. (Dalton & Proctor, 2009, p. 302)

Particularly, with the mandate of the Individuals with Disabilities Education Act (IDEA), enacted in 1975 and most recently amended in 2004, UDL has become an increasingly familiar concept in special education. The federal law ensures that "all students, including those with disabilities, have the right to access, participate, and make meaningful progress in the general education curriculum, with the long-term goal of developing individuals who are lifelong learners and contributing citizens" (Dalton & Proctor, 2009, p. 302).

In literacy education, UDL is manifested through the use of digital text, which offers the read-aloud functionality via text-to-speech (TTS), and synthetic voice or signing on book-on-audio/video (i.e., performance literacy). Performance literacy capsizes the concept of *readability* because access to information is no longer dependent on students' word recognition skills and fluency levels on print; instead, listening or signing comprehension might be a better indicator of the *readability* of the text (Dalton & Proctor, 2009; Edyburn, 2002; McKenna, Reinking, Labbo, & Kieffer, 1999).

Research on this topic (see the review in Strangman & Dalton, 2005) has been interested in employing performance literacy as a compensatory tool either to bypass decoding difficulties and provide access to the content in the print text or to directly improve general reading comprehension of digital text. The results provided a mixed picture of the effectiveness of performance literacy on comprehension, however. A general finding is that performance literacy might be more effective in improving the comprehension of older students compared with younger ones.

Lundberg and Oloffson (1993) found that while TTS improved the comprehension of grades 4 to 6 students with reading disabilities, it had no effect on younger students in grades 2 to 3. It might be possible that older students experienced a larger gap between the readability of the text and their print reading-skill level than the younger ones, or they were more capable of determining when they need TTS support (McKenna, 1998; McKenna & Watkins, 1994). Furthermore, studies have suggested that performance literacy could improve reading engagement, motivate students, particularly adolescent readers, in accessing age-appropriate materials, and provide the opportunities to focus on the content of the text without considering the print reading fluency (e.g., Dalton, Pisha, Eagleton, Coyne, & Deysher, 2002).

Conclusion

At present, the literacy of schooling is mainly based on a hierarchical access to print literacy. Because students are not required to exhibit technology-related literacy skills, the New and Multiple Literacies are considered supplemental activities by many teachers. For example, in a landmark study of thirteen teachers on how the Internet influences literacy and literacy instruction in their K-12 classroom (Karchmer, 2001), one of the fourth-grade teachers wrote that the weak readers in his class did not use the computer at all because their reading abilities made it so difficult to complete a task that they ran out of time easily; they simply did not have time for anything that was "not part of the curriculum." Such a linear media form is increasingly in conflict with the more diverse and interactive media forms made available by digital technologies that are used in the real world of home and community. The use of the New and Multiple Literacies in the classroom can be the bridge between school and the home community.

Meanwhile, we must be careful not to over-romanticize the opportunities provided by the New and Multiple Literacies. Instead of guaranteeing effective learning, technology can only make it easier to create environments that can be manipulated by students in acquiring and consolidating new understanding through accessing, structuring, connecting, storing, retrieving, and processing information to become experts in a given content area (Bransford, Brown, & Cocking, 2000). Just as any other good-intention intervention in the field of education, the New and Multiple Literacies can be easily turned into hindrances instead of propellers of a child's learning if not being implemented appropriately. For example, consider an immigrant child who enters school without any previous formal access to schooling and much less school-based Internet access. This child faces a potentially steep learning curve on Internet-based literacy instruction, which might lead to the creation of "new categories of disabilities" (Dalton & Proctor, 2009). In many cases, at-risk students spend their computer time completing dull drill-and-practice programs instead of engaging in Internet-inquiry projects.

In short, launching a successful practice takes a mixture of leadership, vision, commitment, cooperative planning, knowledge, and time. It took a century from the invention of print to the wide-spread use of print literacy in society (Tyner, 1998). The development of the New and Multiple Literacies to their maturity is expected to take long as well.

SUMMARY

This chapter discusses the definition of literacy, which includes traditional print literacy as well as the New and Multiple Literacies. We investigate the New and Multiple Literacies through different paradigms and modes (media). Then we explore the impact on our understanding of literate thought and knowledge. The chapter concludes with the effects of the New and Multiple Literacies on children with disabilities and those who have traditional language/literacy problems such as ELLs.

A few major points expounded in this chapter are as follows.

- The traditional perception of literacy (i.e., reading and writing) mistakenly identifies the means of communication with the knowledge that is communicated, that is, it confounds the *means* of literacy education with the *ends* of literacy education.
- *Literacy* should be defined broadly as a form of captured information, including traditional print literacy as well as the New and Multiple Literacies.
- There are three co-existing paradigms of the New and Multiple Literacies—learning, change, and power—all of which should work collaboratively for paradigmatic commensurability.
- Some print literacy skills might still be required in certain New and Multiple Literacy activities, whereas many New and Multiple Literacies do not involve any basic print literacy skills. As well, many New and Multiple Literacies require additional literacy skills that are irrelevant to print literacy skills.
- As one medium of the New and Multiple Literacies, Internet literacy requires an integrated sum of numerous sub-skills. For example, while promoting democracy and freedom, the Internet also demands unique skills to access, navigate, critically evaluate, and store information, communicate and share perspectives with each other through e-text, establish online discourse communities, and judge the friendliness or usability of digital tools to work effectively and efficiently, all of which go beyond traditional vocabulary and text comprehension in print literacy.
- As another medium of the New and Multiple Literacies, video gaming might provide players with many advantages over traditional print literacy, such as situated learning, reducing the deleterious consequences of failure, the benefits of affinity groups, and the power of information given on-demand or just-in-time instead of just-in-case.
- Different literacies have different modes of communication, which does not necessarily mean that these different modes of communication result in different ways to access and interpret information during communicative interactions.

- The object reference of the word—not reading and writing skills—is the main instrument of human conscious activity or, in our view, the mental tools of literate thought. Furthermore, the mode of the word is not limited to print, which suggests that literate thought could be mode-independent.
- By adding the additional dimension of technology, the reconceptualized notion of literacy connects the concept of literate thought with the goal of literacy (in a broad sense), which significantly broadens the choices for children with disabilities or those who have traditional language/literacy problems such as ELLs to access and interpret captured information.
- Through the contextualized use of the New and Multiple Literacies in scientific inquiry, students with disabilities and ELLs can develop and practice metacognitive thinking skills while simultaneously enhancing their scientific conceptual understanding.
- As an instructional design framework, Universal Design for Learning (UDL) utilizes the dynamic flexibility of the New and Multiple Literacies to offer new opportunities to meet the individual needs of a wide spectrum of learners—including those with disabilities—to access, participate, and make meaningful progress in the general education curriculum, with the long-term goal of becoming lifelong learners and contributing citizens.
- Launching a successful practice takes a mixture of leadership, vision, commitment, cooperative planning, knowledge, and time. We need to be careful not to over-romanticize the opportunities provided by the New and Multiple Literacies and to realize that the development of the New and Multiple Literacies to their maturity might require a substantial amount of time.

QUESTIONS FOR REFLECTION AND DISCUSSION

1. Discuss the effects of the New and Multiple Literacies on the refinement or reconceptualization of the traditional concept of literacy. Does this reconceptualization comport with the concept of literate thought? Why or why not?

2. Discuss the paradigms of the New and Multiple Literacies.

3. Discuss the skills needed to navigate and utilize information on the Internet versus those needed for traditional script or print literacy.

4. How do the New and Multiple Literacies impact our understanding of literate thought and challenge our assumptions about knowledge?

5. What are the implications of the New and Multiple Literacies for children with disabilities and those with traditional language or literacy problems?

REFERENCES

Bangert-Drowns, R. L. (1993). The word processor as an instructional tool: A meta-analysis of word processing in writing instruction. *Review of Educational Research, 63*(1), 69-93.

Barman, C. R., & Stockton, J. D. (2002). An evaluation of the SOAR-High Project: A Web-based science program for deaf students. *American Annals of the Deaf, 147*(3), 5-10.

Bloome, D., & Paul, P. (2006). This issue: Literacies of and for a diverse society. *Theory into Practice, 45*(4), 293-295.

Bodrova, E., & Leong, D. (1996). *Tools of the mind – The Vygotskian approach to early childhood education.* Columbus, OH: Prentice Hall.

Borron, R. (1978). Modifying science instruction to meet the needs of the hearing impaired. *Journal of Research in Science Teaching, 15*(4), 257-262.

Bransford, J., Brown, A., & Cocking, R. (2000). *How people learn: Brain, mind, experience, and school.* Washington, DC: National Academy Press.

Cawley, J., & Parmar, R. (2001). Literacy proficiency and science for students with learning disabilities. *Reading & Writing Quarterly, 17*, 105-125.

Clanchy, M. T. (1993). *From memory to written record: England 1066-1307* (2nd ed.). Oxford, U. K. and Cambridge, MA: Blackwell.

Cochran-Smith, M. (1991). Word-processing and writing in elementary classrooms: A critical review of related literature. *Review of Educational Research, 61*(1), 107-155.

Coiro, J., Knobel, M., Lankshear, C., & Leu, D. (2009a). Central issues in new literacies and new literacies research. In J. Coiro, M. Knobel, C. Lankshear, & D. Leu (Eds.), *Handbook of research on new literacies* (pp. 1-21). New York: Routledge.

Coiro, J., Knobel, M., Lankshear, C., & Leu, D. (Eds.) (2009b). *Handbook of research on new literacies.* New York: Routledge.

Dalton, B., Pisha, B., Eagleton, M., Coyne, P., & Deysher, S. (2002). *Engaging the text: Reciprocal teaching and questioning strategies in a scaffolded learning environment.* Final report to the U.S. Department of Education, Office of Special Education Programs, Peabody, MA: CAST.

Dalton, B., & Proctor, C. P. (2009). The changing landscape of text and comprehension in the age of new literacies. In J. Coiro, M. Knobel, C. Lankshear, & D. Leu (Eds.), *Handbook of research on new literacies* (pp. 297-324). New York: Routledge.

Donohoe, K., & Zigmond, M. (1988, April). *High school grades of urban LD students and low achieving peers.* Paper presented at the annual meeting of the American Educational Research Association, San Francisco, CA.

Edyburn, D. L. (2002). Cognitive rescaling strategies: Interventions that alter the cognitive accessibility of text. *Closing the Gap, 1,* 10-11.

Freire, P. (1970). *Pedagogy of the oppressed.* New York: Seabury Press.

Freire, P. (1973). *Education for critical consciousness.* New York: Seabury Press.

Freire, P. (1985). *The politics of education.* South Hadley, MA: Bergin & Garvey.

Freire, P., & Macedo, D. (1987). *Literacy: Reading the word and the world.* South Hadley, MA: Bergin & Garvey.

Gee, J. (2003). *What video games have to teach us about learning and literacy.* New York: Palgrave.

Gee, J. (2007). *Good video games and good learning: Collected essays on video games, learning and literacy.* New York: Peter Lang.

Goldberg, A., Russell, M., & Cook, A. (2003). The effect of computers on student writing: A meta-analysis of studies from 1992 to 2002. *Journal of Technology, Learning, and Assessment, 2*(1), 1-24.

Graff, H., J. (1995). *The labyrinths of literacy: Reflections on literacy past and present.* Pittsburgh, PA: University of Pittsburgh Press.

Harnisch, D., & Wilkinson, I. (1989). *Cognitive return of schooling for the handicapped: Preliminary findings from high school and beyond.* Paper presented at the annual meeting of the American Educational Research Association, San Francisco, CA.

Kaestle, C. F. (1991). Studying the history of literacy. In C. F. Kaestle, H. Damon-Moore, L. C. Stedman, K. Tinsley, & W. V. Trollinger, Jr. (Eds.), *Literacy in the United States: Readers and reading since 1880* (pp. 3-32). New Haven, CT and London: Yale University Press.

Karchmer, R. A. (2001). The journey ahead: Thirteen teachers report how the Internet influences literacy and literacy instruction in their K-12 classroom. *Reading Research Quarterly, 36,* 442-467.

Kellner, D. (2000). New technologies/new literacies: reconstructing education for the new millennium. *Teaching Education, 11*(3), 245-265.

Kuiper, E., & Volman, M. (2009). The web as a source of information for students in K-12 Education. In J. Coiro, M. Knobel, C. Lankshear, & D. Leu (Eds.), *Handbook of research on new literacies* (pp. 241-266). New York: Routledge.

Kulikowich, J. (2009). Experimental and quasi-experimental approaches to the study of new literacies. In J. Coiro, M. Knobel, C. Lankshear, & D. Leu (Eds.), *Handbook of research on new literacies* (pp. 179-205). New York: Routledge.

Langer, J. (1995). *Envisioning literature – literacy understanding and literature instruction,* New York, NY: Teacher's College Press.

Lawless, K. A., & Schrader, P. G. (2009). Where do we go now? – Understanding research on navigation in complex digital environment. In J. Coiro, M. Knobel, C. Lankshear, & D. Leu (Eds.), *Handbook of research on new literacies* (pp. 267-296). New York: Routledge.

Livingstone, S., Van Couvering, E., & Thumim, N. (2009). Converging traditions of research on media and information literacies. In J. Coiro, M. Knobel, C. Lankshear, & D. Leu (Eds.), *Handbook of research on new literacies* (pp. 103-132). New York: Routledge.

Lundberg, I., & Oloffson, A. (1993). Can computer speech support reading comprehension? *Computers in Human Behavior, 9*, 283-293.

Luria, A. R. (1982). *Language and cognition.* Washington, DC: V. H. Winston & Sons.

Mayer, R. E. (1997). *Multimedia learning.* Cambridge, UK: Cambridge University Press.

Mayer, R. E. (2001). *Multimedia learning.* Cambridge, UK: Cambridge University Press.

Mayer, R. E. (2009). Multimedia learning. In J. Coiro, M. Knobel, C. Lankshear, & D. Leu (Eds.), *Handbook of research on new literacies* (pp. 359-376). New York: Routledge.

McKenna, M. C. (1998). Electronic texts and the transformation of beginning reading. In D. Reinking, M. C. McKenna, L. D. Labbo, & R. D. Kieffer (Eds.), *Handbook of literacy and technology: Transformations in a post-typographic world* (pp. 45-59). Mahwah, NJ: Lawrence Erlbaum Associates.

McKenna, M. C., Reinking, D., Labbo, L. D., & Kieffer, R. D. (1999). The electronic transformation of literacy and its implications for struggling readers. *Reading and Writing Quarterly, 15*, 111-126.

McKenna, M. C., & Watkins, J. (1994). *Computer-mediated books for beginning readers.* Paper presented at the annual meeting of the National Reading Conferences, San Diego, CA.

Olson, D. (Ed.) (1974). *Media and symbols: the forms of expression, communication, and education,* Chicago, IL: The University of Chicago.

Olson, D. (1989). Literate thought. In C. K. Leong, & B. Randhawa (Eds.), *Understanding literacy and cognition* (pp. 3-15). New York, NY: Plenum Press.

Olson, D. (1994). *The world on paper.* New York, NY: Cambridge University Press.

Ong, W. (1967). *The presence of the word – Some prolegomena for cultural and religious history,* New Haven and London: Yale University Press.

Ong, W. (1977). *Interfaces of the word – Studies in the evolution of consciousness and culture,* Ithaca, NY: Cornell University Press.

Paivio, A. (1986). *Mental representations: A dual coding approach.* Oxford, UK: Oxford University Press.

Paul, P. (1998). *Literacy and deafness: The development of reading, writing, and literate thought.* Needham Heights, MA: Allyn & Bacon.

Paul, P. (2001). *Language and deafness* (3rd ed.). San Diego, CA: Singular/Thomson Learning.

Paul, P. (2006). New literacies, multiple literacies, unlimited literacies: What now, what next, where to? A response to "Blue listerine, parochialism & ASL literacy." *Journal of Deaf Studies and Deaf Education, 11*(3), 382-387.

Paul, P. (2009). *Language and deafness* (4th ed.). Sudbury, MA: Jones & Bartlett.

Paul, P., & Wang, Y. (2006a). Multiliteracies and literate thought. *Theory into Practice, 45*(4), 304-310.

Paul, P., & Wang, Y. (2006b). Literate thought and deafness: A call for a new perspective and line of research on literacy. *Punjab University Journal of Special Education* (Pakistan), *2*(1), 28-37.

Saljo, R. (Ed.) (1988). *The written world – Studies in literate thought and action*, Berlin, Germany: Springer-Verlag.

Stoddart, T., Pinal, A., Latzke, M., & Canaday, D. (2002). Integrating inquiry science and language development for English language learners. *Journal of Research in Science Teaching, 39*(8), 664-687.

Strangman, N., & Dalton, B. (2005). Technology for struggling readers: A review of the research. In D. Edyburn, K. Higgins, & R. Boone (Eds.), *The handbook of special education technology research and practice* (pp. 545-569). Whitefish Bay, WI: Knowledge by Design.

Tapscott, R. (1988). *Growing up digital: The rise of the Net generation*. New York: McGraw-Hill.

Tyner, K. (1998). *Literacy in a digital world: teaching and learning in the age of information*. Mahwah, NJ: Lawrence Erlbaum Associates.

Vygotsky, L. (1962). *Thought and language*. Cambridge, MA: The MIT Press.

Vygotsky, L. (1978). *Mind in society: The development of higher psychological processes*. Cambridge, MA: Harvard University Press.

Vygotsky, L., & Luria, A. R. (1993). *Studies in the history of behavior: Ape, primitive, and child*. Hillsdale, NJ: Lawrence Erlbaum. (Original work published in 1930).

Wang, Y. (2005). *Literate thought: Metatheorizing in literacy and deafness*. Unpublished doctoral dissertation, Ohio State University, Columbus.

Warschauer, M., & Ware, P. (2009). Learning, change, and power: Competing frames of technology and literacy. In J. Coiro, M. Knobel, C. Lankshear, & D. Leu (Eds.), *Handbook of research on new literacies* (pp. 215-240). New York: Routledge.

Wertsch, J. V. (1985). *Vygotsky and the social formation of mind*. Cambridge, MA: Harvard University Press.

Williams, R. (1983). Keywords: A vocabulary of culture and society. London: Fontana.

FURTHER READING

Cuban, L. (2001). *Oversold and underused: Computers in classrooms, 1980-2000*. Cambridge, MA: Harvard University Press.

Cummins, J., & Sayers, D. (1995). *Brave new schools: Challenging cultural illiteracy through global learning networks*. New York: St. Martin's Press.

Hull, G., & Schultz, K. (Eds.). (2002). *School's out! Bridging out-of-school literacies with classroom practice.* New York: Teachers College Press.

Rose, D. H., & Meyer, A. (2002). *Teaching every student in the digital age: Universal design for learning.* Alexandria, VA: Association for Supervision and Curriculum Development (ASCD).

Warschauer, M., & Kern, R. (2000). *Network-based language teaching: Concepts and practice.* Cambridge, UK: Cambridge University Press.

CHAPTER 4

Cognition and Discipline Structures

*Mental models have become a widely used concept in various disciplines.
Unfortunately, the use of the term varies across the different applications,
such that a common notion or even a core meaning is difficult to find.*

Vosgerau, 2006, p. 256

*For some decades a variety of researchers in education and psychology have
been contributing to the development of this captivating general model.
The learning process has been conceptualized in terms of entities—the
"structure of the discipline" that is being learned, and the "cognitive structure" that is built up inside the learner as he or she gradually masters that
particular subject.*

Phillips, 1983, p. 60

There are two broad themes of this chapter, based on the above passages.
One entails a discussion of cognitive (or mental) models that includes the
concepts of structures or processes. The second theme is discipline (or
knowledge) structure, that is, a structure associated with specific content
areas such as science, mathematics, reading, or topics such as baseball, big
bang physics, evolution, and so on. In addition, an implicit third theme
hinted in the second passage above, is the relationship, if any, between the
cognitive/mental structure of the individual and the discipline (knowledge) structure of the content area or topic.

Indubitably, these themes have dominated the development of theories and research in psychology, especially cognitive or social–cognitive
psychology (see Ausubel, 1968; Baars, 1986; Bruning, Schraw, Norby, &
Ronning, 2004; Chomsky, 2006; Flavell, 1985; Held, Knauff, &
Vosgerau, 2006; for a readable history, see Hunt, 1993). There are a

number of interesting stories based on the thinking of historical figures such as Watson, Skinner, Vygotsky, Luria, Piaget, Bandura, and Chomsky (Baars, 1986; Flavell; Hunt, 1993) as well as those associated with models for reading (Adams, 1990, Kintsch, 2004), writing (Hayes, 2004), mathematics (Mayer, 1992), and critico-creative thinking (Kuhn, 2005; Norris, 1992). As discussed later, it is not altogether clear what is meant by a mental or cognitive model or whether there is such a psychological entity that is necessary to describe for the purpose of understanding the learning of or even the teaching of, for example, science or mathematics. Confounding this further is what is meant by the concept of *learning* and whether this is related to the concept of *teaching*—a caveat expressed quite some time ago by Ausubel (1968).

Is the process of learning or teaching cognitive, social, both cognitive and social, or more? Is there a better, more productive way to express this inquiry? Suffice it to say that the themes of this chapter need to be clarified to render a more complete picture of our main construct of literate thought, particularly its development. Specifically, we hope to expand somewhat on the contents of Chapter 2, which emphasized the comprehension model or components of literate thought. Nevertheless, as will be seen in this chapter, this comprehension-based model has been suggested for areas other than literacy such as mathematics and science.

Prior to beginning our discussion, it should be highlighted that a number of scholars have argued that the research and findings in cognitive psychology have been underutilized in practice, especially in education and clinical settings (e.g., Bruning et al., 2004; for additional perspectives on children with disabilities or those who are d/Deaf or hard of hearing, see Mann & Sabatino, 1985; Marschark & Spencer, 2010; Paul, 2009; Paul & Jackson, 1993; Trezek, Wang, & Paul, 2010). On one hand, it might be that practitioners are simply unaware or unclear about the implications of such scientific and scholarly endeavors. On the other hand, as implied by Phillips (1983; Phillips & Soltis, 2004) and others (Ausubel, 1968; Vosgerau, 2006), perhaps it is not clear what can be applied to practice. This latter point not only refers to the controversies and disagreements associated with establishing and conducting research and building models, but also to the underlying meanings or implications of the findings based on the research and models.

We harbor no illusions about our ability to clarify these complicated issues completely in the present chapter. Our hope is to shed some light that will stimulate further reading and reflection. First, we describe briefly what we think any adequate model of cognition needs to address, especially for implications and applications to the murky world of practice. Then we trace a few historical high points from behaviorism models to the present. Next, we discuss the relationship of cognition to disciplinary structure, focusing on three disciplines: literacy (reading & writing), mathematics, and science. Finally, we discuss briefly one of our major underlying themes pertaining to the development of literate thought in literacy and the various disciplines—the Qualitative-Similarity Hypothesis—which should drive theorizing, research, and practice. In essence, our main topics are: nature and relevance of cognitive psychology, cognitive models and structures, cognition and knowledge structures, and the Qualitative-Similarity Hypothesis.

NATURE AND RELEVANCE OF COGNITIVE PSYCHOLOGY

It may seem strange to devote a section of this chapter to the nature and relevance of cognitive psychology or, specifically to that of cognitivism. Nevertheless, it has been argued that models such as information processing or connectionism are restrictive because they are predominantly *inside the head* and do not seriously consider other important avenues of learning, particularly social factors (e.g., with respect to reading, see Tierney, 2008; see also, the various discussions in Israel & Duffy, 2009). A number of scholars—the authors of this book included—aver that it is still fruitful to investigate teaching and learning via the use of cognitive models, and it is not beneficial to abandon cognition completely in favor of only social orientations or models (see also, Hayes, 2004).

In short, research on information processing, particularly short-term or working memory, is still critical for understanding processes such as language and literacy development (Pickering, 2006; Snowling & Hulme, 2005). Such research is also being funded on a federal level (e.g., see *Request for Applications, Special Education Research & Development Center Program, CFDA Number 84.324C; IES 2010, U.S. Department of Education*). It is important to understand how cognitive or mental frameworks, or perhaps general cognitive development, assist individuals in organizing, storing, and retrieving information from memory. In fact, there is a robust line of research demonstrating the interrelations among working memory, phonology, and reading development (Cain & Oakhill, 2007; McGuinness, 2004, 2005; Pickering; Snowling & Hulme; for deafness, see Paul, 2009; Trezek et al., 2010).

Within the realm above, it is also critical to remember that learning or the generation of understanding is a constructive process (Bruning et al., 2004; Donovan & Bransford, 2005; Phillips & Soltis, 2004). Whether one ascribes to cognitive information processing, cognitive constructivism, or some other cognitive or social–cognitive model, there is an interaction between the learner and what is being learned. This is not a passive process; it is active and also extremely productive if learners can utilize their prior knowledge about topics to assist their understanding or learning of new information. The accumulation and utilization of prior knowledge is discussed in Chapter 2 as being critical for the development of literate thought and in Chapter 5 for critico-creative thinking skills. Prior knowledge is also a major component of early and mature reading ability (Israel & Duffy, 2009; National Early Literacy Panel (NELP), 2008; National Reading Panel (NRP), 2000; Ruddell & Unrau, 2004).

An effective cognitive framework cannot really be only an inside-the-head model, especially in light of research on sociocultural factors and the influence of contextualist perspectives (see Bruning et al., 2004; Donovan & Bransford, 2005; Gaffney & Anderson, 2000). There is little doubt that the environment, particularly the social interactions or social contexts, also contributes to the development of an individual's knowledge base. The beneficial effects of an enriching language and literacy milieu are certainly facilitative but are not all encompassing or a panacea. It is also important for parents, teachers, and others to be engaged in the learning process; consider, for example, reciprocal teaching, learning styles, and mediated learning.

The influences of sociocultural and contextualist views have also provided implications for areas such as metacognition, self-regulated learning, and cognitive strategy instruction (Bruning et al., 2004; Israel & Duffy, 2009). Across various disciplines such as mathematics, science, and reading, individuals need to be able to take charge of their learning by developing and utilizing effective strategies for solving problems and thinking in a critico-creative manner. Strategy use and self-regulation are contextual and need to be applied appropriately. Individuals also need to know how, when, and why to use certain strategies in specific situations and contexts. Socioculturalists have demonstrated the importance of learners being able to view themselves within their social worlds (Donovan & Bransford, 2005; Israel & Duffy).

Another area that seems to be neglected in the research on children and adolescents with disabilities and literacy (reading & writing) is the affective domain (see discussions in Israel & Duffy, 2009; Ruddell & Unrau, 2004). Development of cognition is influenced pervasively by the motivation and beliefs of learners. One fruitful line of research, for example, has been based on Bandura's self-efficacy theory (Bandura, 1997). In short, learners must be motivated and interested in the active process of self-regulation and reflection. Learners need to not only have comprehension and other cognitive skills and strategies, but also the desire to organize, plan, and seek solutions to problems.

Last, but certainly not least, learners—particularly those with disabilities and those who are English language learners (ELLs)—need ample opportunities, practice, and time to develop many of the skills and strategies in the areas discussed above (Bruning et al., 2004; Donovan & Bransford, 2005). The goal is for learners to reach a level of automaticity—that is, a repertoire of automatic processes—that permits them to concentrate on higher-level tasks such as reasoning, making inferences, and critico-creative thinking. This automaticity frees up the resources and energy needed for such higher-level thinking in that individuals do not need to pay undue, burdensome attention to details. In the field of reading (discussed later), this is interpreted to mean that good readers have developed rapid, automatic word identification processes and can concentrate on higher-level comprehension processes involving, for example, metacognition and self-regulation (Cain & Oakhill, 2007; Israel & Duffy, 2009; McGuinness, 2004, 2005; National Early Literacy Panel, 2008; National Reading Panel, 2000; Ruddell & Unrau, 2004). Automaticity is necessary for fluency in reading, that is, individuals need to be able to read accurately and quickly.

So, for us, the authors of this book, cognitive psychology or the use of cognitive models has tremendous potential for developing active learners. As discussed above, such models should include the dimensions of affective and social factors with considerations of contextual and constructive issues and processes. There is also some discussion that, perhaps, neither cognitive nor social psychology is paramount. It is critical to utilize the findings from the recent, newly-emerging fields of neuroscience with functional magnetic resonance imagery (fMRIs) and other brain-study techniques that might be more constructive (see readable account in Hunt, 1993). We do think that neuroscience has something to offer; however, we tend to agree with a popular account about the constraints of such approaches (see also Chomsky, 2006):

> Most cognitive psychologists thus believe that a word retrieved from memory cannot be equated with the firing of millions of neurons and the resultant millions or billions of synaptic transmissions, but is the product of the pattern or structure of those firings and transmissions. The neurobiological study of memory, valuable as it is, does not tell us how we learn anything, recognize things we have earlier experienced, or retrieve items from memory as needed—the words we use in speech, to give one example. Such phenomena, or epiphenomena, are governed not by the law of cognitive neuroscience but by those of cognitive psychology. (Hunt, 1993, p. 521)

Table 4-1 provides highlights of an adequate cognitive approach to studying human behavior.

Table 4-1. Highlights of an Adequate Cognitive Approach to the Study of the Mind

- This cognitive approach is not an inside-the-head approach only.
- The approach recognizes that learning or the generation of understanding is a constructive process.
- Learning is active and also extremely productive if learners can utilize their prior knowledge about topics to assist their understanding or learning of new information.
- The environment, particularly the social interactions or social contexts, also contributes to the development of an individual's knowledge base.
- It is also important for parents, teachers, and others to be engaged in the learning process. Consider, for example, reciprocal teaching, learning styles, and mediated learning.
- The influences of sociocultural and contextualist views have also provided implications for areas such as metacognition, self-regulated learning, and cognitive strategy instruction.
- Learners must be motivated and interested in the active process of self-regulation and reflection.
- Learners—particularly those with disabilities and those who are English language learners (ELLs)—need ample opportunities, practice, and time to develop many of the skills and strategies.

COGNITIVE MODELS

Previously we mentioned that there is much debate and confusion surrounding the construct of a cognitive model. We also think it is imperative to discuss briefly what is meant by cognitive-related terms such as structures, processes, and products. In one sense, cognitive structures provide the architectural framework for the construct of cognitive models.

Our plan for this section is as follows. First, we describe selected cognitive terminology and proffer, perhaps iterate, what it means to use one's cognition. Then we trace the development of broad mental frameworks via highlights that represent our schema for presenting this information. Finally, we return to the notion of what it means to develop an adequate cognitive model, and relate this issue to the subsequent discussion of cognition and discipline structures.

Structures, Processes, and Products

The term *cognition* evokes terms or constructs such as *knowledge, intelligence, mental, mind, thinking, reasoning,* and *problem-solving* along with *perception, memory, attention,* and *learning* (Baars, 1986; Bruning et al., 2004; Johnson-Laird, 1988; Pickering, 2006; for an accessible discussion, see Brown, 2006). Nevertheless, terms such as *thinking, mental, mind, knowing,* and *knowledge* are purported to be ambiguous in that they are difficult to define operationally and to assess. We will not touch the debate on the relationship, if any, between cognition and intelligence, which has a long colorful history, especially in the development of intelligence tests (Baars; Hunt, 1993).

In general, cognition is concerned with how the mind works. Much of the working of the mind appears to be on an unconscious level, if we consider the processing of information in the central nervous system. In our view, it thus is best to focus on *structures, processes,* and *products.*

Structures refer to the underlying architecture from which cognitive *processes* spring in the formation of cognitive *products.* It is permissible to think of structures as the hardware (for those who are passionate about computers) as long as one keeps in mind that this hardware is or can be malleable or influenced (e.g., think of *plasticity*). Of course, being malleable or influenced does not really change the contents of the hardware (albeit, the future of neuroscience might be full of surprises!).

In linguistics, some theorists propose innate language structures as responsible for language processes and products (Chomsky, 2006; see also the discussion in Carruthers, Laurence, & Stich, 2005, 2006; Lund, 2003). In reading, one will encounter terms such as *schema, frame,* or *script* that refer to knowledge structures, defined as the manner in which information is stored and organized in the mind. In short, the efficiency of cognitive processes is dependent on the adequacy of the structures. The essence of these structures—that is, whether they are biological, neuro-physiological, social, or some other entity—forms the content of the varying cognitive models ranging from Piaget to Luria to Vygotsky to the computer (Baars, 1986; Bruning et al., 2004; Jarvis, 2000). In fact, the nature of the structures is also influenced by the frameworks associated with the construct of psychology, which is presumed to be the study of the mind (Jarvis).

Cognitive processes, in short, represent the confluence of individuals and their attempts to address or process information. This confluence is manifested by activities such as making decisions, inferences, judgments, analogies, solving problems, and so on. These processes also shed light on the strategies that individuals employ in perceiving and understanding information. As such, some strategies may be more effective than others. For example, in reading, it is argued that using phonics-based strategies are more effective than using sight-word strategies for identifying or recognizing unknown words (although there are a few benefits to the sight-word strategies) (National Early Literacy Panel, 2008; National Reading Panel, 2000). It should be obvious that we cannot observe the processes or strategies associated with cognition directly. We can only make inferences based on our observations of the products.

Cognitive *product* is not a widely used term; however, it refers to the results of the interplay of the structures and processes. Products include the visible perceptions, concepts, decisions, language behaviors, reading behaviors, written language constructions, and so on. In Chomsky's linguistic theory (2006), product might refer to the performance of the speaker/user of the language. Chomsky's argument is that performance is an imperfect reflection of competence (whether this means processes or structures, in our view). Regardless of the manner in which one views constructs such as product or performance, our main point should be clear: Because we cannot directly observe the working of the mind (neuroscience foci, notwithstanding), we can only surmise what might be operating in the structure. This should provide the context for the controversy and debate surrounding cognitive models—our next topic.

A Brief History of the Development of Cognitive Models

It is a challenge to adopt an approach for classifying models of cognition as well as to select and exemplify only a few models. One feasible modern approach is to use broad foci such as associationism (similar to behaviorism or environmentalism) and cognitivism (Baars, 1986; Bruning et al., 2004; Lund, 2003). Still another approach, based mostly on *theoretical approaches* in psychology, is Jarvis' (2000) classification scheme: behavioral, psychodynamic, humanistic, cognitive, cognitive-developmental, social, and biological (either genetics or neurophysiology). One also could use Baars' notion of three general metatheoretical frameworks: introspectionism, behaviorism, and cognitivism.

We prefer the Bruning et al. (2004) model that uses *associationism* and *cognitivism* as long as cognitivism is interpreted broadly to include social and contextual factors. In fact, both associationism (behaviorism) and cognitivism represent a stance (or stances, in some cases) to the most basic philosophical problem in psychology: the mind–body problem (Baars, 1986; Fodor, 1981; Johnson-Laird, 1988). For the most part, nearly all of the associationist or behaviorist theories (or models) denied the existence of the mind or simply stated that it was not observable. Cognitive models were a reaction to those of behaviorism, beginning with the works of George Miller, Noam Chomsky, and others (e.g., David Ausubel, Jerome Bruner, and Ulrich Neisser).

Associationism or behaviorism is often termed a stimulus-response (S-R) paradigm that employs constructs such as *reinforcement, imitation, fading, shaping, antecedents, consequences,* and so on (Baars, 1986; Cooper, Heward, & Heron, 1987; Mann & Sabatino, 1985). The general premise (at least according to radical behaviorists) is that the performance of organisms (people, animals) is predominantly a function of the environment in which they are located along with their history of learning. Behaviorists claim that all performance is learned behavior ranging from simple to complex (sequential accumulation of simple) steps. One assertion, often found in popular accounts (Hunt, 1993), is that a behaviorist can train anyone to assume any particular identity, such as a baker, thief, or candlestick maker.

Associationism or behaviorism is no longer as dominant a force in psychology as it was in the mid-1960s. Nevertheless, its contributions can still be seen in areas such as special education, animal science, and clinical psychology. Applications in education and clinical settings include concepts such as precision or target teaching, classroom management, elimination or reduction of undesirable behavior, and so on.

To cognitivists, it is not enough to simply state that the mind exists; more importantly, it is critical to describe the mind's structures and processes (for an accessible account, see Brown, 2006; see also, Bruning et al., 2004; Held et al., 2006; Pickering, 2006). At the waning of behaviorism came a proliferation of mind-explaining terms such as *frames* (Minsky, 1975), *schemata* (Rumelhart, 1977), and *scripts* (Schank & Abelson, 1977). The two dominant cognitive models up until the 1990s were Piaget's theory of cognitive development and information-processing, based on the computer metaphor (Flavell, 1985; Hunt, 1993).

The information-processing paradigm, in our view, is still fairly dominant, even though it has undergone revisions from other current views (e.g., constructivism and contextualism). According to Brown (2006), this paradigm asserts that (p. 9):

- People interact purposefully within the world.
- Patterns/symbols that are used in such interactions are made meaningful in the real-world context.
- The processes and patterns used in performing cognitive tasks can be identified by psychologists and there is some neurological basis, although this does not control all information processing.
- Cognitive tasks may take time before being computed, although the mind has a limited-capacity processor.

In short, the information-processing paradigm has engendered computational/computer models to understand cognition with common types (used in our fields involving language and literacy) such as semantic networks and connectionist networks. More recent models tend to incorporate the influences of social and social-cognitive factors.

Table 4-2 provides a brief summary of remarks related to terminology and models.

Prelude to Cognition and Knowledge Structures
Similar to Phillips (1983; Phillips & Soltis, 2004), we, the authors, are skeptical of the need to describe adequately the cognitive structures of

Table 4-2. Description of Terminologies and Models

Cognitive Models

- The term *cognition* has evoked terms or constructs such as *knowledge, intelligence, mental, mind, thinking, reasoning,* and *problem-solving* along with *perception, memory, attention,* and *learning.*
- Terms such as *thinking, mental, mind, knowing,* and *knowledge* are purported to be ambiguous (difficult to define operationally and to assess).
- In general, cognition is concerned with how the mind works.

Structures, Processes, Products

- *Structures* refer to the underlying architecture from which cognitive *processes* spring in the formation of cognitive *products.*
- The efficiency of cognitive processes is dependent on the adequateness of the structures.
- The essence of these structures—that is, whether they are biological, neurophysiological, social, or some other entity—forms the content of the varying cognitive models ranging from Piaget to Luria to Vygotsky to the computer.
- Cognitive processes, in short, represent the confluence of individuals and their attempts to address or process information.
- This confluence is manifested by activities such as making decisions, inferences, judgments, analogies, solving problems, and so on.
- These processes also shed light on the strategies that individuals employ in perceiving and understanding information.
- Cognitive *product* is not a widely used term; it refers to the results of the interplay of the structures and processes.
- Products include the visible perceptions, concepts, decisions, language behaviors, reading behaviors, written language constructions, and so on.

Development of Models

- This book uses the Bruning et al. (2004) model—*associationism* and *cognitivism*—as long as cognitivism is interpreted broadly to include social and contextual factors.
- Both associationism (behaviorism) and cognitivism represent a stance (or stances, in some cases) to the most basic philosophical problem in psychology: the mind–body problem.
- For the most part, nearly all of the associationist or behaviorist theories (or models) deny the existence of the mind or simply state that it is not observable.
- Cognitive models were a reaction to those of behaviorism, beginning with the works of George Miller, Noam Chomsky, and others.

(continues)

Table 4-2. Description of Terminologies and Models *(continued)*

- Associationism or behaviorism is often termed a stimulus-response (S-R) paradigm, which employs constructs such as *reinforcement, imitation, fading, shaping, antecedents, consequences,* and so on. The general premise (at least according to radical behaviorists) is that the performance of organisms (people, animals) is predominantly a function of the environment in which they are located along with their history of learning.
- To cognitivists, it is not enough to simply state that the mind exists; more importantly (or, perhaps most importantly), it is critical to describe the mind's structures and processes.
- The two dominant cognitive models until the 1990s were Piaget's theory and information-processing, based on the computer metaphor.
- The information-processing paradigm, in our view, is still fairly dominant, even though it has undergone revisions from other current views (e.g., constructivism and contextualism). More recent models tend to incorporate the influences of social or social–cognitive factors.

---

the mind—as an entity unto itself or, rather, the positing of general mental structures. This does not mean that models such as Piaget's and information-processing are not useful. Nevertheless, these and other general models (e.g., Luria, Vygotsky, etc.) most likely do not tell the full story, even with the inclusion of social or contextualist factors.

What might be needed is a better understanding of the structures (i.e., knowledge) of the disciplines and the capabilities of individuals to acquire and develop their specific discipline's knowledge. For example, as discussed later, if individuals have difficulties in the early reading stage, this might be due to their inadequate development of phonology or phonemic awareness—a critical aspect of early reading structure. By focusing on what is needed to learn to read (and read to learn) or to learn some other content area, we might be in a better position to teach individuals to develop the necessary skills and strategies to be successful.

Having said this, we iterate that focusing on the teaching and learning of disciplines also might not be sufficient, despite our best efforts. In essence, theorists and researchers might still need to understand the workings of the minds of those individuals who continue to experience difficulties with learning. It might be that such individuals do not possess—what we could label as—general cognitive capabilities, which are necessary to acquire selected aspects of content areas or disciplines. In addition, we might need to explore neurocognitive or neurophysiological issues, as in children with dyslexia or autism.

Nevertheless, for the development of literate thought and discipline knowledge, we, the authors, place most of our concerns on the need to understand further the discipline structure and manner (i.e., the necessary processes, strategies, and skills) in which individuals interact with such information to develop proficiency or competency. To us, it does not matter whether a discipline has a coherent or loosely-defined structure. It is still important for individuals to develop conceptual understanding, which is related to the conceptual framework of disciplines. In our view, this is what is meant by applying cognitive psychology to the teaching and learning of content areas. We discuss this further in the ensuing paragraphs.

COGNITION AND KNOWLEDGE STRUCTURES

In this section, we explore briefly the notion of discipline structures, also called *knowledge structures* (Donovan & Bransford, 2005; Phillips, 1983; Phillips & Soltis, 2004). We discuss this construct with respect to literacy (early and mature reading; writing), mathematics, and science. We also acknowledge that a complete understanding of the structure of any discipline has not been accomplished; in fact, we contend that this will always be the case given the pursuit of epistemological endeavors (Phillips & Soltis).

Let's start with a few general questions: Does a discipline, such as mathematics, science, or literacy, have an inherent or conceptual structure? Are some concepts within a discipline easier than others? Why is this the case? If a discipline has a structure, then one can argue that there are certain fundamentals that need to be acquired by individuals to reach a high level of competency or proficiency. Intuitively—and there is some supportive research (see discussions in Donovan & Bransford, 2005; Phillips & Soltis, 2004)—any particular discipline seems to have a structure with concepts on varying difficulty levels. An individual thus may need to understand a piece of information at one level before proceeding to the next. For example, in mathematics, one needs to understand *addition* before one can *multiply*. Nevertheless, this is not as clear as most educators and clinicians hope, especially for disciplines such as reading and writing.

Despite dissension from strong social theorists (e.g., see remarks in Tierney, 2008; see also, the discussions in Phillips, 1983; Phillips & Soltis, 2004), it can be argued that good teaching requires an adequate understanding of specific discipline structures, including methods and concepts, and of the cognitive strategies/skills—at the least—associated with learning that discipline on an expert level. In other words, teachers and clinicians not only should know something about the *psychology of learning* (i.e., understand the particular learning styles, etc., of students and clients), but they also should possess a *deep understanding* of the content areas on which they are planning to focus in the classrooms or clinics. This should enable teachers and clinicians to predict or see the specific areas in which students are experiencing problems with respect to the overall goals of understanding the specific aspects of the content areas (disciplines). Then these professionals can come up with an array of ideas to assist students in overcoming barriers to their understanding. Teachers and clinicians with a deep knowledge of the discipline and of their students/clients can be extremely creative with their instructional suggestions and strategies.

Let us be clear: The discussion above should not be interpreted as an argument *in favor of* a relationship between models of cognition (i.e., models on the cognitive structure of individuals) and knowledge of the discipline. That is a different relationship than what we have described. We examine some of the research reviews in this area, but, similar to Phillips (1983), we tend to be skeptical because cognitive models are psychological (biological, etc.) and discipline models are conceptual. Why should there be a specific relationship between these two entities?

Much of the support for the Qualitative-Similarity Hypothesis (QSH; discussed later) has come from research based on discipline structures with some reference to the performance (i.e., strategies, errors, etc.) of the learner if this pertains to the purported structure of the discipline (Paul, 2009; Paul & Lee, 2010; Wang, Trezek, Luckner, & Paul, 2008). Examples in the field of deafness include the acquisition of the various hand shapes of American Sign Language—and in deafness and other disabilities—the acquisition of English syntactic structures, aspects of the English reading process, and the development of conceptual understanding via the inquiry approach in science (Moores & Martin, 2006; Paul,

2009; Stanovich, 1992; Stanovich, Nathan, & Zolman, 1988; Trezek et al., 2010; Wild, 2008).

In the ensuing sections, we discuss cognition and the construct of discipline structures for literacy, mathematics, and science. In our discussion of the structures of these disciplines, we emphasize what it means to acquire concepts such that one can operate *like* a literacy expert or accomplish the goal of mathematical or scientific literacy. Discussing the purported structures of these disciplines in depth is beyond the scope of this chapter. Rather, we present, briefly, the cognitive underpinnings (i.e., general structures/processes) and cognitive implications for improving instruction. We end with a summary of this issue, leading to our discussion of the QSH.

Cognition and Literacy

The structure of literacy has three broad components: early reading (i.e., learning to read), mature reading (reading to learn), and writing. Although our rendition is based heavily on cognitive models, we have attempted to summarize the major highlights in national reports and syntheses (Adams, 1990; McGuinness, 2004, 2005; NELP, 2008; NRP, 2000; Snow, Burns, & Griffin, 1998) as well as theories, models, and other syntheses (Cain & Oakhill, 2007; Israel & Duffy, 2009; Ruddell & Unrau, 2004). Given the complexity of these broad components, we can only provide a brief overview in this chapter.

Early Reading (or Learning to Read)

It might be difficult for many nonspecialists to understand the acrimonious debates currently raging in attempting to delineate the foundations (requisites), if any, of early reading (see McGill-Franzen, 2010 as well as the rest of the special issue of *Educational Researcher*). Learning to read may seem like a rather straightforward process. This process is not easy for many children, however, and the underlying complexity is not transparent.

To simplify matters (and it is not simple), we discuss both the linguistic or language aspects and the cognitive aspects of learning to read (Cain & Oakhill, 2007; Israel & Duffy, 2009; NELP, 2008; NRP, 2000; McGuinness, 2004, 2005; Ruddell & Unrau, 2004). The linguistic aspect contains two broad sub-areas: English language development and metalinguistic understanding of the aspects of English language related to English print literacy. The major cognitive aspects include non-print areas such as prior knowledge, metacognition (including self-regulation), inferencing, affective factors (e.g., motivation and interest), and specific attributes associated with working memory and attention.

What it means to develop or possess proficiency in the English language is open to debate (e.g., Lund, 2003; McGuinness, 2005; Owens, 2004; Pence & Justice, 2008). Nevertheless, as discussed in Chapter 2, possessing a level of competency is necessary for the development of literate thought. For our purposes here, a level of language competency is also critical for development in early (and mature) reading. Briefly, we are referring to the development of proficiency in the use (pragmatics), content (semantics), and structure (phonology, morphology, syntax) of language.

Much of the structure of English is in place by age 3 or so, except that a few elements of phonology may develop as late as age 7 or 8 (Crystal, 1997, 2006). Beyond the three-word stage, children continue to increase their content (semantics) knowledge, which essentially means vocabulary knowledge as well as idiomatic and metaphorical phrases and uses. This growth in language continues in tandem with cognitive growth, especially knowledge of the world, ranging from prior or background knowledge of specific topics to a wide understanding of cultural literacy (see Chapter 2).

To make initial progress in early reading—especially to learn to read—children need to develop what is called *metalinguistic awareness*. This is interpreted to mean metalinguistic proficiency in language areas that pertain to the literacy process such as awareness of print (pragmatics), sounds (phonemes), letters (graphemes), relationships between letters and sounds (phonics or sound–letter correspondences), word parts (morphemes), word order (syntax), and connected text structures (discourse). For an in-depth discussion of these areas, we refer you to additional sources (Cain & Oakhill, 2007; Israel & Duffy, 2009; McGuinness, 2004, 2005; NELP, 2008; NRP, 2000; Ruddell & Unrau, 2004). We emphasize here that metalinguistic awareness—which means reflecting on language as a product (Olson, 1994, 2004)—is the hallmark of a good beginning reader. This is especially true, for example, if the reader is aware of constructs such as *letter*, *word*, and *sentence*. In addition, the reader needs to know that there are relationships between letters and sounds and that print contains meaning or a message.

Progress in the language areas mentioned above facilitates and is facilitated by cognitive factors such as the ongoing development of prior knowledge, metacognition, and breadth and depth of vocabulary knowledge. Most of these cognitive factors are considered higher-level skills (albeit a case can be made for language factors such as morphology and syntax as well). For readers to use these higher-level skills productively, they must have automatic lower-level skills often associated with word identification, but specifically including alphabet knowledge (knowledge of letters and sounds and the relationships between them) and morphological understanding (word parts). When readers can identify words rapidly and accurately, they can expend the greater part of their efforts and resources on applying higher-level skills to make sense of the text.

Two other cognitive areas need to be mentioned: attention and working memory (Cain & Oakhill, 2007; Snow et al., 1998; Snowling & Hulme, 2005). Readers must focus and sustain their attention to the words on the page. They must be able to move their eyes back and forth, left to right for reading, and to fixate on selected but important information. In addition, they need to pay attention to the comments of their classmates and teachers to receive additional input re the meaning or message in stories or passages. Attention cannot really be separated from other cognitive skills such as making inferences, using metacognitive strategies, applying prior knowledge, and, of course, affective factors such as motivation and interest.

The role of working memory in the development of reading is controversial, but there is much research advocating its importance (Pickering, 2006; Snowling & Hulme, 2005; for d/Deaf children, see Paul, 2009; Trezek et al., 2010; Wang et al., 2008) as well as for the other content areas discussed here such as mathematics and science (e.g., Bruning et al., 2004; Pickering, 2006). Basically, to process syntax and longer discourse structures, readers need to hold specific information long enough in working memory (also short-term memory) to work out the meanings of phrases, sentences, and even the entire passage. Working memory is related to the use of phonology (e.g., phonological code, decoding into sounds, etc.) for reading, mainly because of the properties of English. Slow, laborious reading of words places a huge burden on working memory (an overload) such that it is difficult for readers to remember information and construct a meaning model. Obviously, readers need to extract information from long-term memory as well so that there is an important relation between working memory and long-term memory for construction of meaning from print (Cain & Oakhill, 2007; Snowling & Hulme, 2005; see also, related discussions in Israel & Duffy, 2009; McGuinness, 2004, 2005; Ruddell & Unrau, 2004).

Mature Reading (Reading to Learn)

There is little doubt that English reading is reflective of complex activities involving cognition, language, and socio-emotional issues. It is a daunting task to develop an adequate, complete theoretical model that accounts for the acquisition and development of reading, particularly mature reading skills. In fact, it is not likely that one model will ever be sufficient (Israel & Duffy, 2009; McGuinness, 2004, 2005; Ruddell & Unrau, 2004).

There is no single factor that can explicate the range of difficulties that impede the development of skilled readers. Whatever the perspective, there are several intricate models of the reading process that can range across four major categories: cognitive-processing (e.g., the works of Adams, Rumelhart, as well as Flowers and Hayes), sociocognitive-processing (Ruddell and Unrau), transactional (Rosenblatt), transactional-sociopsycholinguistic (Goodman), and attitude-influence (Mathewson) (see discussions in Israel & Duffy, 2009; Ruddell & Unrau, 2004). With a heavy focus on language and concentrating on reading only, McGuinness (2005), as mentioned previously in this book, has averred that reading can be stated as a *decoding–encoding* entity. *Decoding* refers to word identification or access, and *encoding* can refer, broadly, to the output such as writing, spelling, or overall comprehension or interpretation.

Regardless of the reading model, it is clear that accessing print (i.e., letters, words) needs to be automatic so that readers can expend sufficient energy on the critical higher-level task of comprehension (Israel & Duffy, 2009; McGuinness, 2004, 2005; Snowling & Hulme, 2005). Reciprocal relationships between word identification (access skills) and comprehension occur at every stage of the reading process from beginning (i.e., word and word parts) to advanced (e.g., sentences, paragraphs, story or stories).

In sum, to develop mature or proficient reading skills, individuals need to continue their acquisition of knowledge, vocabulary, metacognitive (e.g., to monitor and evaluate their understanding), and inferencing skills (e.g., retelling, answering questions, syntheses, etc.). To obtain fluency—defined as the point at which most energy and time can be spent on comprehending and interpreting the message—individuals need increased experiences with print as well as deeper and more extensive growth in language and cognitive variables.

Table 4-3 applies some of the principles in this section on reading to the understanding of a short passage.

Table 4-3. Understanding a Short Passage

Comprehension Processes for Constructing Meaning

Passage

She plunked down ten dollars at a window.

She refused to take five dollars from the man standing next to her.

She did let him buy the popcorn and sodas before they found their seats in the dark room.

In this Postmodern Age, a woman wants to be as independent and in charge as much as possible.

Possible Interpretations

To make sense of the above passage, the reader needs to utilize a number of processes ranging from identifying letters to words to sentences, along with understanding social, historical, and contextual factors (discussed in this chapter). For example, drawing on language knowledge, the reader knows that the pronoun *she* refers to a woman of a particular age. The phrase *plunked down* conjures a cognitive image of a specific manner of putting money on a surface at a particular location. To surmise the meaning of *window* requires both linguistic and cognitive–social knowledge. This seems to indicate a specific type of place and possible guesses might be a bank, theatre, or racetrack. The location is not cleared up by the second sentence, although one could hazard a guess. At this point in the text, the reader has constructed an ambiguous model of meaning (and this has happened at a fast pace).

Considering the second sentence on the refusal to take money from the man and the third sentence on permitting the man to buy popcorn and sodas indicates at least two points: 1) they are together, perhaps on a date or they know one another, albeit the location might be disambiguated (theatre, opera house, etc.) by the end of the third sentence (dark room); and 2) the woman seems to exhibit a certain take charge attitude. Perhaps she asked the man for a date? A number of interpretations can be proffered after the last sentence, which are heavily influenced by one's understanding of the term *Postmodern Age* as well as one's feelings and opinions about this social event in one's own social environment.

In short, comprehension of this passage requires the coordination of three broad groups of skills: language, metalinguistics of language terms related to literacy, and cognitive–social factors. This is or should be happening at a fairly fluent pace.

Writing

Describing writing is just as difficult as describing reading. Writing, similar to reading, is not a unitary skill; that is, there is no single all-encompassing factor or variable that can account for or explain all of written language development. For sure, writing involves the juggling and integration of a number of mental strategies and skills, placing a huge demand on cognition.

It is interesting that many individuals do not view themselves as good writers. As synthesized by Bruning et al. (2004):

> Writing is such a complex cognitive task that it involves almost all of the processes and concepts we have discussed in earlier chapters, including working and long-term memory, procedural and declarative knowledge, motivation, self-regulation, and beliefs and attitudes. No wonder students can find writing assignments intimidating. (p. 291)

Theories and models on writing have been influenced by theories and models on reading. It thus has been argued that reading and writing consist of a number of similar subprocesses (Lipson & Wixson, 1997; McCarthey & Raphael, 1992). Reading facilitates the development of writing, and writing facilitates the development of reading. The nature of this facilitation process, albeit accepted, is not well understood.

In any case, good readers have the potential to become good writers. Good writers (of a particular genre) are already good readers (of the same genre). If an individual does not read well, it is not likely that s/he can write well. If an individual does not write well, s/he may or may not be a good reader; obviously, this is a complex relationship (Adams, 1990; Hayes, 2004). Based on these remarks, it seems that children and adolescents need to be given numerous opportunities to write and that writing and reading should be taught together in the early grades, at the least (Adams, 1990; Ehri, 2006; Pearson, 2004).

The foundations for being a good reader must be fairly, but not completely, established before one can become a good writer. We support the view that reading and writing can develop simultaneously—especially during the emergent literacy years (e.g., Hayes, 2004). We argue, however, that a specific level of proficiency in writing cannot be higher than the corresponding level of proficiency in reading. In short, writing requires all of the factors (e.g., language, cognitive, experiential) expounded for reading plus more. The *more* relates to the rendition of information involving both lower-level (e.g., grammar, spelling, etc.) and higher-level (e.g., planning, audience, purpose, and drafting) skills.

In essence, the process of writing is said to consist of several linguistic and cognitive stages such as planning, composing (also translating), and revising (also reviewing) (Flower & Hayes, 1980; Hayes, 2004). Writers operate on several levels, which include activities such as selecting topics, planning and organizing ideas, making decisions on what information to include, and engaging in self-monitoring during the stages of composing and revising their productions (Hayes, 2004; Hillocks, 1986; Montague, 1990). Similar to the processes of reading, writers cannot expend too much effort and time on the lower-level aspects of writing such as mechanics (e.g., spelling, grammar, punctuation, etc.). These lower-level skills should become automatic processes so that writers can focus on the higher-level skills such as organization, intent, and audience (Graves, 1994; Routman, 2005).

The early acquisition of reading and writing occurs in tandem with the emerging language development of children. One can see steady, incremental increases in quantity and quality during this period (Routman, 2005; Ruddell & Haggard, 1985; Saada-Robert, 2004). In essence, the early writings of children seem to resemble the level of their corresponding spoken language development (Avery, 2002; Sulzby & Teale, 1987, 2003).

From age nine and beyond, there is an exponential growth in the development of writing, reflecting the increasing language and cognitive demands of reading materials, that is, at about the third- or fourth-grade level. Despite the close relationship between the development of writing and that of spoken language, children's written language samples are still more complex and intricate than their spoken language utterances. Due to varying factors (see also, Chapters 1 and 2), children (and most other writers) tend to produce complex language structures more often in their writings than in their spoken language utterances.

Mature (and perhaps critico-creative) writing development requires an increase in the facility, range, and depth of higher-level skills (Hayes, 2004). That is, individuals need to increase their sophistication in language use, involving the use of vocabulary, figurative and analogical language, and other areas for language composition. These language composition skills entail the ability to integrate the language components (e.g., morphology, syntax, semantics, pragmatics) to formulate, refine, and, eventually, to express thoughts in writing.

Finally, there needs to be a further development of cognitive areas such as knowledge, inferencing, synthesizing, and so on, especially with respect to writing on expository topics such as science, social studies, and other academic content areas. The problems with reading and writing expository materials have been well documented in the research literature on literacy (Hayes, 2004; Pearson, 2004) as well as with children with disabilities and those who are English language learners (e.g., see related discussions in Chapters 6 to 9). Expository writing is critical for success in education at pre-postsecondary and postsecondary levels.

Table 4-4 provides an example of both narrative and expository writing, and **Table 4-5** provides highlights of the discussion of reading and writing.

Now that we have discussed the relation of cognition (e.g., cognitive strategies, skills) to the development of literacy, we turn our attention to the content areas of mathematics and science in the ensuing sections.

Cognition and Mathematics

To understand the paradigm shift in developing mathematics knowledge and in mathematics education, consider the following scenario.

Scenario

The teacher spent an enormous amount of time helping her class understand the basic computation operations of addition and subtraction. Students were repeatedly engaged in playing math games in which the goal was to answer quickly and accurately. One day, the teacher observed the following performance across several students:

$$
\begin{array}{cccc}
65 & 73 & 88 & 91 \\
-44 & -55 & -77 & -54 \\
\hline
21 & 22 & 11 & 43 \\
\end{array}
$$

One possible interpretation is that students have overgeneralized the computational principles by focusing, mainly, on the surface level features. This works for the first and third problems, but not for the second and fourth ones above. This overgeneralization or dependence on surface language features is also prevalent in the research literature on word problems. Consider the following:

Scenario

Mary has 10 more marbles than Joan. Joan has 5 marbles. What is the total number of marbles? The answer is 20; however, a common wrong answer is 15.

Table 4-4. Example of Narrative and Expository Writing

Narrative Writing

When the fierce and extraordinary Ayn Rand was fifty-two years old, about to become world famous, and more than thirty years removed from her birthplace in Russia, she summed up the meaning of her elaborate invented, cerebral world this way: "My philosophy, in essence, is the concept of man, as a heroic being, with his own happiness as the moral purpose of his life, with productive achievement as his noblest activity, and reason as his only absolute." (Heller, 2009, p. 1)

Expository Writing

In the 1950s and 1960s cognitive psychology took over from behaviourism as the dominant force in psychology. One of the major reasons for this was the development of the computer. Initially the contribution of the computer to psychology was in giving psychologists a way of thinking about mental or cognitive processes. The use of the computer as a tool for thinking about how the human mind handles information is known as the **computer analogy**. *By the end of the 1960s psychologists had taken the computer analogy to its next logical step and put together programmes called* **computer stimulations** *that carried out simple cognitive processes such as storing information.* (Jarvis, 2000, p. 79)

Questions for Further Discussion

1. What are the characteristics of a narrative passage? Expository passage?
2. What are a few similarities and differences between the narrative and the expository passage?
3. Discuss the language and cognitive demands made by each passage.
4. Does proficiency in one type (i.e., reading and writing narrative passages) mean that one is also proficient in the other type (i.e., reading and writing expository passages)? Why or why not?

Again, the focus is on the computational surface level not on understanding the conceptual framework of the problem.

As a result of the above scenarios, researchers and educators have argued for a paradigm shift from traditional mathematics instruction focused on computation procedures and memorization, to an emphasis on understanding mathematical methods and concepts at different difficulty levels (Battista, 2001; English & Halford, 1995; Mayer, 1992). The thrust of this paradigm shift has been due to the impetus of cognitive psychology, particularly the models of cognitive and social constructivism. Instead of the simple acquisition of isolated concepts and procedural skills (e.g., addition, subtraction, etc.), teachers should assist students in developing a conceptual understanding of mathematics problems. Solving word problems has set the stage for the kind of thinking in which students should engage, that is, a problem-solving paradigm.

Table 4-5. Highlights of Reading and Writing

Reading

- There are two broad time periods: early reading (or learning to read) and mature reading (or reading to learn).
- In learning to read, there are two broad categories of factors: linguistic and cognitive.
- The linguistic or language aspect contains two broad sub-areas: English language development and metalinguistic understanding of the aspects of English language related to literacy (print).
- The cognitive aspect includes non-print areas such as prior knowledge, metacognition (including self-regulation), inferencing, affective factors (e.g., motivation and interest), and specific attributes associated with working memory and attention.
- A level of language competency is critical for development in both early and mature reading stages. Briefly, this refers to the development of proficiency in the use (pragmatics), content (semantics), and structure (phonology, morphology, syntax) of language.
- To make initial progress in early reading—especially when learning to read—children must develop *metalinguistic awareness*. This is interpreted as metalinguistic proficiency in language areas that pertain to the literacy process, such as awareness of print (pragmatics), sounds (phonemes), letters (graphemes), relationships between letters and sounds (phonics or sound–letter correspondences), word parts (morphemes), word order (syntax), and connected text structures (discourse).
- Progress in the language areas mentioned above facilitates and is facilitated by cognitive factors such as the ongoing development of prior knowledge, metacognition, and breadth and depth of vocabulary knowledge.
- There is little doubt that English reading is reflective of complex activities involving cognition, language, and socio-emotional issues.
- No single factor can explicate the range of difficulties that impede the development of skilled readers.
- To develop mature (proficient) reading skills, individuals must continue their acquisition of knowledge, vocabulary, metacognitive (e.g., to monitor and evaluate their understanding), and inferencing skills (e.g., retelling, answering questions, syntheses, etc.). To obtain fluency—that is, the point at which most energy and time can be spent on comprehending and interpreting the message—individuals need increased experiences with print as well as deeper and more extensive growth in language and cognitive variables.

Writing

- Writing, similar to reading, is not a unitary skill. There is no single all-encompassing factor or variable that can account for or explain all of written language development.

Table 4-5.   Highlights of Reading and Writing *(continued)*

- Writing involves the juggling and integration of a number of mental strategies and skills, placing a huge demand on cognition.
- Theories and models on writing have been influenced by theories and models on reading. It has been argued that reading and writing consist of a number of similar subprocesses.
- Reading facilitates the development of writing, and writing facilitates the development of reading. The nature of this facilitation process, albeit accepted, is not well understood.
- A specific level of proficiency in writing cannot be higher than the corresponding level of proficiency in reading. In short, writing requires all of the factors (e.g., language, cognitive, experiential) expounded for reading plus more. The *more* relates to the rendition of information involving both lower-level (e.g., grammar, spelling, etc.) and higher-level (e.g., planning, audience, purpose, and drafting) skills.
- The process of writing is said to consist of several linguistic and cognitive stages such as planning, composing (also translating), and revising (also reviewing). Writers operate on several levels, which include activities such as selecting topics, planning and organizing ideas, making decisions on what information to include, engaging in self-monitoring during the stages of composing, and revising their productions.
- Writers cannot expend too much effort and time on the lower-level aspects of writing such as mechanics (e.g., spelling, grammar, punctuation, etc.). These lower-level skills should become automatic processes so that writers can focus on the higher-level skills such as organization, intent, and audience.
- Further development of cognitive areas such as knowledge, inferencing, synthesizing, and so on, must be done especially with respect to writing about expository topics such as science, social studies, and other academic content areas.

Problem-solving is exemplified because it requires procedural and conceptual knowledge and skills. There should be a reasonable balance between procedural and conceptual understanding or between skills and processes, similar to the arguments in the field of script literacy (Battista, 2001; De Corte, Verschaffel, & Eynde, 2000; English & Halford, 1995). Within the constructivist realm, students are said to be active in the construction and self-regulation of their mathematical knowledge. This is true whether students are solving simple addition problems or complex problems in algebra, geometry, or calculus.

Problem solving is an important aspect of mathematics education because it facilitates the development of a deep understanding of mathematical ideas as well as the application of sub-skills and conceptual knowledge. This approach encourages students to make sense of the problems that they are attempting to solve (Mayer & Hegarty, 1996; Rittle-Johnson, Siegler, & Alibali, 2001). The goal of this approach seems to be quantitative literacy in which students are encouraged to conceptualize the problems and apply this approach in other aspects of their lives (in and out of school).

The thrust and influence of cognitive research have been on the understanding of mental processes that students use in attempting to solve mathematics problems. A number of theorists and researchers (e.g., Kintsch & Greeno, 1985; Mayer & Hegarty, 1996) asserted that there is a need to apply a comprehension-based model to understanding problem solving (see the influence of Kintsch to literacy comprehension in Chapter 2). Procedural or operational knowledge (e.g., counting algorithms) is important, but only in the context of a conceptual framework on the mathematics problem. Performing the correct operation is not problem solving; however, applying the correct algorithms to the solution of a problem after conceptualizing and setting it up requires both lower-level (computational) and higher-level (establishing a mental model, planning) skills. In this sense, students are thinking strategically and making a decision on the manner in which the problem can be solved.

Problem solving has been examined via several cognitive perspectives such as text processing (Kintsch, 1998, 2004; Kintsch & Greeno, 1985), information processing (Mayer, 1992; Van Der Schoot, Arkema, Horsley, & Van Lieshout, 2009), and reading comprehension (Pape, 2004). Despite the range of models, the common element seems to be the need for students to develop a mental, conceptual understanding of the mathematics problem and then use this understanding to guide the selection of procedures and operations to solve the problem.

Similar to other content areas, including reading and writing, it is critical for students to continue their growth in the language and concepts of mathematics. This acquisition of conceptual and procedural knowledge contributes to the facilitation of solving deeper, more complex problems in mathematics. The focus should be on conceptual understanding because there is a growing consensus that mathematics is deeply conceptual, not procedural (Schoenfeld, 1992; Siegler, 1996).

What does this mean with respect to the cognitive implications for instruction? We assume that our readers can predict a few ideas; nevertheless, we end this section with a list from Bruning et al. (2004, pp. 336-337) highlighting the main implications (for further details, please consult the source):

1. All mathematics should be taught from a comprehension-based problem-solving perspective.

2. Mathematics instruction should focus on processes, structures, and decisions, not on answers.

3. Build on students' informal knowledge.

4. Teachers need to spend time verbally modeling mathematics problem-solving behavior.

5. Assist students in verbalizing and, if possible, visualizing processes used in solution attempts.

6. Use students' errors as a source of information on students' understanding.

7. Provide a mixture of problem types.

8. Teachers themselves need appropriate levels of mathematics skills.

Cognition and Science

It should come as no surprise that many of the cognitive instructional implications, strategies, and arguments for understanding and developing mathematics knowledge in students also apply to developing scientific knowledge. Reform in science seems to be similar to the reform in mathematics. The national science education reform is a response to the shifted goal of education away from knowing *that* and towards knowing *how* (Dreyfus & Dreyfus, 1986; Kuhn, 1970, 1996; Stoddart, Pinal, Latzke, & Canaday, 2002). Instead of rote learning, students are directed towards more conceptual ways of searching for information and pursuing their understanding of the material.

If the focus is on obtaining factual knowledge, then *knowing that* is a rule-governed, rigid understanding of the subject matter. Strictly speaking, students simply memorize information, regurgitate it on paper-and-pencil tests, and recite it when called on in classrooms. These parrot-type imitative activities do not facilitate the development and understanding of what it means to be a scientist. Science is not simply the accumulation of facts and definitions, ranging from simple to complex.

With a focus on conceptual knowledge or understanding—that is, on *knowing how*—students can think like a scientist and apply these principles to—once again—solving problems in science. Thinking like a scientist entails some version of the scientific method such as stating the problem or hypothesis, gathering background information, testing the hypothesis, presenting the results, and explaining the findings. These activities can be accomplished—most effectively in some scholars' eyes—in inquiry-based science instruction, which emphasizes the more generalizable conceptual knowledge over factual information (although some factual information is important within a conceptual framework) (Carin, Bass, & Contant, 2005; Wild, 2008). Within such a conceptual approach, students act as involved performers instead of detached observers, and their comprehension of the subject matter is contextually contingent and grounded in experience (Cawley & Parmar, 2001; Stoddart et al., 2002).

In the ensuing sections, we highlight briefly the inquiry approach, which seems to be the hallmark of this revolution in science education and an approach that is most conducive to the development of a scientific literacy. Then we proffer a few remarks about science education and children with disabilities. Given the language and literacy issues of these children (see Chapters 6 to 8) as well as those who are English language learners (Chapter 9), there is a tendency to think—erroneously—that these issues need to be resolved before engaging the above students in science extensively (see also, Chapter 3). There is no doubt that language and literacy issues contribute to the problem of understanding information, but there is more to science, for example, than the ability to read and write well.

Inquiry Process

To help students develop scientific literacy and understand scientific concepts and methods, students need to approach science as a problem-solving technique via the use of constructivist, inquiry-based approaches. The inquiry process has no age restriction; it should be a part of the curriculum at all education levels from preschool to secondary education. Of course, it is important for students in middle and high school (and even elementary) to be able to access science texts. Nevertheless, the focus should not be on the information in the texts only because this induces memorization of facts and definitions.

As a critical component targeted in the *National Science Education Standards* (National Research Council [NRC], 1996), scientific inquiry provides mechanisms for students to explore and offer explanations based on evidence. The *Standards* define scientific inquiry as "a set of interrelated processes by which scientists and students pose questions about the natural world and investigate phenomena" (NRC, 1996, p. 214). To engage in effective scientific inquiry, it is critical to design inquiry-based instructional environments.

We recognize that scientific inquiry is a complicated and complex concept. A review of the literature reveals several other terms used to describe or define inquiry-based science instruction such as the following, which is not exhaustive: *inquiry-based science* (Keys & Bryan, 2001), *inquiry-oriented science* (Mastropieri, Scruggs, Boon, & Butcher, 2001), *inquiry learning* (Mastropieri, Scruggs & Butcher, 1997), *project-based science* (Schneider, Krajcik, Marx, & Soloway, 2002), *activity-based science* (Mastropieri & Scruggs, 1994), *discovery teaching* (Odubunmi & Balogun, 1991), and on and on.

If we adhere to the model of Carin et al. (2005), we can list several cognitive-based process skills for conducting inquiry-based investigations. Carin et al. delineate these skills for middle school classrooms; however, with a few modifications, they are applicable to classrooms at all educational levels. These cognitive skills include the following: observing, measuring, classifying, inferring, hypothesizing, controlled investigation, predicting, explaining and communicating (**Table 4-6**).

Carin et al.'s (2005) model represents another perspective on the use of the scientific approach, mentioned previously. For example, the gathering of information is heavily dependent on sharp observation skills. Repeated observations and checking the data are critical for reliability and validity. As students grow in conceptual understanding, their observation skills deepen and morph into the use of categories (e.g., schemata) for understanding the information.

The skills of measuring and classifying information facilitate the development of a hypothesis (and prediction), especially in a pure inductive-type approach. To sharpen the hypothesis, students need to fine-tune their classification skills. There are two classification systems. The first is *binary classification* where students are asked to divide objects into two groups based upon similar properties. In the second system, students may also engage in *multistage classification* systems in which objects are sorted, based upon similar properties, a multiple number of times until a hierarchy of sets and subsets are formed. Classification helps students to obtain an understanding of the properties and functions of objects in their environment.

After observing, measuring, and classifying, students can make an inference. An *inference* is an interpretation based upon prior knowledge and

Table 4-6.   Process Skills of Inquiry Learning

Process of Science	Methods
Observing	Gather information using all appropriate senses and instruments that extend the senses.
Measuring	Quantify variable using a variety of instruments and standard and nonstandard units.
Classifying	Group objects or organisms according to one or more common properties.
Inferring	Draw a tentative conclusion about observations based on prior knowledge.
Hypothesizing	Make a statement about a possible relationship in the natural world that might be found through investigation.
Controlled Investigation	Investigate by deliberately manipulating one variable at a time and observing the effect on a responding variable, while holding all other variables constant.
Predicting	Make a forecast of a possible outcome of an investigation based on known patterns in data.
Explaining	Logically link evidence and scientific knowledge to make sense of puzzling events.
Communicating	Record and present the results of investigations to others in multiple ways.

Source: Adapted from Carin et al. (2005).

experiences (more cognitive skills!). Students should proffer inferences based upon observations, measurements, concepts and assumptions.

The next step in this inductive framework is to formulate a hypothesis. The *hypothesis* refers to a possible relationship that might occur between the natural world and the investigations to be made. Students can communicate their hypotheses in either a written or spoken form. In fact, it is strongly recommended that students engage in a wide variety of communication techniques.

After the above stages, students are ready to conduct controlled investigations, involving the manipulations of variables in a systematic manner. For example, students may examine the phases of the moon at night. To obtain relevant and adequate data, they should conduct periodic examinations and report on others' examinations from different vantage points or locations.

During these investigations, students can offer a prediction about their observations and evidence. This enhances the importance of using evidence to support predictions. The evidence (or data) can be represented in a variety of ways such as via the use of graphs, recorded calculations, pictures, and so on (Carin et al., 2005).

Upon completion of the investigation or experiment, students may offer explanations. *Explanations* require the linking of collected data to scientific phenomena. Finally, there is a need to communicate the findings. For example, students may take a test, complete a presentation, write a report, and so on.

The inquiry-based approach above (and other types of constructivist activities) is considered effective for helping students to confront their naïve scientific assumptions and beliefs. In other words, to confront misunderstandings and to proceed toward conceptual understanding similar to that of a scientist, students need to think like a scientist via the use of discovery processes and an understanding of scientific language and methods. Similar to other content areas and literacy, growth requires an increase in higher-level cognitive skills such as enhancing and utilizing prior knowledge, metacognition, and self-regulation as well as developing motivation and interest. The comprehension-based model, which is the basis for literate thought, literacy, and mathematics (discussed previously) is also applicable to the development of scientific understanding.

Children with Disabilities

How does reform in science relate to children with disabilities? In a seminal comprehensive review of science education for students with disabilities, Mastropieri and Scruggs (1992) concluded that science education typically has received little emphasis in special education classrooms, involving children with disabilities. Specifically, they reported that there has been little or no dialogue on the relevance and adequateness of inquiry-based science instruction. Scruggs, Mastropieri, and Boon (1998) reviewed the inquiry-based practices in special education science classrooms and found that the use of inquiry-based instruction was scarce; its merits thus were poorly understood with respect to children with disabilities.

There is a need to either adapt or develop well-designed science-instructional materials and to determine what science-instructional techniques are effective—that is, based on evidence-based research—for children with disabilities. For children with language difficulties (in fact, for nearly all children with disabilities), it might be necessary to use techniques that have been effective in literacy; examples are graphic organizers, semantic mapping, and other related inferential strategies (see related discussions in Chapters 6 to 9). Similar to the research in literacy, it is suspected that the above techniques might assist students with the development of higher-level cognitive skills such as prior knowledge, metacognitive, and problem-solving skills. In a nutshell, much research still needs to be conducted to address both science instruction and the effectiveness of inquiry-based learning for children with disabilities, including children with specific disabilities involving vision, hearing, and cognition (e.g., Lang, 2006; Wild, 2008).

There is no doubt that research and instruction need to continue on language and literacy development of children with disabilities. Nevertheless, this does not mean that concomitant work cannot ensue on the instruction of science. At first blush, it seems unrealistic to assume that children who are struggling with the language of communication and instruction (e.g., English) will be able to access and understand the language of science. In the absence of strong empirical evidence, we have sufficient bravado to argue that teachers need to work on both broad areas simultaneously, to say the least.

Summary

In the above sections, we describe—albeit briefly—the relationship of cognition (i.e., structures, strategies, skills) to the structures of disciplines such as literacy, mathematics, and science. Understanding the structure of a discipline is an ongoing process for both learners and experts or scholars. To be effective teachers or clinicians, individuals need to have a deep understanding of discipline structure and the psychology of learning as they pertain to students who endeavored to acquire knowledge in these content areas.

If disciplines have structures, ranging from coherent to loosely-structured, then there must be some fundamentals that are necessary for everyone who wants to develop discipline knowledge. Discipline knowledge is not a mere accumulation of facts or definitions; it is an understanding of facts, methods, and concepts within an overall conceptual framework. It might be feasible to apply a comprehension-based model to growth in discipline knowledge in that a continued growth is dependent on the continual development of cognitive-based areas such as prior or world knowledge, metacognition, and motivation and interest.

There is little doubt that language is at the core of any discipline and particularly of the ones discussed here: literacy, mathematics, and science. Nevertheless, there is more to discipline knowledge than just the language for communication and thought or even the language of the discipline. With respect to children with disabilities (Chapters 6 to 8) and children who are English language learners (Chapter 9), teachers and clinicians cannot simply wait until these individuals have obtained proficiency in the majority language of society. And, as discussed in the next section, the evidence for fundamentals in any discipline most likely applies to everyone, albeit there are some important considerations due to the concept of individual differences.

QUALITATIVE-SIMILARITY HYPOTHESIS

Thus far, we have discussed issues regarding the psychological framework of cognitive models and the conceptual framework of discipline areas as well as the relationships between these two entities. Clearly, we are somewhat skeptical about a direct relationship between these two entities. We do contend, however, that disciplines have a conceptual framework that may range from structured to ill-structured, even within the disciplines. More importantly, we argue that there are fundamentals that all individuals need to know and understand to achieve a level of proficiency in a specific topic or discipline. Individual differences notwithstanding, our views can be best stated within our proclivity for a construct labeled the *Qualitative-Similarity Hypothesis* (QSH; Paul, 1998, 2001, 2008a, 2008b, 2009; Paul & Lee, 2010; Paul, Wang, Trezek, & Luckner, 2009; Wang et al., 2008; for a related discussion, see Stanovich, 1986, 1992; Stanovich, Nathan, & Zolman, 1988 and the concept of *developmental lag*).

The basic assumption of the QSH is that the language and literacy development of children and adolescents with disabilities or even those who are learning English, especially as a second language, is similar to that of individuals who are typical (or with typical development) or who are native language users. In other words, those individuals with disabilities or ELLs proceed through stages, produce errors, and use strategies that are *developmentally* similar to what has been observed for individuals who are typical, albeit usually younger. Although the rate of development is quantitatively slower, it is presumed that, with extensive and intensive instruction or intervention, these individuals will eventually achieve at a level that matches the chronological age of others who are typical.

Within the QSH framework, we argue—again—that there are certain fundamentals that are necessary for *all* individuals in the acquisition process relative to a specific content area or discipline. This does not mean that all children with disabilities, for example, come to the process of learning on an even playing field. There is wide variation in the psychosocial lives of these children that impacts their development (for literacy, see Paul, 2008b). For children with specific disabilities such as deafness, blindness, and even learning, there may be additional non-academic needs that need to be addressed. There are tremendous variations that contribute to the construct of individual differences in development and learning. In our view, the presence of individual differences or the need to differentiate instruction does not necessarily weaken the support for the QSH, but this does lead to refinements based on specific research findings.

In addition to the above, the QSH does not demand a one-size-fits-all with respect to the fundamentals, or more specifically, to the delivery of instruction. For example, although the fundamentals remain essentially the same, the instruction needs to be differentiated given the individual needs of children. Let's use reading as an example.

The National Reading Panel (2000; see also, the NELP, 2008) provides recommendations for the development of reading—presumably in all children who are attempting to learn to read English. Among the various areas, the NRP has argued that phonemic awareness and the use of phonics are important to build upon emergent literacy skills (McGuinness, 2004, 2005). Specifically, the need is for children to learn the alphabetic principle.

For a number of children, it might not be feasible to use traditional approaches to enhance phonemic awareness and the development of the alphabetic principle, especially via phonics (e.g., for d/Deaf or hard of hearing children, see Trezek et al., 2010; Wang et al., 2008; see also, Chapters 6–8). That is, children may not benefit adequately from typical phonics instruction. Alternative approaches, for example, for d/Deaf or hard of hearing children, include Cued Speech/Language and Visual Phonics, which have been proffered by several researchers with some documented success (LaSasso, Crain, & Leybaert, 2010; Trezek et al., 2010; Wang et al., 2008).

Much of the discussion and research on the QSH has been undertaken on language and literacy development. There is a long history of this research, including for children who are English language learners. The impetus for the QSH, described mostly in the research on deafness, has been the work of Stanovich via his constructs of the Matthew Effects and the Developmental Lag Hypothesis (Stanovich, 1986, 1992; Stanovich, Nathan, & Zolman, 1988). These constructs are discussed in the ensuing section.

Matthew Effects and the Developmental Lag Hypothesis

Stanovich (1986) formed the construct of the *Matthew Effects*, which influenced a line of research especially for children with garden-variety disabilities and for those with specific disabilities such as dyslexia. Based on this line of research, Stanovich and his collaborators developed a framework coined the *Developmental Lag Hypothesis*, which is roughly similar to our QSH (see also, Stanovich, 1992; Stanovich et al., 1988).

The Matthew Effects is based on the premise that there is an optimal, perhaps critical, period for developing literacy skills. The Matthew Effects is interpreted as "*The rich get richer* and *the poor stay the same or become poorer*," which relates to the development and growth of reading and reading skills. If individuals have *learned to read* during an optimal period—usually by the end of third grade—then they will read to learn. And they will or can get "richer"—that is, develop more advanced skills and knowledge—if they read voraciously and widely.

On the other hand, if individuals do not learn to read during the optimal period, then they will be "poor," unable to read to learn adequately or to acquire much knowledge. Their growth may become stagnated or they may become even more deficient linguistically and cognitively because they cannot or will not read much at all. There is no reciprocal relationship between reading and cognition or between reading and language development or even among language, cognition, and reading—especially given the language and cognitive demands of literacy materials beyond the third grade. As poor or struggling literacy users become older, the lag between them and that of good literacy users becomes greater.

Research on the Matthew Effects led to the construction of the Developmental Lag Hypothesis with strong and weak versions (Stanovich, 1992; Stanovich et al., 1988). In the strong version of this hypothesis, it is asserted that children can catch up to their typically-reading peers if reading instruction is focused, sustained, and extensive, particularly addressing areas such as phonological and phonemic awareness. In the weak version, it has been found that some children, for whatever reason, will not catch up or reach the level of their typical counterparts—albeit in theory they should.

The weak version engendered another view labeled the *Deficit Hypothesis* (Francis, Shaywitz, Stuebing, Shaywitz, & Fletcher, 1996; O'Brien, Mansfield, & Legge, 2005; O'Shaughnessy & Swanson, 1998; Reimer, 2006; Snowling, Defty, & Goulandris, 1996). It is often associated with children with severe dyslexia and severe cognitive delays, who seem to have barriers that cannot be overcome psychologically, that is, via intense instruction or intervention. It should be noted that the weak version is not asserting that these children develop differently per se or that these children cannot make *any* progress in literacy.

Both versions of the Developmental Lag Hypothesis as well as the QSH assert that the acquisition of literacy skills is developmentally similar to typical literacy users. In addition, struggling literacy users may or may not catch up developmentally as they mature and acquire more advanced skills. There are fundamentals that are necessary for all individuals in learning English language and literacy. Based on the findings of the NRP (2000), NELP (2008), and extant interpretations and literacy theories discussed previously (Israel & Duffy, 2009; McGuinness, 2004, 2005; Ruddell & Unrau, 2004), these fundamentals include an understanding or competence in English (i.e., proficiency and processing) plus print access skills (e.g., decoding) and comprehension skills (e.g., vocabulary, prior knowledge, and metacognition).

Application to Children with Disabilities

Debates are ongoing as to whether the QSH or the Developmental Lag Hypothesis applies to all or most children with disabilities. Another perspective is to pose this question: Do the findings of the NRP (2000) or NELP (2008) apply to children with specific disabilities such as learning disabilities, autism, emotional disabilities, intellectual disabilities, visual and hearing disabilities? Much of the work on literacy does mention children with disabilities, but many of these children have not been part of the investigations.

With a focus on the NRP, a special journal issue on reading and children with disabilities seems to conclude that the recommendations and finding could apply, but additional considerations (and research) are also needed (Paul, 2008a, 2008b; c.f., Tierney, 2008). There have not been similar research reviews focusing on the findings of the NELP (2008). However, based on the main tenets of the QSH and even the Developmental Lag Hypothesis, it is argued here that the results are applicable, even for children who are English language learners.

Even if the NRP or the NELP recommendations (or any other set of literacy recommendations) do apply, this is not a one-size-fits-all process, given the complexity of working with children with a range of disabilities. There may be a need for alternative instructional approaches to ensure that the fundamentals (e.g., foundations) are acquired. These types of approaches are necessary to prevent Stanovich's *Matthew Effects*.

We shall take this one step further—given the focus of this book. We have applied the QSH and Developmental Lag Hypothesis to the development of language and literacy variables with respect to subsequent development of early and advanced print (i.e., script) literacy skills thus far. While we are strong proponents of script literacy, we are even stronger proponents of literate thought *in any mode or in as many modes as possible.* In our view, there is a need for focusing also on the use of performance literacy (see Chapters 1 and 2) and the New and Multiple Literacies (see Chapter 3) for the development of literate thought, including critico-creative thinking skills (Chapter 5). At the very least, this focus should enhance the development of language proficiency and processing skills (including listening comprehension, etc.), which are also important for early and advanced script literacy skills. Ongoing language comprehension development, whether through-the-air or in a captured form (e.g., performance literacy as in audio- and videobooks without print), is necessary for all children and especially for children with disabilities and those who are ELLs.

As mentioned repeatedly, despite our best efforts, a number of children will not be able to become mature, critical readers and writers of English print. It is also true that a number of children may not become literate thinkers in any mode. Nevertheless, we are bold to assert (and actually predict via future research endeavors) that developing literate thought in a performance literacy mode or a mode that suits the through-the-air capabilities of children will yield greater success than attempts to develop literate thought in a script literacy mode only.

Finally, it is necessary to conduct research on the QSH or Developmental Lag with respect to other content areas such as mathematics or science. There seems to be some research in these areas, but much more is needed for children with disabilities or those who are ELLs. Despite the dearth of evidence-based research, we assert that future research endeavors will justify the basic tenets of the QSH or Developmental Lag for all content areas.

SUMMARY

This chapter explores the nature of two broad themes and their interactions: cognitive models and discipline structures. We provide a brief introduction to models, structures, processes, and products. In addition, we discuss the contributions of cognitive psychology to the acquisition of discipline knowledge in three areas: literacy, mathematics, and science. The major themes are nature and relevance of cognitive psychology, cognitive models and structures, cognition and discipline structures, and the Qualitative-Similarity Hypothesis (QSH).

A summary is as follows:

- A number of scholars—the authors of this book included—aver that it is still fruitful to investigate teaching and learning via the use of cognitive models, and it is not beneficial to abandon cognition completely in favor of only social orientations or models.
- An effective cognitive framework cannot really be only an inside-the-head model, especially in light of research on sociocultural factors and the influence of contextualist perspectives. The influences of sociocultural and contextualist views have also provided implications for areas such as metacognition, self-regulated learning, and cognitive strategy instruction.
- Cognitive structures refer to the underlying architecture from which cognitive *processes* spring in the formation of cognitive *products*. It is permissible to think of structures as the hardware.
- Cognitive *processes*, in short, represent the confluence of individuals and their attempts to address or process information.
- Cognitive *product* is not a widely used term; however, it refers to the results of the interplay of the structures and processes.
- To discuss the nature and development of cognitive models, we use the Bruning et al. (2004) framework—*associationism* and *cognitivism*—in which cognitivism is interpreted broadly to include social and contextual factors.
- Similar to other scholars, we (the authors) tend to be skeptical of the need to describe adequately the cognitive structures of the mind as either an entity unto itself or the positing of general mental structures. What might be needed is a better understanding of the structures of the disciplines and the capabilities of individuals to acquire and develop their specific discipline knowledge.

- In this chapter, we discuss cognition and the construct of discipline structures for literacy, mathematics, and science. In our discussion of the structures of these disciplines, we emphasize what it means to acquire concepts such that one can operate *like* a literacy expert or accomplish the goal of mathematical or scientific literacy.
- Understanding the structure of a discipline is an ongoing process for both learners and experts or scholars. To be effective teachers or clinicians, individuals need to have a deep understanding of discipline structure and the psychology of learning as they pertain to students who endeavor to acquire knowledge in these content areas.
- Discipline knowledge is not a mere accumulation of facts or definitions; it is an understanding of facts, methods, and concepts within an overall conceptual framework.
- It might be feasible to apply a comprehension-based model to growth in discipline knowledge in that a continued growth is dependent on the continual development of cognitive-based areas, such as prior or world knowledge, metacognition, and motivation and interest.
- The basic assumption of the QSH is that the development of children and adolescents with disabilities or even those who are English language learners (ELLs) is similar to that of individuals who are typical or who are native language users (for comparison with ELL individuals). In other words, these individuals proceed through stages, produce errors, and use strategies that are *developmentally* similar to what has been observed for individuals (usually younger) who are typical.
- Despite the dearth of evidence-based research, we assert that future research endeavors will justify the basic tenets of the QSH or Developmental Lag for all content areas.

QUESTIONS FOR REFLECTION AND DISCUSSION

1. Discuss a few highlights of the nature and relevance of cognitive psychology.

2. Describe the following concepts: *structures*, *processes*, and *products*. Do these concepts facilitate an understanding of cognitive models? Why or why not?

3. What is discipline or knowledge structure? Why do the authors favor a better understanding of discipline (or content) knowledge over the development of general cognitive models?

4. Discuss a few major points in the sections on cognition and the construct of discipline structures for literacy, mathematics, and science.

5. Describe the Qualitative-Similarity Hypothesis. What are the implications for teaching and learning situations?

REFERENCES

Adams, M. (1990). *Beginning to read: Thinking and learning about print.* Cambridge, MA: The MIT Press.

Ausubel, D. (1968). *Educational psychology: A cognitive view.* New York: Holt, Rinehart, & Winston.

Avery, C. (2002). *And with a light touch: Learning about reading, writing and teaching with first graders.* Portsmouth, NH: Heinemann.

Baars, B. (1986). *The cognitive revolution in psychology.* New York: The Guilford Press.

Bandura, A. (1997). *Self-efficacy: The exercise of control.* New York: Freeman.

Battista, M. (2001). Research and reform in mathematics education. In T. Loveless (Ed.), *The Great curriculum debate: How should we teach reading and math?* (pp. 42-84). Washington, DC: Brookings Institution Press.

Brown, C. (2006). *Cognitive psychology.* Thousand Oaks, CA: SAGE.

Bruning, R., Schraw, G., Norby, M., & Ronning, R. (2004). *Cognitive psychology and instruction* (4th ed.). Upper Saddle River, NJ: Pearson/Merrill/Prentice Hall.

Cain, K., & Oakhill, J. (Eds.). (2007). *Children's comprehension problems in oral and written language.* New York: The Guilford Press.

Carin, A., Bass, J., & Contant, T. (2005). *Methods for teaching science as inquiry* (9th ed.). Upper Saddle River, NJ: Pearson/Merrill/Prentice Hall.

Carruthers, P., Laurence, S, & Stich, S. (Eds.). (2005). *The innate mind: Structure and contents.* New York: Oxford University Press.

Carruthers, P., Laurence, S, & Stich, S. (Eds.). (2006). *The innate mind: Volume 2: Culture and cognition.* New York: Oxford University Press.

Cawley, J., & Parmar, R. (2001). Literacy proficiency and science for students with learning disabilities. *Reading & Writing Quarterly, 17,* 105-125.

Chomsky, N. (2006). *Language and mind* (3rd ed.). New York: Cambridge University Press.

Cooper, J., Heward, W., & Heron, T. (1987). *Applied behavior analysis.* Columbus, OH: Merrill Publishing Co.

Crystal, D. (1997). *The Cambridge encyclopedia of language (2nd ed)*. New York: Cambridge University Press.

Crystal, D. (2006). *How language works*. London, England: Penguin Books.

De Corte, E., Verschaffel, L., & Eynde, P. O. (2000). Self-regulation: A characteristic and a goal of mathematics education. In M. Boekerts, P. R. Pintrich, & M. Zeidner (Eds.), *Handbook of self-regulation* (pp. 687-726). San Diego, CA: Academic Press.

Donovan, M., & Bransford, J. (Eds.). (2005). *How students learn: History, mathematics, and science in the classroom*. Washington, DC: The National Academies Press.

Dreyfus, H., & Dreyfus, S. (1986). *Mind over machine: The power of human intuition and expertise in the era of the computer*. New York: Free Press.

Ehri, L. (2006). Alphabetics instruction helps students learn to read. In R. M. Joshi & P. G. Aaron (Eds.), *Handbook of orthography and literacy* (pp. 649-677). Mahwah, NJ: Erlbaum.

English, L., & Halford, G. (1995). *Mathematics education: Models and processes*. Mahwah, NJ: Lawrence Erlbaum Associates.

Flavell, D. (1985). *Cognitive development* (2nd ed.). Englewood Cliffs, NJ: Prentice-Hall.

Flower, L., & Hayes, J. (1980). The dynamics of composing: Making plans and juggling constraints. In L. Gregg & E. Steinberg (Eds.), *Cognitive processes in writing* (pp. 31-50). Hillsdale, NJ: Erlbaum.

Fodor, J. (1981). The mind-body problem. *Scientific American, 244*, 114-123.

Francis, D., Shaywitz, S., Stuebing, K., Shaywitz, B., & Fletcher, J. (1996). Developmental lag versus deficit models of reading disability: A longitudinal, individual growth curve analysis. *Journal of Educational Psychology, 88*(1), 3-17.

Gaffney, J., & Anderson, R. (2000). Trends in reading research in the United States: Changing intellectual currents over three decades. In M. Kamil, P. Mosenthal, P. D. Pearson, & R. Barr (Eds.), *Handbook of reading research* (Vol. III) (pp. 53-74). Mahwah, NJ: Erlbaum.

Graves, D. (1994). *A fresh look at writing*. Portsmouth, NH: Heinemann.

Hayes, J. (2004). A new framework for understanding cognition and affect in writing. In R. Ruddell & N. Unrau (Eds.), *Theoretical models and processes of reading* (5th ed.) (pp.1399-1430). Newark, DE: International Reading Association.

Held, C., Knauff, M., & Vosgerau, G. (Eds.). (2006). *Mental models and the mind: Current developments in cognitive psychology, neuroscience, and philosophy of mind*. New York: Elsevier.

Heller, A. (2009). *Ayn Rand and the world she made*. New York: Doubleday.

Hillocks, G. (1986). *Research on written composition: New directions for teaching*. Urbana, IL: National Conference on Research in English.

Hunt, M. (1993). *The story of psychology*. New York: Doubleday.

Israel, S., & Duffy, G. (Eds.). (2009). *Handbook of research on reading comprehension*. New York: Routledge.

Jarvis, M. (2000). *Theoretical approaches in psychology*. Philadelphia, PA: Routledge.

Johnson-Laird, P. (1988). *The computer and the mind: An introduction to cognitive science*. Cambridge, MA: Harvard University.

Keys, C., & Bryan, L, (2001). Co-constructing inquiry-based science with teachers: essential research for lasting reform. *Journal of Research in Science Teaching, 38*(6), 631-645.

Kintsch, W. (1998). *Comprehension: A paradigm for cognition*. Cambridge, UK: Cambridge University Press.

Kintsch, W. (2004). The construction-integration model of text comprehension and its implications for instruction. In R. Ruddell & N. Unrau (Eds.), *Theoretical models and processes of reading* (5th ed.) (pp. 1270-1328). Newark, DE: International Reading Association.

Kintsch, W., & & Greeno, J. (1985). Understanding and solving arithmetic word problems. *Psychological Review, 92*, 109-129.

Kuhn, D. (2005). *Education for thinking*. Cambridge, MA: Harvard University Press.

Kuhn, T. (1970). *The structure of scientific revolutions*. Chicago: University of Chicago Press.

Kuhn, T. (1996). *The structure of scientific revolutions* (3rd ed.). Chicago: University of Chicago Press.

Lang, H. (2006). Teaching science. In D. Moores & D. Martin (Eds.), *Deaf learners: Developments in curriculum and instruction* (pp. 57-66). Washington, DC: Gallaudet University Press.

LaSasso, C., Crain, K., & Leybaert, J. (Eds.). (2010). *Cued speech and cued language for deaf and hard of hearing children*. San Diego, CA: Plural Publishing.

Lipson, M., & Wixson, K. (1997). *Assessment and instruction of reading and writing disability: An interactive approach* (2nd ed.). New York, NY: Longman.

Lund, N. (2003). *Language and thought*. New York: Routledge.

Mann, L., & Sabatino, D. (1985). *Foundations of cognitive process in remedial and special education*. Rockville, MD: Aspen.

Marschark, M., & Spencer, P. (2010). The promises(?) of deaf education: From research to practice and back again. In M. Marschark & P. Spencer (Eds.), *The Oxford handbook of deaf studies, language, and education* (Vol. 2) (pp. 1-14). New York: Oxford University Press.

Mastropieri, M., & Scruggs, T. (1992). Science for students with disabilities. *Review of Educational Research, 62*(4), 377-411.

Mastropieri, M., & Scruggs, T. (1994). Text versus hands-on science curriculum. *Remedial and Special Education, 15*(2), 72-86.

Mastropieri, M., Scruggs, T., Boon, R., & Butcher, K. (2001). Correlations of inquiry learning in science. *Remedial and Special Education, 22*(3), 130-137.

Mastropieri, M., Scruggs, T., & Butcher, K. (1997). How effective is inquiry learning for students with mild disabilities? *The Journal of Special Education, 31*(2), 199-211.

Mayer, R. (1992). Mathematical problem solving: Thinking as based on domain-specific knowledge. In R. Mayer (Ed.), *Thinking, problem solving, cognition* (pp. 455-489). New York: Cambridge University Press.

Mayer, R., & Hegarty, M. (1996). The process of understanding mathematics problems. In R. Sternberg & T. Ben-Zeev (Eds.), *The nature of mathematical thinking* (pp. 29-53). Mahwah, NJ: Erlbaum.

McCarthey, S., & Raphael, T. (1992). Alternative research perspectives. In J. Irwin & M. Doyle (Eds.), *Reading/writing connections: Learning from research* (pp. 2-30). Newark, DE: International Reading Association.

McGill-Franzen, A. (Ed.) (2010). Guest editor's introduction. *Educational Researcher, 39*(4), 275-278.

McGuinness, D. (2004). *Early reading instruction: What science really tells us about how to teach reading.* Cambridge, MA: The MIT Press.

McGuinness, D. (2005). *Language development and learning to read: The scientific study of how language development affects reading skill.* Cambridge, MA: The MIT Press.

Minsky, M. (1975). A framework for representing knowledge. In P. H. Winston (Ed.), *The psychology of computer vision* (pp. 211-277). New York: McGraw Hill.

Montague, M. (1990). *Computers, cognition, and writing instruction.* Albany, NY: State University of New York Press.

Moores, D., & Martin, D. (Eds.). (2006). *Deaf learners: Developments in curriculum and instruction.* Washington, DC: Gallaudet University Press.

National Early Literacy Panel (NELP). (2008). *Developing early literacy: Report of the National Early Literacy Panel – A scientific synthesis of early literacy development and implications for interventions.* Washington, DC: The Institute for Literacy and National Center for Family Literacy.

National Reading Panel (NRP). (2000). *Report of the National Reading Panel: Teaching children to read – An evidence-based assessment of the scientific research literature on reading and its implications for reading instruction.* Jessup, MD: National Institute for Literacy at EDPubs.

National Research Council (NRC). (1996). *National science education standards.* Washington, DC: National Academy Press.

Norris, S. (Ed.). (1992). *The generalizability of critical thinking: Multiple perspectives on an educational ideal.* New York: Teachers College Press, Columbia University.

O'Brien, B., Mansfield, J., & Legge, G. (2005). The effect of print size on reading speed in dyslexia. *Journal of Research in Reading, 28*(3), 332-349.

Odubunmi, O., & Balogun, T. A. (1991). The effect of laboratory and lecture teaching methods on cognitive achievement in integrated science. *Journal of Research in Science Teaching, 28*(3), 213-224.

Olson, D. (2004). The cognitive consequences of literacy. In T. Nunes & P. Bryant (Eds.), *Handbook of children's literacy* (pp. 539-555). Boston, MA: Kluwer Academic Publishers.

Olson, D. (1994). *The world on paper.* Cambridge: Cambridge University Press.

O'Shaughnessy, T., & Swanson, H. (1998). Do immediate memory deficits in students with learning disabilities in reading reflect a developmental lag or deficit?: A selective meta-analysis of the literature. *Learning Disability Quarterly, 21*(2), 123-148.

Owens, R. (2004). *Language disorders: A functional approach to assessment and intervention* (4th ed.). Boston, MA: Pearson Education.

Pape, S. (2004). Middle school children's problem-solving behavior: A cognitive analysis from a reading comprehension perspective. *Journal of Research in Mathematics Education, 15*, 187-219.

Paul, P. (1998). *Literacy and deafness: The development of reading, writing, and literate thought.* Needham Heights, MA: Allyn & Bacon.

Paul, P. (2001). *Language and deafness* (3rd ed.). San Diego, CA: Singular/Thomson Learning.

Paul, P. (2008a). (Ed.). Reading and children with disabilities. *Balanced Reading Instruction, 15*(2).

Paul, P. (2008b). Introduction: Reading and children with disabilities. Reading and children with disabilities. *Balanced Reading Instruction, 15*(2), 1-12.

Paul, P. (2009). *Language and deafness* (4th ed.). Sudbury, MA: Jones & Bartlett Learning.

Paul, P., & Jackson, D. (1993). *Toward a psychology of deafness: Theoretical and empirical perspectives.* Needham Heights, MA: Allyn & Bacon.

Paul, P., & Lee, C. (2010). Qualitative-similarity hypothesis. *American Annals of the Deaf, 154*(5), 456-462.

Paul, P., Wang, Y., Trezek, B., & Luckner, J. (2009). Phonology is necessary, but not sufficient: A rejoinder. *American Annals of the Deaf, 154*(4), 346-356.

Pearson, P. D. (2004). The reading wars. *Educational Policy, 18*(1), 216-252.

Pence, K., & Justice, L. (2008). *Language development from theory to practice.* Upper Saddle River, NJ: Pearson/Merrill/Prentice Hall.

Phillips, D. (1983). On describing a student's cognitive structure. *Educational Psychologist, 18*(2), 59-74.

Phillips, D., & Soltis, J. (2004). *Perspectives on learning.* New York: Teachers College Press.

Pickering, S. (Ed.). (2006). *Working memory and education.* Boston, MA: Elsevier.

Reimer, J. (2006). Developmental changes in the allocation of semantic feedback during visual word recognition. *Journal of Research in Reading, 29*(2), 194-212.

Rittle-Johnson, B., Siegler, S., & Alibali, M. (2001). Developing conceptual understanding and procedural skill in mathematics: An iterative process. *Journal of Educational Psychology, 93*, 345-362.

Routman, R. (2005). *Writing essentials: Raising expectations and results while simplifying teaching.* Portsmouth, NH: Heinemann.

Ruddell, R., & Haggard, M. (1985). Oral and written language acquisition and the reading process. In H. Singer & R. Ruddell (Eds.), *Theoretical models and processes of reading* (3rd ed.) (pp. 63-80). Newark, DE: International Reading Association.

Ruddell, R., & Unrau, N. (Eds.). (2004). *Theoretical models and processes of reading* (5th ed.). Newark, DE: International Reading Association.

Rumelhart, D. (1977). Toward an interactive model of reading. In S. Dornic (Ed.), *Attention and performance VI* (pp. 573-603). New York, NY: Academic Press.

Saada-Robert, M. (2004). Early emergent literacy. In T. Nunes & P. Bryant (Eds.), *Handbook of children's literacy* (pp. 575-598). Boston, MA: Kluwer Academic Publishers.

Schank, R., & Abelson, R. (1977). *Scripts, plans, goals, and understanding*. Hillsdale, NJ: Erlbaum.

Schneider, R., Krajcik, J., Marx, R. W., & Soloway, E. (2002). Performance of students in project-based science classrooms on a national measure of science achievement. *Journal of Research in Science Teaching, 39*(5), 410-422.

Schoenfeld, A. (1992). Learning to think mathematically: Problem solving, metacognition, and sense making in mathematics. In D. A. Grouws (Ed.), *Handbook of research on mathematics teaching and learning* (pp. 334-370). New York: Macmillan.

Scruggs, T., Mastropieri, M., & Boon, R. (1998). Science education for students with disabilities: a review of recent research. *Studies in Science Education, 32*, 21-44.

Siegler, R. (1996). *Emerging minds: The process of change in children's thinking*. New York: Oxford University Press.

Snow, C., Burns, S., & Griffin, P. (Eds.). (1998). *Preventing reading difficulties in young children*. Washington, DC: National Academy Press.

Snowling, M., Defty, N., & Goulandris, N. (1996). A longitudinal study of reading development in dyslexic children. *Journal of Educational Psychology, 88*(4), 653-669.

Snowling, M., & Hulme, C. (Eds.). (2005). *The science of reading: A handbook*. Malden, MA: Blackwell.

Stanovich, K. (1986). Matthew effects in reading: Some consequences of individual differences in the acquisition of literacy. *Reading Research Quarterly, 21*, 360-407.

Stanovich, K. (1992). Speculations on the causes and consequences of individual differences in early reading acquisition. In P. Gough, L. Ehri, & R. Treiman (Eds.), *Reading acquisition* (pp. 307-342). Hillsdale, NJ: Erlbaum.

Stanovich, K, Nathan, R., & Zolman, J. (1988). The developmental lag hypothesis in reading: Longitudinal and matched reading-level comparisons. *Child Development, 59*, 71-86.

Stoddart, T., Pinal, A., Latzke, M., & Canaday, D. (2002). Integrating inquiry science and language development for English language learners. *Journal of Research in Science Teaching, 39*(8), 664-687.

Sulzby, E., & Teale, W. (1987). *Young children's storybook reading: Longitudinal study of parent-child interaction and children's independent functioning*. Final Report to the Spencer Foundation. University of Michigan, Ann Arbor.

Sulzby, E., & Teale, W. (2003). The development of the young child and the emergence of literacy. In J. Flood, D. Lapp, J. Squire, & J. Jensen (Eds.), *Handbook of research on teaching the English language arts* (2nd ed., pp. 300-313). Mahwah, NJ: Erlbaum.

Tierney, R. (2008). Reading and children with disabilities: Searching for better guidance. *Balanced Reading Instruction, 15*(2), 89-98.

Trezek, B., Wang, Y., & Paul, P. (2010). *Reading and deafness: Theory, research and practice*, Clifton Park, NY: Cengage Learning.

Van der Schoot, M., Arkema, A. H. B., Horsley, T. M., & Van Lieshout, E. C. D. M. (2009). The consistency effect depends on markedness in less successful but not successful problem solvers: An eye movement study in primary school children. *Contemporary Educational Psychology, 34*, 58-66.

Vosgerau, G. (2006). The perceptual nature of mental models. In C. Held, M. Knauff, & G. Vosgerau (Eds.), *Mental models and the mind: Current developments in cognitive psychology, neuroscience, and philosophy of mind* (pp. 255-275). New York: Elsevier.

Wang, Y., Trezek, B., Luckner, J., & Paul, P. (2008). The role of phonology and phonological-related skills in reading instruction for students who are deaf or hard of hearing. *American Annals of the Deaf. 153*(4), 396-407.

Wild, T. (2008). *Students' with visual impairments conceptions of causes of seasonal change.* Unpublished doctoral dissertation. The Ohio State University.

FURTHER READING

Bransford, J., Brown, A., & Cocking, R. (Eds.). (2000). *How people learn: Brain, mind, experience, and school.* Washington, DC: National Academy Press.

Greene, R. (1992). *Human memory: Paradigms and paradoxes.* Mahwah, NJ: Erlbaum.

Hofer, B., & Pintrich, P. (Eds.). (2002). *Personal epistemology: The psychology of beliefs about knowledge and knowing.* Mahwah, NJ: Erlbaum.

Stanovich, K. (2000). *Progress in understanding reading: Scientific foundations and new frontiers.* New York: Guilford Press.

Sternberg, R., & Ben-Zeev, T. (Eds.). (1996). *The nature of mathematical thinking.* Mahwah, NJ: Erlbaum.

CHAPTER 5

Critico-Creative Thinking

. . . critical thinking is the careful application of reason in the determination of whether a claim is true. Notice that it isn't so much coming up with claims, true or otherwise, that constitutes critical thinking; it's the evaluation of claims, however we come up with them. You might say that our subject is really thinking about thinking—we engage in it when we consider whether our ideas really make good sense. Of course, since our actions usually depend on what thoughts or ideas we've accepted, whether we do the intelligent thing also depends on how well we consider those thoughts and ideas.

Moore & Parker, 2009, p. 3

How does one teach critical thinking? Years ago, educators emphasized general principles of thinking that could be applied to any area of study. This was part of the reason so many of us studied Latin in high school. Today, however, there is broad agreement that critical thinking skills are best learned in the context of a particular discipline rather than in the abstract. Cognitive psychologists have found that in order to think like an expert in a discipline, one must have a considerable base of knowledge in that discipline. Further, critical thinking skills learned in one discipline do not always transfer to another.

McBurney, 2002, p. 2

Our focus in this chapter is on critico-creative thinking, which on the surface seems to entail two broad concepts, critical thinking and creative thinking. As we discussed in Chapters 1 and 2, literate thought entails the ability to think critically and creatively as well as logically, rationally, and reflectively. This is the basis for solving problems, making decisions, and rendering judgments. Lest we be accused of circular reasoning, let it be known that we are aware of the slippery, ill-defined nature of our concepts and descriptions. We also recognize that it is not altogether clear what is meant by critical or creative thinking or even by literate thought, for that matter.

For sure, we argue that literate thought involves critico-creative thinking or that critico-creative thinking is a component of being a literate thinker. In fact, as implied by the first passage above, it is related to metacognition (see the *thinking about thinking* phrase). We also contend that the ability to engage in critico-creative thinking is not an all-or-nothing phenomenon—there are levels of engagement or development. Nevertheless, some fundamentals (with threshold levels) are involved such as attitude (or demeanor), language proficiency, cognitive ability, and content knowledge, which are explored later.

But, we are ahead of ourselves here. First, we address the title of this chapter. Then, we proffer a few implications of the two passages at the beginning. At first blush, the title and passages, and a bit of reflection on these items, suggest major questions such as:

- What is critico-creative thinking?
- Are there general skills across the curriculum or topics or are there skills specific to a discipline or content area?
- Is it possible to teach, evaluate, and conduct research on critico-creative thinking skills?
- Is being a critico-creative thinker a good thing (or should this be the goal of education)?

Along the way, we also examine several corollaries to the above questions such as the manner in which critico-creative thinking can be taught or evaluated and whether there is really such an entity as critico-creative thinking. Our major themes for this chapter thus are the nature, characteristics, and forms of critico-creative thinking; general and domain-specific views; and issues of generalizability, evaluation, and instruction.

On a daily basis, we are exposed to problem-solving or decision-making situations that seem to require, at the least, a judgment or evaluation on our part. We make decisions on what car or house to purchase, whether to vote for one candidate or another or support one position or another, the best way to catch a mouse in our basement, and so on. In schools, teachers require students to engage in lower- and higher-level critico-creative activities such as drawing conclusions, finding the main ideas, solving word problems in mathematics, or composing an essay that begins with the phrase "What if," as in "What if the South had won the Civil War?"

To obtain a sense of the complexity of critico-creative thinking, consider the following scenario:

Scenario

In a newspaper, the following cartoon appeared. A couple was standing by a window in their home, watching a snowstorm that was happening in late May in Georgia. The man turned to the woman and remarked: "This proves that global warming is a false entity."

Whether the above cartoon is humorous depends on your sense of humor as well as your understanding of the complexities of global warming. We shall put aside for now the notion of *proof* in the passage, as this requires an understanding of research. For starters, however, we assume that this cartoon demonstrates a misunderstanding between the concepts of *weather* and *climate* as well as patterns or trends in the climate. And, of course, there is more. Our question is this: What is required to analyze critically this cartoon (or to appreciate the depth of the humor)? To begin the response to our question, we need to discuss our first theme: the nature, characteristics, and forms of critico-creative thinking.

NATURE, CHARACTERISTICS, AND FORMS

We prefer to use the term *critico-creative thinking* rather than just critical or creative thinking (see also, the discussions in Bruning, Schraw, Norby, & Ronning, 2004; Flage, 2004; Moore & Parker, 2009; Porter, 2002; Ruggiero, 2001, 2002). Critical and creative thinking are interrelated or can be considered as complementary components of *good thinking*. It is difficult to imagine how individuals can engage in one aspect without the other because they are so intertwined.

If individuals think creatively, then they will generate (or synthesize) new ideas and thoughts. During this generation, individuals also engage in an evaluation of these items (Moore & Parker, 2009; Porter, 2002; Ruggiero, 2001, 2002). It is certainly possible to separate the two; however, it is more likely that both processes have been undertaken (or should be undertaken). Of course, one can certainly be creative without being critical in the sense we are discussing here (evaluating the merits of one's ideas).

Nevertheless, in solving problems, resolving conflicts, making decisions, and so on, we proceed in a back-and-forth maneuver, repeatedly at times, involving critical and creative dimensions. Even though some scholars separate the various aspects of thinking—that is, critical, creative, problem-solving, and decision-making (Bruning et al., 2004)—we prefer to consider all of these aspects within the purview of the critico-creative thinking domain. In addition, we contend that there are levels ranging from activities such as identifying the main idea or summarizing a passage to complex evaluations, as in comparing and contrasting several sources as well as ascertaining the validity of the sources. In essence, if teachers actually want to improve the ability of their students to engage in literate thought, the focus should be on both the critical and creative aspects of thinking (Moore & Parker, 2009; Porter, 2002; Ruggiero, 2001, 2002).

Regardless of whether one believes in general aspects (i.e., generalizations across domains or subjects) or in specific, disciplinary, or domain aspects, the underlying values and attitudes associated with critico-creative thinking remain constant across content areas or subjects. Of course, the knowledge base of the domain (or, rather, domain knowledge) will vary as will specific skills and processes, as discussed later (Moore & Parker, 2009; Porter, 2002; Ruggiero, 2001, 2002). Essentially, teachers should encourage students to develop a *questioning spirit*—that is, students should know how and when to question information and should wonder if there are additional views. For any topic or subject, students should recognize when additional information is necessary, what types of information are required to answer questions, and to generate multiple, alternative, or possible solutions or answers. Most of life's problems and puzzles are deep and complex and do not have a simple answer or solution.

Despite the fact that critico-creative thinking is difficult to describe or define, most books provide examples suggesting that such thinkers are able to display any number of the following attributes or characteristics, which are not exhaustive (Bruning et al., 2004; Moore & Parker, 2009; Porter, 2002; Ruggiero, 2001, 2002):

- compare and contrast, conceptualize, construct, identify, paraphrase, synthesize, summarize, and evaluate or judge

- understand the logical connections between ideas and identify their relevance and importance
- delineate inconsistencies and mistakes in reasoning and arguments
- solve problems systematically and logically
- analyze and justify one's own beliefs and values, especially with respect to other competing beliefs and values

With respect to the last attribute above, a distinction should be made between what is considered the weak form and strong form of critico-creative thinking, as discussed in the subsequent section.

Weak and Strong Forms

These two forms of critico-creative thinking, weak and strong, were mentioned in Chapter 1. We reiterate and elaborate here with examples from two broad areas. For one area, there is no right or wrong position or, rather, the merits of the position cannot be evaluated empirically or scientifically (albeit one can use these methods as part of the evaluation). This includes debates on topics such as abortion, death penalty, religion, philosophy, and so on. Setting aside the arguments about epistemology (and metaphysics!) (Martin, 1992; Noddings, 1995; Pring, 2004; Ritzer, 2001), another broad area entails the use of research or science, and the evaluation of positions that occurs within the purview for doing science or research. This area entails issues such as evaluating effective practices or methods, delineating the causes of cancer, theorizing about the beginning of the universe, and so on.

Let us consider the issue of abortion and relate this to the use (i.e., our rendition) of both the weak and strong forms of critico-creative thinking. Individuals are utilizing a weak form if they simply argue for their position, either for or against abortion, and virtually ignore the arguments on the other side. The main objective is to defend one's view against the arguments of others. There might be an attempt to reveal the fallacies or weaknesses in the opposition; however, there is no admission that one's own position also contains similar or related fallacies or weaknesses. In essence, within the framework of the weak form, one's view does not actually change or evolve (see related discussions in Applegate, Quin, & Applegate, 2008; Browne & Keeley, 2007; Flage, 2004; Kuhn, 2005).

Within the framework of the strong form, the goal is to examine critically all prominent views—including contradictory ones—associated with abortion. Given the nature of this topic, one should probably acknowledge that there is no empirical or scientific resolution, especially because arguments are emanating from different worldviews. Strong-form proponents might even emphasize areas of agreement or disagreement and possible compromises. Essentially, it is recognized that this conflict can only be managed—not resolved.

After much dialogue and reflection, strong-form proponents can state their current position, which should always be tentative and may change in light of what proponents see as a better argument, not necessarily as a result of science or research, albeit this can be part of the argument, even for the abortion issue (e.g., research on attitudes, preferences, etc. of women; see related discussions in Applegate, Quin, & Applegate, 2008; Browne & Keeley, 2007; Flage, 2004; Halpern, 1997; Kuhn, 2005). It is possible that the strong form can lead to a refinement or further development of one's thinking. Utilizing a strong form, one can even see and admit the *sources* of disagreements and recognize the *merits* of different views.

A similar analogy can be made for the second broad area involving research or science. Albeit, the resolution appears to be easier or clearer, given the so-called *scientific approach*, this can be an illusion. There is much complexity and dissension that fuel the debates in this area. Most of this revolves around contentious issues such as the nature of the scientific method, the orientation of the discipline, the relevancy and interpretation of the data, the nature of the data, and so on. Several of these concepts were explored in Chapter 4 about the structure of the discipline. We shall return to a few of them in a later section of this chapter covering the generalizability of critico-creative thinking skills.

A Brief Summary

Prior to discussing more complex issues and nuances associated with critico-creative thinking, we provide a brief summary of our initial thoughts. We hope that it is clear that critico-creative thinking is not merely the accumulation or simple recall of a range of information or positions. (Being good at *Jeopardy* or *Trivial Pursuit* is not the same as being good at critico-creative thinking.) It is not necessary to have an encyclopedic memory or even one that remembers and retrieves a substantial amount of information.

It is important to possess a sufficient amount of knowledge or information about topics or domains and to understand or to be able to contextualize such knowledge or information. Then it is incumbent to utilize and evaluate the information to perform activities, for example (as discussed previously) to solve problems, make decisions, or to state a theoretical position.

In short, *critico-creative thinking* can and should facilitate the acquisition and conceptualization of knowledge and information whereby we can test and refine our hypotheses, models, ideas, and arguments. It has been suggested that this type of thinking can even enhance our processes used during work, school, and in our social intercourses and institutions (Applegate, Quin, & Applegate, 2008; Browne & Keeley, 2007; Flage, 2004; Halpern, 1997; Kuhn, 2005).

The last topic discussed here is the *tone* for critico-creative discussions or arguments. Although we suspect that possessing a considerate, respectful demeanor can be present in all forms of critico-creative dialogues, we contend that it is most prevalent in discourses involving the strong form, as discussed above. What we mean by considerateness and respectfulness has been captured nicely by a philosopher of religion, who commented on the emotional-laden task of discussing the merits of religious or non-religious belief systems (Taliaferro, 2009):

> I will not, for example, advance brazen and I believe unsupported charges that either religious belief or skepticism about religion is ignorant, hateful, and greedy. . . . A spirit of generosity is called for in the philosophy of religion because there are good arguments for almost every position. There are good reasons for theism as well as for atheism, good reasons for being a Christian, and good reasons for being a Buddhist, and good reasons for being a skeptic.
>
> I propose what may be called 'the golden rule in philosophy': that one should treat other philosophies as one would like one's own to be treated. (p. x)

Table 5-1 provides highlights of the characteristics and forms of critico-creative thinking.

The next theme to explore is whether critico-creative thinking is based on universal intellectual attributes and skills that transcend a range of disciplines or content areas (i.e., the *general view*) or whether it is contained within a particular area (i.e., *domain-specific view*). As you might guess, there is no simple answer. Nevertheless, there are enormous implications here—notwithstanding the issue of whether critico-creative thinking skills can actually be generalized, evaluated, or taught.

Table 5-1.   Characteristics and Forms of Critico-Creative Thinking

---

Characteristics

- Critical and creative thinking are interrelated or can be considered as complementary components of good thinking.
- In solving problems, resolving conflicts, making decisions, and so on, individuals proceed in a back-and-forth maneuver, repeatedly at times, involving critical and creative dimensions.
- Teachers should encourage students to develop a *questioning spirit*—that is, students should know how and when to question information and should wonder if there are additional views.
- Critico-creative thinking can and should facilitate the acquisition and conceptualization of knowledge and information whereby we can test and refine our hypotheses, models, ideas, and arguments.
- Some of the lower-level and higher-level skills of critico-creative thinking include: categorizing or classifying, comparing and contrasting, conceptualizing, evaluating or judging, paraphrasing, reasoning, synthesizing, and summarizing.

Forms

- There are two forms of critico-creative thinking: weak and strong.
- Individuals are utilizing a weak form if they simply argue for their position and virtually ignore the arguments on the other side. The main objective is simply to defend one's view against the arguments of others.
- Within the framework of the weak form, one's view does not actually change or evolve.
- Within the framework of the strong form, the goal is to examine critically all prominent views—including contradictory ones.
- After much dialogue and reflection, strong-form proponents can state their current position, which should always be tentative and may change in light of what proponents see as a better argument.
- It is possible that the strong form can lead to a refinement or further development of one's thinking on the topic. Utilizing a strong form, one can even see and admit the *sources* of disagreements and recognize the *merits* of different views.
- Possessing a considerate, respectful demeanor can be present in all forms of critico-creative dialogues; however, this demeanor is most prevalent in discourses involving the strong form.

GENERAL OR DOMAIN-SPECIFIC

There are two broad views on critico-creative thinking. One view can be labeled the *general view*—that is, an individual possesses general critico-creative thinking skills, which can be applied or transferred to any content, topic, domain, or disciplinary area (Bruning et al., 2004; Moore & Parker, 2009; Norris, 1992; Willingham, 2007). On a surface level, possessing general skills means being aware of the various sides or perspectives of an issue; able to provide evidence (logical or scientific) for a specific position; open to new data from different perspectives; and recognizing that any such conclusion, based on serious analysis, is tentative. Being a good critico-creative thinker in, for example, solving economic problems, thus would transfer or generalize to being good in solving philosophical problems.

The second view on critico-creative thinking can be labeled the *domain-specific view* (or *domain knowledge view*). In short, this view is specialized or confined to a particular discipline such as science, mathematics, or language development or to a specific topic such as masonry or tennis (Bruning et al., 2004; Moore & Parker, 2009; Norris, 1992; Willingham, 2007). A few scholars contend that it is even more specialized or confined due to the divisions within a discipline (e.g., in science this would mean biology, physics, chemistry, etc.; in psychology it involves developmental, cognitive, and neuroscience).

It can be asserted that the domain-specific view refers to the case of thinking like a scientist, thinking like a mathematician, thinking like a psychologist or to thinking like an expert on the topic (Bruning et al., 2004; McBurney, 2002). Furthermore, it is averred that if one becomes adept in thinking like a psychologist (or an expert on a topic), this does not mean that one has those specific skills that are commensurate to thinking like a mathematician or to thinking expertly about a range of other domains or topics. That is, within this position, the skills in one area do not transfer or generalize to another area.

In the next section, we probe deeper into the generalizability problem of the two broad views.

The Generalizability Problem

As discussed by, for example, Norris (1992) and Johnson (1992), the feasibility of generalizability is confounded by several contentious issues (see also, Bruning et al., 2004). One major issue is disagreements regarding the definition or description of critico-creative thinking. Additional challenges arise in considering the understanding of other concepts such as *transfer* and *comprehension*.

The Definition or Description Issue

On one hand, understanding the definition or description of critico-creative thinking can assist us in discussing what aspects are general (transferable) and what aspects might be domain-specific. On the other hand, however, the definition challenge is compounded by what was discussed in Chapter 4: the nature of the psychological structure of the individual and the nature of the knowledge structure of the discipline as well as the relationship between these two entities. Delineating the skills and attributes within the individuals (i.e., the psychological dimension) may not facilitate our understanding of the knowledge structure of the discipline (i.e., the conceptual dimension). In addition, the knowledge structure varies from discipline to discipline.

Are critico-creative thinking skills related to the domain-specific conceptual structure of a discipline only? If so, then the definition/description and evaluation of such skills must be contextualized with respect to the degree to which individuals understand the conceptual structure of the discipline. Given the contentious debate on the nature of conceptual structure, the difficulty of evaluating such skills is influenced by philosophical issues such as epistemology and methodology, as discussed also in Chapter 4.

The Transfer Issue

Another perspective on the problem of generalizability can be seen in the notion of transfer, which is also difficult to define or research and, for the most part, tends to be simplified or misinterpreted. As an example, consider the debate on transfer in the research on second language learning of English (Cummins, 1984, 1989; see reviews in Paul, 2009, and Trezek, Wang, & Paul, 2010, for d/Deaf and hard of hearing students). It is often assumed that second-language learners use skills from their first language (i.e., transfer of skills) in order to learn the second language. If an individual is a good reader/writer in his/her first language, s/he thus has the potential to become a good reader/writer in the second language.

In the above example, the issue of transfer is debatable and complex and is in need of further research. There seems to be some consensus that second-language learners understand the general processes of reading/writing (e.g., relationship between letters and sounds; need for making inferences, etc.) in their first language. Nevertheless, it has been argued that this transfer is actually limited because second-language learners still need to learn the structure of the second language to read and write well in that language (Israel & Duffy, 2009; Klingner, Vaughn, & Boardman, 2007; Ruddell & Unrau, 2004; for d/Deaf and hard of hearing students, see Paul, 2009; Trezek et al., 2010).

Thus far, we seem to be providing evidence against a strong version of the general view of critico-creative thinking skills—based on the generalizability problem, particularly the issue of transfer. Nevertheless, there are a few general skills that can be transferred across the curriculum, so to speak. The effectiveness of the transfer might be contingent on the level of proficiency in the new topic or domain. Perhaps the best evidence can be found in the literature on developing critical reading skills, mostly involving metacognitive or self-regulative aspects (Gunning, 2008; Klingner et al., 2007), as discussed briefly in the next section.

Critical Reading: Support for Transfer

With respect to reading, keep in mind that we are referring to the concept of script literacy (see Chapter 2), namely, information that has been captured in print. At the very least, individuals need to access and interpret such information. To be a critical reader, individuals also must evaluate the content. To be succinct, we would say that critical reading means the use of critico-creative thinking skills in the print domain on a variety of levels (e.g., paraphrasing, summarizing, evaluating, etc.).

Gunning (2008) argues that there are general critical reading skills that can be taught and used across a range of topics in print. These skills are within the cognitive domain of reading such as locating and recalling, integrating and interpreting, and critiquing and evaluating. Gunning devotes chapters of his book to the development of specific strategies, among these are learning to think deductively and inductively, locating and comprehending details, obtaining the main idea, drawing and supporting conclusions, asking questions, determining the importance of information, and summarizing and synthesizing. It is asserted that these general critical skills are applicable to whatever students or individuals read.

As a sidebar, we argue that if there are general strategies and skills, as proposed by Gunning (2008) and others (Klingner et al., 2007; Kuhn,

2005; Moore & Parker, 2009), then these can also be applied to any form of captured information (discussed in Chapter 2). In fact, they can be developed in both the through-the-air mode and in a captured mode. A few of these strategies are illustrated later in the section on instruction.

The presence or use of general skills or strategies can only go so far in the development of critico-creative thinking skills. As asserted by a number of theorists and researchers, the development of adequate critico-creative thinking is contingent on a deep level of knowledge associated with a topic or discipline—that is, with respect to the *domain-specific view* (Israel & Duffy, 2009; Ruddell & Unrau, 2004; Snowling & Hulme, 2005; Willingham, 2007). This deep level of knowledge can be labeled as the *comprehension* issue, discussed in the next section (see also, our discussion of comprehension in Chapter 2).

The Comprehension Issue

Comprehension is part of a larger *communicative interactive* process involving authors/speakers or signers and readers/listeners or receivers of the message (Cain & Oakhill, 2007; Israel & Duffy, 2009; Ruddell & Unrau, 2004). As discussed later in this book on disabilities/conditions (Chapters 6–8) and on English language learners (Chapter 9), it is difficult to develop general comprehension skills if individuals do not have competency in a language for communication and thought, yet alone competency in the language of print.

Comprehension occurs inside the head and cannot be observed—only inferred. For our purposes here regarding generalizability within domain-specific areas, it is important to distinguish between surface-level comprehension and deep-level comprehension (Israel & Duffy, 2009; Willingham, 2007; for d/Deaf and hard of hearing students, see Paul, 2009; Trezek et al., 2010). This distinction can be illustrated by the following example.

> *The Reconstruction of the South after the Civil War was a mixed blessing. Depending on where you live, you were most likely to view this process as either positive or negative—beneficial or destructive. According to some scholars, this is what we should expect at the conclusion of any war. The rebuilding of the infrastructure on the losing side is fraught with controversies and, sometimes, corruption.* (Trezek et al., 2010, p. 15)

On a surface level, readers need to understand language issues such as letters and sounds (i.e., decoding processes), words, phrases, and sentences. In short, readers need a working knowledge of the structure of English, which includes phonology, morphology, syntax, and semantics. This working knowledge can assist with paraphrasing or summarizing the specific information in the text or passage.

It would also help to possess some general knowledge about the Civil War, but this actually proceeds beyond surface-level comprehension. To obtain a deeper understanding of this passage—an understanding that is necessary for applying higher-level critico-creative thinking skills—individuals need knowledge of the situations that occur with the aftermaths of wars as well as knowledge of different wars. Some scholars (e.g., see discussion in Israel & Duffy, 2009) argue that it is also important to be aware of the biases that come with the reporting of history from the framework or mindset of a writer, who also is influenced by social and contextual factors (e.g., education; location of residence; era in which the history is written; etc.). Individuals thus need to be able to compare the perspective of one writer with those of others on the concept of reconstruction after one war or several wars (Trezek et al., 2010). In addition, it is important to evaluate the quality of the source of information (e.g., in newspapers, history books, Web sites, etc.). Taken together, the above leads to a deeper understanding (or deep-level comprehension) of the passage on the aftermath of the Civil War.

Surface- and deep-level comprehension is affected by several groups of factors, mentioned previously in this book, such as text (e.g., language structure, genre), reader (e.g., age, language and cognitive abilities, prior knowledge, metacognitive skills, motivation, and interest), context (e.g., classroom literacy practices, teacher–student interactions), and task (e.g., test-taking, pleasure reading, retelling, sharing, scanning, etc.). As mentioned in Chapter 1, we believe that it is pertinent to highlight the concept of prior knowledge (in the reader area above), which is also a major component of literate thought. Prior knowledge refers to background knowledge or experiences associated with topics or contents of reading passages as well as of those discussed in through-the-air communicative interactions.

Individuals need, at least, a working prior knowledge of the metalanguage, or specialized vocabulary, associated with specific topics, disciplines, or academic content areas (i.e., domain-specific view). That is, to develop conceptual understanding in science, mathematics, or social studies, a knowledge of jargon or specific terminologies, often labeled as *rare* or *technical* vocabulary expressed in complex sentence constructions or expositions, is necessary (Israel & Duffy, 2009; Willingham, 2007). This prior knowledge facilitates the ability to think, explore, and engage in scholarly debates similar to, for example, a scientist or mathematician. This is what is meant by the phrases, thinking like a scientist, or thinking like a mathematician, or even thinking like an expert on, or thinking intelligently about a topic.

The ability to use prior knowledge effectively is also enhanced by a general understanding of the metalanguage of topics associated with the larger mainstream culture, often labeled as *cultural literacy* (Hirsch, Kett, & Trefil, 2002). The more students know about the wider cultural concepts, the easier it will be for them to become good readers and writers or, broadly, good, critical literate thinkers. The use of terminology from other disciplines tends to deepen and broaden knowledge of a particular topic (Hirsch et al.). Both a specialized and broad metalanguage contributes to the acquisition of prior knowledge and is essential for the overall development of critico-creative and literate thinking abilities.

Summary

Although there are ongoing empirical and philosophical debates on the general versus the domain-specific views of critico-creative thinking (see Bruning et al., 2004; Kuhn, 2005; Norris, 1992), we tend to agree that much of the evidence—albeit contentious—favors the domain-specific view (Bruning et al.; McBurney, 2002; Willingham, 2007). This means that it is difficult to evaluate and teach *general* critico-creative skills; rather, most endeavors should be attempted within a *domain-specific* area or topic (Bruning et al.; Willingham). The goal in education thus should be to assist students in thinking like a historian, scientist, or even a mathematician while they are acquiring and understanding information and knowledge in these areas. We should emphasize that we are not proposing that students become experts in the disciplines—that is not realistic.

Having stated the above, we do not want to rule out the need to develop an overall, general critico-creative demeanor—for lack of a better descriptor. Individuals will encounter a number of topics about which little might be known but nevertheless are important. Consider what it means to engage in a participatory democracy and be exposed to controversial issues such as global warming, abortion, disability rights, and so on.

The inquiry and argument approach (Kuhn, 2005) is certainly one commendable approach to developing *general* critico-creative skills. Understanding the meanings of opinions and facts, what constitutes a good argument, and evaluating the quality of one's sources of information are also important general skills. Being open to different perspectives and recognizing whether an issue can or cannot be settled empirically is also laudable. In short, we and others (Applegate et al.; Browne & Keeley, 2007; Bruning et al., 2004; Flage, 2004; Halpern, 1997; Moore & Parker, 2009) argue that general critico-creative thinking skills, complemented by a serious inquiry into and understanding of the topic or area, should facilitate the production of a more tolerant, inclusive, informed, participatory citizenry.

Willingham (2007) seems to support both general and domain-specific approaches (albeit Willingham favored domain-specific ones as most amendable to instruction):

> Virtually everyone would agree that a primary, yet insufficiently met, goal of schooling is to enable students to think critically. In layperson's terms, critical thinking consists of seeing both sides of an issue, being open to new evidence that disconfirms your ideas, reasoning dispassionately, demanding that claims be backed by evidence, deducing and inferring conclusions from available facts, solving problems, and so forth. Then, too, there are specific types of critical thinking that are characteristics of different subject matter: That's what we mean when we refer to "thinking like a scientist" or "thinking like a historian". (p. 8)

Table 5-2 summarizes the general and domain-specific views.

Table 5-2. Highlights of General and Domain-Specific Views

General View

- Individual possesses general critico-creative thinking skills, which can be applied or transferred to any content, topic, domain, or disciplinary area.
- On a surface level, possessing general skills means: being aware of the various sides or perspectives of an issue; being able to provide evidence (logical or scientific) for a specific position; being open to new data from different perspectives; and recognizing that any such conclusion, based on serious analysis, is tentative.

(continues)

Table 5-2. Highlights of General and Domain-Specific Views (continued)

Domain-Specific View
- This view is specialized or confined to a particular discipline such as science, mathematics, or language development, or to a specific topic such as masonry or tennis.
- This view refers to the case of thinking like a scientist, thinking like a mathematician, thinking like a psychologist, or to thinking like an expert on the topic.
- If one becomes adept in thinking like a psychologist (or expert on a topic), this does not mean that one has those specific skills that are commensurate to thinking like a mathematician or to thinking expertly about a range of other domains or topics. That is, within this position, the skills in one area do not transfer or generalize to another area.

The Problem of Generalizability Associated with the Two Views
- Generalizability is confounded by several contentious issues. One major issue is disagreements regarding the definition of critico-creative thinking. Additional challenges arise in considering the understanding of other concepts such as *transfer* and *general* as well as *comprehension*.
- The presence or use of general skills or strategies can only go so far in the development of critico-creative thinking skills.
- The development of adequate critico-creative thinking is contingent on a deep level of knowledge. This can be stated as the *comprehension* issue.
- Understanding the definition or description of critico-creative thinking can assist in discussing what aspects are general (transferable) and what aspects might be domain-specific.
- The definition challenge is compounded by the nature of the psychological structure of the individual and the nature of the knowledge structure of the discipline as well as the relationship between these two entities.
- Although there are ongoing debates, both empirical and philosophical, on the general versus the domain-specific views of critico-creative thinking, much of the evidence—albeit contentious—favors the domain-specific view.
- It is difficult to teach and evaluate *general* critico-creative skills; rather, such endeavors should be attempted within a content area or topic.

EVALUATION ISSUES

In this section, we examine the difficulty of evaluating the two broad views of critico-creative thinking skills, including whether such dispassionate foci (e.g., see Willingham's quote above) are even desirable or possible (Martin, 1992; Noddings, 1995; Ritzer, 2001). One issue is whether evaluations can be considered to be objective or are, in fact, always subjective. Another is whether dispassionate (i.e., objective) approaches should actually be the main goal of all critico-creative thinking endeavors. We argue that the concept of evaluation is intertwined with the epistemological framework of the evaluator. We hope that our discussion here exemplifies the nature of our instructional examples, presented later.

Role of Epistemology

It has been asserted that the nature and evaluation of critico-creative thinking is both empirical and philosophical (actually, non-empirical) (Norris, 1992; see also, Bruning et al., 2004; Kuhn, 2005). Succinctly stated, if the stance is empirical, then this most likely means that the individual favors the use of a type of standard epistemology that focuses on objective methodology, as is often undertaken with the scientific method or approach. If the stance is non-empirical, then it might be that the individual adheres to multiple epistemologies that are not based on the scientific method (Martin, 1992; Noddings, 1995; Ritzer, 2001). In general, multiple epistemologies are based mostly on social constructivism (and even postmodernism) and vary according to the norms, beliefs, and mores of the specific sociological group. Such approaches have been utilized in the various studies such as African American, Feminist, Gay/Lesbian/Bisexual/Transsexual/Intersexual, Deaf, and Disabilities Studies (Noddings; Ritzer).

Within the purview of a scientific focus, it should be possible to reach objective agreement. That is, there is a separation between the subject (e.g., researcher, teacher, student, evaluator) and the object (i.e., the statement, etc., being evaluated and analyzed) such that the evaluation is not confounded by the extreme bias of the observer (or, rather, the bias can be minimized or controlled). The evaluation is thus objective or dispassionate, and independent evaluations (i.e., conducted by different individuals) should yield similar findings. This is considered the hallmark of the scientific approach most often associated with the natural or so-called *hard* sciences such as physics, chemistry, and biology (Noddings, 1995; Ritzer, 2001).

On the other hand, if individuals argue that there cannot ever be a separation of the subject and object, then there is no real objectivity with the evaluation. In general, this is the assertion of researchers and scholars who subscribe to an interpretative, critical, or social constructivist framework

(Noddings, 1995; Ritzer, 2001). Several scholars considered this to be the case for the human or so-called *soft* disciplines such as sociology, education, humanities, philosophy, and—in several instances—some of psychology. It is possible to conduct empirical/scientific research within the above disciplines, but this type of research is rejected as not being relevant.

As indicated by Norris (1992) and others (Kuhn, 2005; Moore & Parker, 2009; Noddings, 1995; Ritzer, 2001; Vaughn, 2010), whether or not critico-creative thinking is empirical is contingent on the question that is being asked and the description of the framework being investigated. For example, if an individual explains the concepts of arguments, premises, and conclusions (the general view), then it should be possible to evaluate the merits of such syllogisms or analogies (see examples in the instruction section of this chapter). The fact that there may be disagreements, as is often the case in both general and domain-specific views, does not render the evaluation moot or necessarily subjective. Disagreements might result in the formulation of different arguments with different premises and different conclusions, which can then be evaluated.

Nevertheless, if there are disagreements regarding the conceptual framework of a topic or discipline (i.e., within the domain-specific view), then there are bound to be disagreements on the notion of an objective evaluation. As demonstrated in our instructional section, we believe that it is possible to evaluate critico-creative thinking skills objectively but not completely. If there is no objective stance, then there is no such entity as critico-creative thinking, and this, to us—and others (e.g., see Kuhn, 2005)—seems unacceptable.

We do sympathize somewhat with the argument by Martin (1992) that not all instances of critico-creative thinking should be dispassionate or objective or even generalizable. Martin's concern is that this distance (i.e., objectivity or dispassionateness) should not be predominantly valued, especially in the social sciences and humanities or even in the natural sciences. For Martin, objectivity and dispassion dispel with the uniqueness, feelings, and problems of individuals. This is similar to the current debate in the United States regarding the appropriate demeanor of a Supreme Court Justice (circa 2010). That is, there seems to be a tension between selecting someone who engages in abstract evaluations and one who recognizes the need to tailor or differentiate rulings according to the situations of affected individuals.

We cannot respond adequately to Martin's (1992) assertions and problems with evaluations and instruction, given our space limitations. We do argue that there needs to be a framework for teaching and evaluating such skills, however; guidelines for improving and strengthening critico-creative skills have to be in place, regardless of the controversies. To address Martin's concerns, it should be possible to develop multiple-perspectives guidelines that acknowledge the various voices associated with different social groups regarding controversial issues such as abortion, religion, and so on.

Evaluation of the General View

In a number of texts on critico-creative or critical thinking, there are evaluation schemes for *general* areas such as analogies, syllogisms, forming hypotheses, identifying the supporting statements, writing a persuasive essay, developing definitions, and so on (Moore & Parker, 2009; Ruggiero, 2002; Vaughn, 2010). Consider the following syllogisms, which can be evaluated as being valid or invalid (Porter, 2002).

Valid Syllogism
If Emily is a doctor, then she can cure bronchitis.
Emily is a doctor.
Therefore, she can cure bronchitis. (p. 164)

Invalid Syllogism
If Emily is a doctor, then she can cure bronchitis.
Emily is not a doctor.
Therefore, Emily can't cure bronchitis. (p. 165)

In short, Emily still might have a cure for bronchitis even though she is not a doctor (she could be one of those wise grandmothers).

There are numerous other examples of evaluation for the general view. For instance, Ruggiero (2002) presents a scheme for evaluating *arguments*. He lists four steps and demonstrates each one. The merits of arguments are based on the evaluation of the four steps by the individual, which are:

- *Step 1:* Understand the argument
- *Step 2:* Seek out competing views
- *Step 3:* Sort out disagreements
- *Step 4:* Make your judgment (p. 68)

As mentioned previously, there are levels of thinking that can be evaluated. For example, in the area of critical reading, the instructor can determine if students can perform tasks such as finding the main idea, listing supporting statements, making inferences, and drawing conclusions. Higher-level skills would be critiquing and evaluating positions or arguments, listing similarities and differences across passages, creating questions for balanced purposes (i.e., perspectives on an issue), and making judgments on the accuracy or completeness of the passage as well as stating and defending one's positions or views. All of these activities fall within the purview of metacognitive or self-regulating strategies.

Evaluation of the Domain-Specific View

By far, most of the difficulties with evaluations are associated with those involving domain-specific areas such as psychology, science, or mathematics (McBurney, 2002) or specific topics (Bruning et al., 2004). And it is possible, as discussed in Chapter 4, that these difficulties vary with the perception of the structure or conceptual framework of a discipline. In addition, there is variability on whether a specific discipline is a science or not (Pring, 2004; Ritzer, 2001).

It is important to facilitate the thinking skills of students so that they can think like a psychologist or think like a scientist, despite the controversy on what these statements mean. Such facilitation requires that students obtain a *basic* understanding of the research methodologies, issues, metalanguage, and paradigms/theories/metatheories associated with a particular field (McBurney, 2002). For a complex, deep understanding, students need to be able to read and critique journal articles and scholarly books; however, this would be the typical case for graduate students in universities.

Even a basic understanding can be difficult for many typical students in middle and high schools because of the metalanguage and, particularly, because of the use of what can be called *academic language* (e.g., see discussions in Israel & Duffy, 2009). It is even more of a challenge for students who have disabilities/conditions or who are English language learners.

It is possible to utilize some of the techniques associated with the general view to assist students with domain-specific areas. This would only be a modest beginning, however. As every history, literature, and so on instructor knows—students have difficulty not only with the academic or specialized language, but also with the manner in which terminology is used in the domain-specific areas. We always cringe whenever we hear our university students make any of the following remarks:

- I have a good theory about that.
- This proves that this method works.
- I want to know how to teach reading, not just vocabulary or prior knowledge.

Table 5-3 presents a few highlights on the evaluation issue.

INSTRUCTIONAL ISSUES

It is easy to find instructional examples and strategies for developing critico-creative thinking skills ranging from simple to complex. Searching the Internet via Web sites and key word searches yields advertisements, games, and a grab bag of ideas, activities, and suggestions, some, of

---

Table 5-3. Evaluation Issues

- Can evaluations be considered objective or are they always subjective?
- Should dispassionate (i.e., objective) approaches be the main goal of all critico-creative thinking endeavors?
- The concept of evaluation is intertwined with the epistemological framework of the evaluator.
- It has been argued that the nature and evaluation of critico-creative thinking is both empirical and philosophical (actually, non-empirical).
- If the stance is empirical, then this most likely means that the individual favors the use of a type of standard epistemology, focusing on objective methodology, as often is used with the scientific method or approach.
- If the stance is non-empirical, then it might be that the individual adheres to multiple epistemologies that are not based on the scientific method.
- A number of texts on critico-creative or critical thinking present evaluation schemes for *general* areas such as analogies, syllogisms, forming hypotheses, identifying the supporting statements, writing a persuasive essay, developing definitions, and so on.
- Most of the difficulties with evaluations are associated with those involving domain-specific areas such as psychology, science, or mathematics, or specific topics. These difficulties vary with the perception of the structure or conceptual framework of a discipline.

course, at a price. A preponderant number of books focus on *how to* with respect to teaching a range of these skills (Halpern, 1997; Moore & Parker, 2009; Porter, 2002; Ruggiero, 2001, 2002; Vaughn, 2010).

Our examples and components of critico-creative skills are selective and are influenced by our interests both professional and personal. Readers are directed to the sources listed previously for a more comprehensive treatment of informal and formal techniques such as syllogisms (arguments, premises, and conclusions), inductive and deductive reasoning, use of analogies, formulation of questions, judging information, statements, or theories, finding the main idea with supporting statements, differentiating between opinions and facts, interpreting Venn diagrams, and so on.

The exercises below require lower-level, mostly language-oriented skills such as paraphrasing, summarizing, and synthesizing, as well as higher-level ones such as critiquing, evaluating, and generalizing. The appropriateness of these and other activities depends on the language, cognitive, and experiential levels of students, especially those with disabilities or conditions. Finally, it should be remembered that these activities can be developed to be used in through-the-air or captured modes or both.

Simple Instructional Activities

Exercise 1

Ask children to consider the following passage:

A cat was lying on the bed.
It was sleeping.
Soon, the cat was lying under the bed.

Start with a few easy questions:

1. What was on the bed?
2. What was it doing?

Now focus on the last sentence of the passage:

3. How did the cat get under the bed? OR
4. Why did the cat go under the bed?

(continues)

Exercise 1 *(continued)*

The answers to questions 3 and 4 are not in the short blurb; these hence require an inference based on the children's experiences (and imagination or problem-solving skills). Most children will answer question 3 with: "The cat jumped off the bed and went under the bed (or under it)." It might be worthwhile, however, to encourage additional responses by inquiring: "Besides jumping off, how else could the cat get under the bed?" Hopefully, someone answers: "An adult (mother, father, etc.) came in, took the cat off the bed, and put it under the bed" or ". . . put the cat under the bed."

There is little doubt that question 4 is more complicated and may be somewhat related to question 3. Again, there are several possibilities: "An adult put the cat on the floor because she did not want the cat on the bed. Then the cat went under the bed" or: "There was a loud noise. The noise caused the cat to jump off the bed and go under it to hide."

A little easier rendition of this exercise might be to provide responses for children to evaluate as *true, maybe,* or *false.*

For example:

A cat was lying on the bed.
It was sleeping.
Soon, the cat was lying under the bed.

Statement	True, Maybe, False?
1. The cat got off the bed.	True (or Maybe!)
2. The cat rolled off the bed accidentally.	Maybe
3. The girl took the cat off the bed.	Maybe
4. The bed threw the cat under it.	False (except in *fairy tales*)

If children have difficulty answering the above questions, then the blurb can be made more explicit as in the following, and questions can be posed:

A cat was lying on the bed.
It was sleeping.
There was a loud noise.
The noise caused the cat to jump off the bed.
The cat went under the bed.
Soon, the cat was lying under the bed.

Exercise 2

Give the students the following problem:

The book says that there are 7 days in a week, 4 weeks in a month, and 52 weeks in a year. If there are 7 days in a week and 4 weeks in a month, then the month of May has 28 days (7 × 4).

1. *Is this correct?*
2. *What's wrong with this approach?*

There should be a discussion about the difficulty of remarking that *4 weeks equals a month*, given that months typically have 30 or 31 days, and February either has 28 or 29 (in a leap year). A month could have 28, 29, 30, or 31 days, which is 4 weeks (so to speak) plus 1 to 3 more days. The same discussion can be applied to the statement of 52 weeks in year. How do we get 52 when 4 weeks × 12 months is 48?

Complex Instructional Activities

Common activities such as locating the main idea, finding supporting statements, stating the conclusion, and so on can be found in popular texts on reading and critical reading (Gunning, 2008; Klingner et al., 2007). Our focus here is on developing metacognitive skills—that is, encouraging students to reflect on and evaluate the information and the nature of the questions/activities to offer possible answers or solutions.

Exercise 1

Say to the student: You have just read a story about bats, but your friends have not read it yet. You want to tell your friends what the story is mainly about. How much will it help to say to them that . . . (based on information from Paul, 1998).

1. *This story is about the eating, hunting, and flying habits of different kinds of bats.*
    a. *This will help a lot.*
    b. *This might help a little bit.*
    c. *This will not help at all.*

(continues)

Exercise 1 *(continued)*

2. *This story is about the ways that bats are different from birds.*
   a. *This will help a lot.*
   b. *This might help a little bit.*
   c. *This will not help at all.*
3. *This story is about the way bats see in the dark.*
   a. *This will help a lot.*
   b. *This might help a little bit.*
   c. *This will not help at all.*

Exercise 2

Blue Jeans

Today you are going to read a story like the stories you read previously at school. This story is about Levi, the man who invented blue jeans in 1849. Think about what life was like during the gold rush of California in the 1850s, and how blue jeans were made. Think about why gold miners and other people needed strong pants like blue jeans.

Below are several ideas. For each idea, decide whether or not you might find it in the story (that you have not read yet!). Circle the best answer. **Explain or defend** *your answer. Your choices are:*

Yes	=	*The idea would be in this story.*
Maybe	=	*The idea might be in this story.*
No	=	*The idea would not be in this story.*

1. *Gold was discovered in California.*   *Yes   Maybe   No*
2. *People traveled to California in the 1850s
   by bus.*   *Yes   Maybe   No*
3. *Levi was a miner.*   *Yes   Maybe   No*
4. *Levi went to K-Mart to find material for
   his jeans.*   *Yes   Maybe   No*
5. *This story happened in France.*   *Yes   Maybe   No*
6. *Gold miners used their pockets to hold gold.*   *Yes   Maybe   No*
7. *Gold miners liked blue jeans because they
   needed strong pants.*   *Yes   Maybe   No*

(continues)

Exercise 2 *(continued)*

8. *People who went to California to find gold*
   decided to stay there.   *Yes Maybe No*
9. *Levi put rivets on the pockets of the blue jeans*
   so that the pockets would be stronger.   *Yes Maybe No*
10. *Levi became famous because he invented socks.*   *Yes Maybe No*

Exercise 3

Students have read two factual expository, persuasive passages about the beginning of the universe: *steady state* and *Big Bang*. They then are asked to read the following narrative passage.

Birth of the Universe

Prior to the 1960s, the thinking of cosmologists on the creation of the universe was heavily influenced by a theory called steady state. Succinctly put, steady-state theorists argued that this world had no beginning and no end. Because matter is regenerated, the universe will go on forever and ever. Philosophically, this notion appealed to the atheists, but it was despised somewhat by the theologians. The joy of the atheists, however, was short-lived.

Evidence collected during the late 1960s and early 1970s suggested that the universe came into being with a big bang. Some Big Bang theorists argued that the universe had a beginning and will come to an end as a result of its expansion. The theologians interpreted this as evidence for Judgment Day whereas the atheists simply ignored this view. The cosmologists labeled it the open universe Big Bang Theory.

Although the open-universe theory is in vogue, some theorists argue that it is still possible for the world to fall back upon itself, producing a big crunch. This view is known as the closed-universe Big-Bang Theory. This idea still makes the theologians happy and the atheists uncomfortable. The opposite would be true if there is enough evidence for an oscillating-universe Big-Bang Theory. In this view, the universe is said to begin with a big bang, end with a big crunch, and then begin all over again with another big bang. All knowledge of the previous universe disappears with each big bang.

(continues)

Exercise 3 *(continued)*

Future theorists might construct yet another theory regarding the begin-ning and end of the universe. Soon, the theologians and the atheists will be arguing again. The Big-Bang theorists insist that no informed person can dispute the fact that the universe began with a big bang. The problem is how the universe will end.

So, on and on it goes. Atheists versus theologians. Philosophers versus sci-entists. Open universe versus closed universe. At one point, nearly everyone agreed that the steady-state theory was dead.

How do you feel about all this? Perhaps you believe the same way that Walt Whitman felt in his poem, "When I heard the learned astronomer," that we read last week in our literature book. Remember that Whitman ended the poem with these lines:

> *How soon unaccountable, I became tired and sick,*
> *Till rising and gliding out I wander'd off by myself,*
> *In the mythical moist night air, and from time to time,*
> *Look'd up in perfect silence at the stars.*
>
> Whitman, 1980, p. 226

The following are questions for students to discuss based on the three passages: *steady state, Big Bang,* and *birth of the universe.* As can be seen, these questions require a range of skills beyond the simple ones of paraphrasing or summarizing. Students need to compare and contrast, evaluate, and critique. In some cases, much of the informa-tion needed is in the passages; however, in other cases, students need to access or assess their prior knowledge of the topics or situations. To obtain a glimpse of specific techniques that can be used to teach com-prehension and other critico-creative skills, readers are referred to other sources (Gunning, 2008; Klingner et al., 2007; Pearson & Johnson, 1978).

Questions

1. In *Birth of the Universe* (BU), what do atheists and theologians be-lieve about Hawking's theory of the universe in the passage about Big Bang (BB)?
2. In BU, the steady-state theory appealed to the atheists. True or false? Why or why not? Is this clear in the passage on steady state (SS)?
3. Is the description of steady state in BU similar to or different from that of the SS passage? In what way(s)?

(continues)

Exercise 3 *(continued)*

4. What are the names of the three Big Bang theories discussed in BU? Are these descriptions similar to or different from the passage on BB?
5. Do any of the three passages relate how atheists feel about the concept of God? If so, describe these beliefs.
6. In BU, are theologians happy with the oscillating universe Big Bang Theory? Why or why not?
7. Would agnostics like the steady-state theory as described in SS? Why or why not?
8. Which of the theories do you think Walt Whitman would have favored? Why do you think that?
9. Which theory do you believe is most true? Why?
10. What questions do you have about these passages?

SUMMARY

The intent of this chapter is to introduce readers to the nature, characteristics, forms, and broad views of critico-creative thinking. It is argued that critico-creative thinking is a component of literate thought. In addition, we discuss problems with generalizability and evaluation. Finally, a few instructional examples were provided.

A few major points are as follows:

• Critical and creative thinking are interrelated; they can be considered as complementary components of good thinking. It is difficult to imagine how individuals can engage in one aspect without the other because they are so intertwined.

• In solving problems, resolving conflicts, making decisions, and so on, we proceed in a back-and-forth maneuver, repeatedly at times, involving critical and creative dimensions.

• Regardless of whether one believes in general aspects (i.e., generalizations across domains or subjects) or in specific disciplinary or domain aspects, the underlying values and attitudes associated with critico-creative thinking remain constant across content areas or subjects.

- Individuals are utilizing a weak form of critico-creative thinking if they simply argue for their position and virtually ignore the arguments on the other side. The main objective is to defend one's view against the arguments of others.
- Within the framework of the strong form, the goal is to examine critically all prominent views—including contradictory ones. After much dialogue and reflection, strong-form proponents can state their current position, which should always be tentative and may change in light of what proponents see as a better argument.
- Critico-creative thinking can and should facilitate the acquisition and conceptualization of knowledge and information whereby we can test and refine our hypotheses, models, ideas, and arguments.
- There are two broad views of critico-creative thinking. One can be labeled the *general view*—that is, an individual possesses general critico-creative thinking skills that can be applied or transferred to any content, topic, domain, or disciplinary area. The second can be labeled the *domain-specific view* (or *domain knowledge view*). In short, this view is specialized to a particular discipline such as science, mathematics, or language development or to a specific topic such as masonry or tennis.
- The feasibility of generalizability is confounded by several contentious issues. One major disagreement is the definition of critico-creative thinking. Additional challenges arise in considering the understanding of other concepts such as *transfer* and *comprehension*.
- Although both empirical and philosophical debates are ongoing about the general versus the domain-specific views of critico-creative thinking, much of the evidence favors the domain-specific view.
- The concept of evaluation of critico-creative skills is intertwined with the epistemological framework of the evaluator. The nature and evaluation of critico-creative thinking is both empirical and philosophical.
- Most of the difficulties with evaluations are associated with those involving domain-specific areas such as psychology, science, mathematics, or specific topics.
- Critico-creative instructional exercises might require lower-level skills, mostly language-oriented, such as paraphrasing, summarizing, and synthesizing, as well as higher-level ones such as critiquing, evaluating, and generalizing. The appropriateness of these and other

activities depends on the language, cognitive, and experiential levels of students, especially those with disabilities or conditions. These activities can be developed to be used in through-the-air or captured modes or both.

In Chapter 6, we discuss literate thought with respect to the population of individuals who have language and literacy difficulties.

QUESTIONS FOR REFLECTION AND DISCUSSION

1. Discuss a few major points in the section on the nature, characteristics, and forms of critico-creative thinking.

2. Describe and give an example of the weak and strong forms of critico-creative thinking. Does the use of a particular form vary with a specific situation? In your view, which form is or should be preferable for educational purposes? Why?

3. Compare and contrast the general view and the domain-specific view. How does the problem of generalization relate to these views? What are the issues?

4. What is a general critico-creative demeanor? What are some aspects? Why is this demeanor important?

5. Discuss the difficulty of evaluating the two broad views of critico-creative thinking.

REFERENCES

Applegate, M., Quin, K., & Applegate, A. (2008). *The critical reading inventory: Assessing students' reading and thinking.* Upper Saddle River, N.J.: Pearson/Merrill/Prentice Hall.

Browne, M. N., & Keeley, S. (2007). *Asking the right questions: A guide to critical thinking.* Upper Saddle River, NJ: Pearson/Prentice Hall.

Bruning, R., Schraw, G., Norby, M., Ronning, R. (2004). *Cognitive psychology and instruction* (4th ed.). Upper Saddle River, NJ: Pearson/Merrill/Prentice Hall.

Cain, K., & Oakhill, J. (Eds.). (2007). *Children's comprehension problems in oral and written language.* New York: Guilford Press.

Cummins, J. (1984). *Bilingualism and special education: Issues in assessment and pedagogy.* San Diego, CA: College-Hill Press.

Cummins, J. (1989). A theoretical framework for bilingual special education. *Exceptional Children, 56*, 111-119.

Flage, D. (2004). *The art of questioning: An introduction to critical thinking.* Upper Saddle River, NJ: Pearson/Prentice Hall.

Gunning, T. (2008). *Developing higher-level literacy in all students: Building reading, reasoning, and responding.* Boston, MA: Pearson/Allyn & Bacon.

Halpern, D. (1997). *Critical thinking across the curriculum: A brief edition of thought and knowledge.* Mahwah, NJ: Erlbaum.

Hirsch, E.D., Kett, J., & Trefil, J. (Eds.). (2002). *The new dictionary of cultural literacy* (3rd ed.). Boston, MA: Houghton Mifflin Company.

Israel, S., & Duffy, G. (Eds.). (2009). *Handbook of research on reading comprehension.* New York: Routledge.

Johnson, R. (1992). The problem of defining critical thinking. In S. Norris (Ed.), *The generalizability of critical thinking: Multiple perspectives on an educational ideal* (pp. 38-53). New York: Teachers College Press, Columbia University.

Klingner, J., Vaughn, S., & Boardman, A. (2007). *Teaching reading comprehension to students with learning difficulties.* New York: Guilford Press.

Kuhn, D. (2005). *Education for thinking.* Cambridge, MA: Harvard University Press.

Martin, J. (1992). Critical thinking for a humane world. In S. Norris (Ed.), *The generalizability of critical thinking: Multiple perspectives on an educational ideal* (pp. 163-180). New York: Teachers College Press, Columbia University.

McBurney, D. (2002). *How to think like a psychologist: Critical thinking in psychology* (2nd ed.). Upper Saddle River, NJ: Prentice Hall.

Moore, B., & Parker, R. (2009). *Critical thinking* (9th ed.). Boston, MA: McGraw-Hill.

Noddings, N. (1995). *Philosophy of education.* Boulder, CO: Westview Press.

Norris, S. (Ed.). (1992). *The generalizability of critical thinking: Multiple perspectives on an educational ideal.* New York: Teachers College Press, Columbia University.

Paul, P. (1998). *Literacy and deafness: The development of reading, writing, and literate thought.* Needham Heights, MA: Allyn & Bacon.

Paul, P. (2009). *Language and deafness* (4th ed.). Sudbury, MA: Jones & Bartlett Learning.

Pearson, P. D., & Johnson, D. (1978). *Teaching reading comprehension.* New York: Holt, Rinehart, & Winston.

Porter, B. (2002). *The voice of reason: Fundamentals of critical thinking.* New York: Oxford University Press.

Pring, R. (2004). *Philosophy of educational research* (2nd ed.). New York: Continuum.

Ritzer, G. (2001). *Explorations in social theory: From metatheorizing to rationalization.* Thousand Oaks, CA: SAGE.

Ruddell, R., & Unrau, N. (Eds.). (2004). *Theoretical models and processes of reading* (5th ed.). Newark, DE: International Reading Association.

Ruggiero, V. (2001). *The art of thinking: A guide to critical and creative thought* (6th ed.). New York: Longman.

Ruggiero, V. (2002). *Becoming a critical thinker* (4th ed.). New York: Houghton Mifflin.

Snowling, M., & Hulme, C. (Eds.). (2005). *The science of reading: A handbook.* Malden, MA: Blackwell.

Taliaferro, C. (2009). *Philosophy of religion: A beginner's guide.* Oxford, UK: Oneworld.

Trezek, B., Wang, Y., & Paul, P. (2010). *Reading and deafness: Theory, research and practice.* Clifton Park, NY: Cengage Learning.

Vaughn, L. (2010). *The power of critical thinking: Effective reasoning about ordinary and extraordinary claims* (3rd ed.). New York: Oxford University Press.

Whitman, W. (1980). *Leaves of grass.* New York: The New American Library.

Willingham, D. (2007). Critical thinking: Why is it so hard to teach? *American Educator*, Summer, 8-19.

FURTHER READING

Dawes, R.M. (1994). *House of cards: Psychology and psychotherapy built on myth.* New York: Free Press.

Gellner, E. (1992). *Postmodernism, reason, and religion.* London: Routledge.

Koslowski, B. (1996). *Theory and evidence: The development of scientific reasoning.* Cambridge, MA: The MIT Press.

Munz, P. (1985). *Our knowledge of the growth of knowledge.* London: Routledge & Kegan Paul.

Nickerson, R.S. (1986). *Reflections on reasoning.* Hillsdale, NJ: Lawrence Erlbaum.

CHAPTER 6

Children with Language/Learning Disabilities

I shall contend that what the particular practices and concepts of reading and writing are for a given society depends upon the context; that they are already embedded in an ideology and cannot be isolated or treated as 'neutral' or merely 'technical'. I shall demonstrate that what practices are taught and how they are imparted depends upon the nature of the social formation. The skills and concepts that accompany literacy acquisition, in whatever form, do not stem in some automatic way from the inherent qualities of literacy, as some authors would have us believe, but are aspects of a specific ideology.

Street, 1984, p. 1

With respect to the development of literate thought or any other reflective thinking framework, it is critical to understand the possible implications of the above passage. Street (1984) proposed that models of literacy should be considered as *ideological* models instead of traditional, narrow, culture-specific, *autonomous* models, which associate literacy with a specific technology, for example, writing systems. In Street's view, technology itself is a social product that resulted from political and ideological processes.

Freeing literacy from the confinement of technology, the ideological model of literacy should raise the New and Multiple Literacies to an equal status with traditional script literacy (see also, Chapter 3). Regardless if the product is a poem, a novel, a painting, a song, a dance, a podcast (i.e., an audio or video file published on the Internet and

179

available for download) or a wiki (i.e., a Web site that allows the users to contribute and edit the content), it thus is a genuine type of literacy as long as it carries accessible meaning/information for the construction or manipulation of reality.

The ability to read and write is only one avenue for accessing and manipulating information (Paul, 2009; Paul & Wang, 2006a, 2006b; Wang, 2005). As we have argued repeatedly, there are a number of paths for accessing and manipulating information from a variety of information carriers such as CDs, DVDs, audiobooks, MP3s, and the Internet. Or, in our purview, there are multiple paths to the goal of literate thought.

This reconceptualized concept of literacy also validates multiple modes of literacy as viable mental tools for developing literate thought. Legitimizing script literacy as the only mode of literacy in school, while ostracizing others, can become a form of oppression and might cause cognitive impoverishment, as mentioned in Chapter 1 (Paul, 2009; Paul & Wang, 2006a, 2006b; Wang, 2005). This is especially true for those individuals for whom script literacy is not easily accessible, as is the case for many children with language/learning disabilities—and is the focus of this chapter.

As discussed in this chapter and throughout the subsequent ones on other populations of children, there is a connection between the development of language and that of literacy—albeit literacy is more than just language development. More importantly, there is a connection between the development of language and that of literate thought. To provide some understanding of these connections, we begin with the discussion of children with language/learning difficulties, and use reading as the major exemplar.

The chapter explicates the different terms associated with children with language/learning disabilities, indicating that there are several subgroups within this broad population. We synthesize the literature on the development of English language and literacy for these subgroups of children to illustrate, in part, the range and depth of their difficulties. Next, the application of the concepts of the New and Multiple Literacies to these children is examined. Finally, based on our understanding of language and literacy needs, we conclude with specific implications for developing literate thought in children with language and reading disabilities.

TERMS ASSOCIATED WITH LANGUAGE/LEARNING DISABILITIES

Various terms have been used to refer to individuals who have traditional language/literacy problems. *Learning disability* is a general term typically used to encompass a collection of different types of learning problems, such as those present in reading, in mathematics, or in social/behavioral learning. *Language/learning disability* is used to describe specifically spoken and written language deficits. *Reading disability* is an even narrower descriptor for different kinds of deficits in learning to read. Historically, individuals with reading disability have been referred to as those with *congenital word blindness, dyslexia, developmental dyslexia,* or *specific reading disabilities* (Catts & Kamhi, 2005). Sometimes, the word *developmental* is added in front of these labels to clarify that the disability has arisen from the initial learning period instead of being an acquired problem.

Figure 6-1 provides a summary of these terms used to refer to individuals who have traditional language/literacy problems.

As one of the most confusing and misunderstood terms, *dyslexia*, etymologically means difficulty with words (e.g., Catts & Kamhi, 2005). Currently, the most widely used definition of dyslexia is proposed by the International Dyslexia Association (IDA):

> Dyslexia is a specific learning disability that is neurobiological in origin. It is characterized by difficulties with accurate and/or fluent word recognition and by poor spelling and decoding abilities. These difficulties typically result from a deficit in the phonological component of language that is often unexpected in relation to other cognitive abilities and the provision of effective classroom instruction. Secondary consequences may include problems in reading comprehension and reduced reading experience that can impede growth of vocabulary and background knowledge. (Lyon, Shaywitz, & Shaywitz, 2003, p. 2)

The above phonological-based definition clarifies the previously documented common misunderstanding of dyslexia as a visual-based reading disability. Furthermore, the current definition suggests that phonological difficulties might lead to problems in accuracy and fluency, which in turn might result in problems in vocabulary and background knowledge, all of which can influence reading and understanding connected text (Lyon et al., 2003).

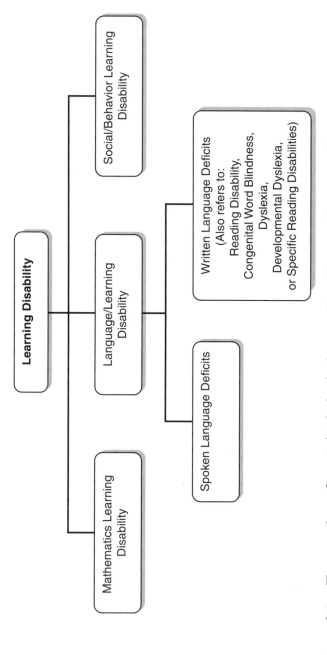

Figure 6-1.   Terms used to refer to individuals who have traditional language/literacy problems.

Our focus in this chapter is on children with written language (i.e., reading disabilities) and spoken language deficits. In a comprehensive review of the literature on reading instruction, the National Reading Panel ([NRP]; 2000; see also, McGuinness, 2004, 2005; Snow, Burns, & Griffin, 1998) identified three broad reasons for reading difficulties: 1) problems in understanding and utilizing the alphabetic principle to acquire fluent and accurate word reading (i.e., decoding) skills; 2) failure to obtain the verbal knowledge and strategies that are exclusively required for comprehension of written materials; and 3) absence or loss of initial motivation to read, or failure to develop a mature appreciation for the rewards of reading.

Certainly, a process as complex as reading can never be fully explained by such a simple tripartite framework, which oversimplifies the range of difficulties children might encounter in learning to read. For example, although many children either have a primary difficulty in learning to identify words in text with accuracy and fluency or have a deficit mainly with constructing the meaning of text, some children might have difficulties in both. Furthermore, many children with problems in decoding skills also suffer from a lack of motivation for reading (e.g., see Torgesen, 2005). Nevertheless, categorizing reading difficulties into three broad groups, as mentioned above, assists in the classification of numerous research studies and avoids the pitfall of *one-size-fits-all* instructional practices.

Accordingly, the NRP (2000) categories provide the guidelines for the next section, which is divided into four parts to discuss the development of language and literacy for four groups of children with language/learning disabilities: 1) children with deficits in word recognition; 2) children with deficits in written language comprehension; 3) children who are less engaged and less intrinsically motivated in reading; and 4) children with deficits in spoken language (i.e., speech). It should be emphasized that the boundaries of these categories can be blurred in cases where a reader might have difficulties in multiple areas. This review should pave the way for our discussion of the utility of the New and Multiple Literacies as a major avenue for developing literate thought.

CHILDREN WITH DEFICITS IN WORD RECOGNITION

The ability to comprehend written text is critically dependent on the reader's ability to identify words with sufficient fluency, that is, accuracy and speed in identifying words and to read the text smoothly with appropriate expression (McGuinness, 2004, 2005; NRP, 2000). Fluency in word recognition is a prerequisite for adequate reading comprehension. Furthermore, language comprehension processes as well as higher-level cognitive processes affecting language comprehension do not become fully operative in text comprehension unless such fluency has been acquired (Adams, 1990; Hoover & Gough, 1990; Vellutino, 2003). After explicating the significance and strategies of word recognition, a summary of the research on children with language and literacy difficulties is presented.

Significance of Word Recognition Fluency

Word recognition fluency is closely related to the limited capacity of working memory, which is involved in understanding meanings in written text, for example, remembering meanings of words within the sentence, retrieving information from preceding text, parsing the sentence, and so on (Perfetti, Landi & Oakhill, 2005; Snowling & Hulme, 2005). *Working memory* is one or more systems of limited capacity responsible for the temporary storage and processing/manipulating of modality-specific information necessary to handle tasks that require comprehension, learning, and reasoning (Baddeley, 1986, 1990). Phonological working memory, a subsystem of working memory that is specialized for holding and manipulating phonological information, is directly linked to reading due to the need to keep the contents active (i.e., in memory) until the end of a clause or sentence. The emerging view is that the use of a phonological code in working memory is most efficient for processing and understanding a language based on an alphabet system (e.g., English) (Adams, 1990; McGuinness, 2004, 2005; Perfetti et al., 2005; Snow et al., 1998; Snowling & Hulme, 2005).

Strategies in Word Recognition

At least five different strategies can be used in word recognition (Ehri, 2002; Torgesen, Otaiba & Grek, 2005). The first strategy refers to identifying and blending together the individual phonemes in words as in *phonological decoding*. The prerequisite of phonological decoding is *phonemic awareness*, which involves the ability to recognize that words are made up of *phonemes*. Phonemic awareness activities teach children to notice, think about, and work with the more than 40 phonemes that comprise the alphabetic system of the English language. These activities include phoneme 1) isolation, 2) identity, 3) categorization, 4) blending, 5) segmentation, 6) deletion, 7) addition, and 8) substitution (Armbruster, Lehr, & Osborn, 2001).

Another critical component in phonological decoding is phonics skills, which help children learn and use the *alphabetic principle*, defined as the understanding that there is a predictable relationship between letters (graphemes) and sounds (phonemes). When a beginning reader with phonological decoding skills encounters a less familiar word during reading, he or she will first identify the letters in the word with their sounds (phonemes), and then blend the phonemes together to attach the meaning to the word.

As beginning readers become more experienced readers, an advanced level of phonological decoding can be used in word recognition: identifying and blending together familiar *spelling patterns*. Processing chunks of letters as units instead of individual letters improves decoding speed. Some common spelling patterns include: *prefixes* (i.e., word parts that are fixed to the beginnings of words) and *suffixes* (i.e., word parts that are fixed to the ending of words), *base words* (i.e., words from which many other words are formed), and *root words* (i.e., words from other languages that are the origin of many English words) (Trezek, Wang, & Paul, 2010).

The third strategy in word recognition is recognizing words in whole units as *sight words*, which is also referred as *orthographic processing*. After a reader encounters a meaningful word multiple times, the orthographic processor instantly handles the orthographic pattern as a whole; simultaneously, the word's meaning and phonological image are stimulated (Adams, 1990). The key to fluent text reading is to build a large vocabulary of sight words, permitting the reader to concentrate effectively on constructing the meaning of text (Perfetti, 1985; Torgesen, Rashotte, & Alexander, 2001). Sight word reading should be emphasized in reading practices after or along with acquiring sufficient phonological decoding skills; otherwise, memorizing every word by sight becomes a heavy burden for beginning readers.

A fourth way for word recognition is to *make analogies to known words*. For example, when confronted by an unfamiliar word like *hardware*, a reader might notice its similarity to a known word *software* and make the slight adjustment to pronunciation required for the different initial phonemes to eventually stimulate the meaning and phonological image of the word *hardware*. The prerequisite for an effective use of an analogy strategy to identify unknown words is to obtain a beginning level of phonological decoding skill (Ehri & Robbins, 1992). Also, it is essential that the analogous word is stored in memory as a sight word.

The last word recognition strategy is to *use context clues* to guess a word's identity. Context clues can be the pictures on the page or the meaning of the passage. However, context clues by themselves can never be an effective reading strategy, especially considering that only about 10% of the words that are most critical to the meaning of passages can be guessed accurately from context alone (Gough & Walsh, 1991). Furthermore, Torgesen and colleagues (2005) identified two more themes from the research on the use of context clues to aid word recognition: 1) context clues are not used by good readers as a major source of information about words in text; and 2) poor readers actually rely on context clues for word identification more than skilled readers.

To reach a sufficient level of word recognition fluency, beginning readers should first develop phonemic awareness and phonics skills to decode unfamiliar words at the phoneme level. As they become more mature readers, they can notice and blend together familiar spelling patterns. After encountering a word multiple times, these readers can recognize the word in a whole unit as a sight word at the automaticity level with almost no expenditure of attention or effort. A large bank of sight word vocabulary is the key to fluent text reading.

Not all words in the sight word vocabulary bank have to be acquired through the phonemic level, spelling pattern level, and whole word level sequence. For example, some irregular, high-frequency words can be acquired directly through the whole word level (e.g., *was*, *were*); however, as mentioned previously, whole word reading should not be the only strategy for word recognition due to the limitation of human memory. Other strategies to improve word recognition fluency include making analogies to known words and using context clues. These two strategies should be used after the reader has a sizable sight word vocabulary bank; otherwise, reading is just a guessing game.

Table 6-1 summarizes these five strategies in developing word recognition fluency, all of which should be taught directly to the students, especially students with language and literacy difficulties.

Summary of Research

Based on an extensive review of the literature, Vellutino (2003) concluded: "reader differences in the acquisition of fluent word recognition

Table 6-1.	Five Strategies for Developing Word Recognition Fluency

Strategy 1:	Identifying and blending together the individual phonemes in words.
Strategy 2:	Identifying and blending together familiar spelling patterns in words.
Strategy 3:	Recognizing words in whole units as sight words.
Strategy 4:	Making analogies to known words.
Strategy 5:	Using context clues to guess a word's identity.

skills are the primary and most common source of variability in reading comprehension in elementary school children" (p. 53). It should be noted that *early* elementary school children is a more accurate phrase for this synthesis by Vellutino.

As an example, in a longitudinal study of approximately 600 monolingual children, Catts, Hogan and Adlof (2005) found that 75% of the variance in reading comprehension for children in second, fourth, and eighth grades can be explained by their performance on measures of word recognition and listening comprehension. Furthermore, the researchers found that, in second grade, word recognition accounted for more variance in reading comprehension than does listening comprehension (67% vs. 9%). But in the fourth grade, listening comprehension accounted for more variance than word recognition (21% vs. 13%). By eighth grade, listening comprehension accounted for almost all of the variance whereas word recognition accounted for only a minimal amount (72% vs. 2%).

From the beginning, many children with deficits in word recognition have difficulties in phonological decoding, which results in an inadequate sight word vocabulary as well (Catts & Kamhi, 2005). For some of these children who may have entered school delayed in phonological development, their word recognition difficulties can be resolved with improved phonics skills. The biological or constitutional basis of reading difficulties in children with dyslexia makes it difficult to dramatically alter their reading skills, however. In many cases, the degree of reading failure in older children with severe phonologically based reading disabilities was *stabilized* instead of *remediated*, or *normalized* compared to their peers over the years (Kavale, 1988; McKinney, 1990; Schumaker, Deshler, & Ellis, 1986; Torgesen, 2005). The notion of and difficulties with listening comprehension, as mentioned above, is an area that might be impacted by utilizing non-print avenues for presenting and discussing information (see also, Chapter 2).

CHILDREN WITH DEFICITS IN WRITTEN LANGUAGE COMPREHENSION

Snowling and Hulme (2005) asserted that, "reading is parasitic on language" (p. 397). Furthermore, they suggested that while decoding is parasitic on phonology, comprehension is parasitic on syntax, semantics, and pragmatics as well as phonology. These points have also been asserted by others (e.g., McGuinness, 2004, 2005). Children who decode well but have specific difficulties in written language comprehension (i.e., poor comprehenders) present a very different language profile from that of children with deficits in word recognition (i.e., poor decoders).

Snowling and Hulme (2005) remarked further:

> Although poor comprehenders' phonological skills are normal, they show deficits in a wide range of language skills outside of the phonological domain that are not simply a facet of low IQ. In particular, their vocabulary knowledge is impoverished and they have especially poor understanding of the meanings of abstract and low-frequency words. The assets and deficits of poor comprehenders point to a likely problem at the level of semantic representation, in contrast to the problems of phonological representation characteristic of dyslexic children. (p. 400)

In general, children with deficits in written language comprehension typically have impoverished vocabulary knowledge and show a range of deficits during reading comprehension processes, which include impairments in metalinguistic awareness, prior knowledge, as well as the use of cognitive and metacognitive strategies. These areas are discussed in the following paragraphs. Keep in mind that it is also possible to work on these areas, analogously, in non-print modes.

Vocabulary

Vocabulary refers to words that need to be known to comprehend and communicate effectively; this includes *listening, speaking, reading,* and *writing vocabulary* (Armbruster et al., 2001). The scientific research on vocabulary instruction concludes that although some vocabulary must be taught directly, the majority of words are learned indirectly (NRP, 2000; Snow et al., 1998; Stahl & Nagy, 2006). Children's indirect vocabulary learning occurs in various contexts: engaging daily in oral language, listening to adults read to them, and reading extensively on their own. Direct vocabulary instruction for children should provide students with specific word instruction and teach word-learning strategies. In addition, *word consciousness* (i.e., an awareness of and interest in words involving both a cognitive and an affective perspective toward words) should be fostered to help students develop their vocabulary (Stahl & Nagy).

In a landmark study, Hart and Risley (1999) concluded that a significant factor in a child's spoken vocabulary was the amount of parent–child interactions per hour. Furthermore, what mattered was not only the quantity of the interactions, but also the quality of the interactions such as language diversity, affirmative feedback, responsiveness, and so on. The significant differences in children's oral vocabulary size at age 3 were closely related to their cognitive and academic outcomes at ages 9 and 10 in areas of reading and writing vocabulary, listening, syntax, and reading comprehension in the longitudinal research of the subsequent years.

Collectively, the best strategy in vocabulary instruction is providing children with a language-rich environment whereby they can directly or indirectly interact with language in both oral (i.e., non-print or through-the-air) and written forms. Before a child produces his or her first word at an average age of 11 months, he or she has been listening to an average of 700 to 800 utterances per hour, half of which are results of overhearing conversations not directed to the child. Incidental language learning cannot be ignored in building the vocabulary knowledge of the child.

Metalinguistic Awareness

Other than limited vocabulary knowledge, children with deficits in written language comprehension typically have impairments in reading comprehension processes, where metalinguistic awareness plays an important role. *Metalinguistic awareness* refers to an awareness of language structures including syntactic awareness and pragmatic awareness (Vellutino, 2003). There are several types of metalinguistic awareness.

Syntactic awareness, for example, means sensitivity to grammatical form in terms of errors that violate conventional usage in spoken and written language. Syntactic awareness is an implicit reflection of a child's knowledge of spoken language conventions. *Pragmatic awareness* refers to sensitivity to the various ways language is used for purposes of communication. It is reflected in a child's awareness of conventions in using language in social situations, which include the desire to understand the intent of the speaker/writer in initiating a dialogue, turn taking during the dialogue, different types of meanings conveyed in the dialogue signaled in speech by intonation, pause, and intensity and in print by punctuation marks, and so forth.

These two components of metalinguistic awareness are critical in the reading comprehension process:

> Syntactic awareness is important for monitoring comprehension in terms of word recognition errors that produce ungrammatical and/or meaningless sentences. Pragmatic awareness is important for comprehending and keeping track of the ideas exchanged during a dialogue in listening and reading and for understanding the goals and purposes of the dialogue. (Vellutino, 2003, p. 61)

Prior Knowledge

Another important factor in the reading comprehension process is *prior knowledge*, which refers to a person's knowledge stored in long-term memory. As discussed in Chapters 1 and 2, prior knowledge, particularly topic-specific prior knowledge is a critical aspect of developing a major requisite of literate thought—metalanguage. Metalanguage refers to knowledge of the technical or specialized vocabulary associated with topics in passages as well as knowledge of broad cultural topics, that is, cultural literacy.

During a reading task, prior knowledge "is activated to interpret new experiences and knowledge, relate them to what is already known, and incorporate them into the already existing storehouse of information in long-term memory" (McAnally, Rose & Quigley, 2007, p. 11). Children's comprehension and memory of text are positively correlated with their ability to relate the ideas in text to their prior knowledge (Anderson, 1984; Dewitz, Carr, & Patberg, 1987; Pearson & Fielding, 1991).

One common framework for categorizing prior knowledge is to classify it as part of one or two components: passage-specific prior knowledge and topic-specific prior knowledge. *Passage-specific prior knowledge*, also known as *discourse knowledge*, refers to knowledge of the unique properties (e.g., language and its use) associated with different types of texts including knowledge on the structural and organizational characteristics of narrative texts (i.e., stories) versus expository and informational texts (Vellutino, 2003). Passage-specific prior knowledge helps the child to organize information in the text in ways that facilitate comprehension. For example, a child with extensive experience with narrative texts has an understanding that the author's primary purpose is to entertain the reader and that the narrative text typically has a central theme (i.e., story line), a beginning section to introduce the theme, a middle section to expand and develop the theme (i.e., plot development), and an end section to provide a conclusion or resolution of conflict. Alternatively, a child with extensive experience with expository and informational texts has an understanding that the author's primary purpose is to deliver information on a particular topic of interest and that the content of such text is usually organized sequentially and hierarchically, often with headings and subheadings, and provides detailed, factual information on the topic. Compared with good comprehenders, poor comprehenders (i.e., children who have specific difficulties in written language comprehension) tend to struggle with appreciating different types of discourse structure, which leads to their difficulty in navigating through different types of texts.

Topic-specific prior knowledge reflects information that is either not explicitly in the text or cannot be inferred from existing text information. It includes world knowledge and domain specific knowledge. *World knowledge* refers to knowledge of events and activities that occur in everyday life involving actual people and factual things that exist in real time and authentic places. It includes not only autobiographical knowledge on events and activities that occur in the child's daily life, but also knowledge on events, places, activities, persons, and things that are not or might not be a part of the child's daily life, that is, cultural literacy. *Domain specific knowledge* refers to knowledge that is unique to a particular content area such as science, social studies, mathematics, sports, entertainment, and so on.

When discussing world knowledge and domain specific knowledge, Vellutino (2003) concluded:

> Knowledge of both types is stored in complex mental structures called "schemata". Such schemata aid children's comprehension by helping them to draw inferences about the . . . concepts encountered in texts that are related to knowledge they have already acquired. Thus, children who have acquired a great deal of world knowledge and/or domain specific knowledge, and well-elaborated schemata representing both types of knowledge, are better equipped to comprehend and profit from text drawing upon such knowledge than children who have acquired less world knowledge or domain-specific knowledge. (p. 64)

Cognitive and Metacognitive Strategies

Whether they engage in through-the-air or print discourses, the possession of vocabulary and prior knowledge is necessary, but not sufficient—especially for the development of comprehension or even of literate thought. Children and adolescents need to know how, what, and when to apply such information. Obviously, as discussed in Chapter 5, this is also important for critico-creative thinking. Essentially, there is a need to use or develop cognitive and metacognitive strategies.

Cognitive strategies are consciously controlled mechanisms or procedures for accomplishing goals such as understanding what is being read, studying for an exam, or solving a problem. General cognitive strategies include critical analysis, inference, reasoning, problem solving and so on (which are also part of the ability to engage in literate thought). Particularly relevant to comprehension, *metacognitive strategies* are routines and procedures allowing individuals to monitor and evaluate their ongoing performance in accomplishing a cognitive task (Dole, Nokes, & Drits, 2009). Metacognitive strategies are employed by good readers to think about and maintain control over their reading.

Comprehension monitoring is a critical part of metacognition. Readers who are aware of when they understand and when they do not and then utilize the appropriate strategies to resolve the problems in their understanding are utilizing comprehension monitoring strategies. For example, in using comprehension monitoring, good readers may clarify the purpose of reading and preview the text before reading; examine their understanding, modifying their reading speed to correspond to the difficulty of the text; and finally, verify their understanding of the text afterward (Armbruster et al., 2001). The NRP (2000; see also, McGuinness, 2004, 2005) identified the following effective comprehension monitoring strategies: 1) identifying where the difficulty arises, 2) identifying what the difficulty is, 3) reiterating via paraphrasing the difficult sentence or passage, 4) looking back through the text, and 5) looking forward in the text for information that might assist in resolving the difficulty.

Substantial research evidence has shown that good comprehenders tend to use cognitive and metacognitive strategies more often and more effectively than poor comprehenders. Furthermore, cognitive and metacognitive strategies should be taught directly to children, even for beginning readers and especially for individuals with reading difficulties, to maximize reading success (Baker & Brown, 1984; Israel, 2008; Palincsar & Brown, 1984; Pearson & Fielding, 1991; Pressley, 2000).

Table 6-2 summarizes the areas in vocabulary knowledge and reading comprehension processes that are challenging for children with deficits in written language comprehension.

Table 6-2. Challenging Areas for Children with Deficits in Written Language Comprehension

Vocabulary

Listening Vocabulary:	The words we need to know to understand what we hear.
Speaking Vocabulary:	The words we use when we speak.
Reading Vocabulary:	The words we need to know to understand what we read.
Writing Vocabulary:	The words we use in writing.

Reading Comprehension

Metalinguistic Awareness:	An awareness of language structures.
Syntactic Awareness:	The sensitivity to grammatical form in terms of errors that violate conventional usage in spoken and written language.
Pragmatic Awareness:	The sensitivity to the various ways language is used for purposes of communication.
Prior Knowledge:	A person's knowledge stored in long-term memory.
Passage-specific Prior Knowledge:	Also *discourse knowledge*, the knowledge on the unique properties of different types of texts (narrative vs. expository and informational); knowledge of items (language, topics) within the text.
Topic-specific Prior Knowledge:	Reflects information that is either not explicitly in the text or cannot be inferred from existing text information.
World Knowledge:	Knowledge of events and activities that occur in everyday life involving actual people and factual things that exist in real time and authentic places.
Domain Specific Knowledge:	Knowledge that is unique to a particular content area such as science, social studies, mathematics, sports, entertainment and so on.
Cognitive Strategies:	Consciously controlled mechanisms or procedures for accomplishing cognitive goals such as understanding what is being read, studying for an exam, or solving a problem.
Metacognitive Strategies:	Routines and procedures allowing individuals to monitor and evaluate their ongoing performance in accomplishing a cognitive task.
Comprehension Monitoring:	An awareness of the readers when they understand what they read and when they do not, and the ability to utilize the appropriate strategies to 'fix' the arising problems in their understanding.

Summary of Research

Reading printed texts can be one key source for building new vocabulary, increasing syntactic and pragmatic awareness, advancing discourse-, world-, and domain-specific knowledge, and acquiring cognitive and metacognitive strategies. Children with limited reading experiences therefore often begin to fall behind their peers in language development, which, in turn, further impairs their reading comprehension abilities. Furthermore, "as a result of their limited reading experiences, poor readers who do not necessarily have a developmental language disorder will soon develop language problems" (Catts & Kamhi, 2005, p. 97). Catts and Kamhi also remarked: "Children from low socioeconomic status backgrounds and/or those with language impairments may be at increased risk for reading disabilities if they have not had home literacy experiences" (p. 95).

Finally, as mentioned in Chapter 1, Stanovich (1986, 1988) coined the term *Matthew effects* to describe this phenomenon of *the rich get richer and the poor get poorer* in reading. This concept has been used to justify the inclusion of non-print modes for poor or struggling readers to address, at the least, their impoverished acquisition of knowledge (Paul, 2009; Paul & Wang, 2006a, 2006b).

CHILDREN WHO ARE LESS ENGAGED AND LESS INTRINSICALLY MOTIVATED IN READING

To become successful readers, children and adolescents need to be sufficiently engaged and motivated to read frequently. As noted by Miller and Faircloth (2009):

> To become strategic, students needed both skill and will. Will represented the motivational intent to become engaged with reading, to continue reading to reach goals, and to persist through difficulties. Motivation was no longer a simple incentive to energize a set of predetermined behaviors; instead, it resulted from learner's expectancies, values, and beliefs. Ultimately, motivation determined the extent to which students became engaged or disengaged in the learning process. Students would be unsuccessful if they acquired the necessary cognitive and metacognitive abilities yet lacked the motivation to become engaged (or vice versa). (p. 308)

It thus is not enough to simply possess knowledge on the various reading strategies (i.e., *declarative knowledge*), knowledge on how to employ reading strategies (i.e., *procedural knowledge*), or knowledge on when and why to apply certain strategies (i.e., *conditional knowledge*). Readers must have the willingness or motivation to actually use the various strategies (Dole et al., 2009).

Children who are less engaged and less intrinsically motivated might suffer from their deficits in word recognition fluency or written language comprehension, or both, and lack confidence in their abilities. They might get caught in a downward spiral of failure or *swamp* of negative expectations, lowered motivation, and limited practice, which makes it even harder for them to *get back on the right road* (Spear-Swerling & Sternberg, 1994). Teachers should encourage students to become more actively engaged in their learning, and teach or persuade them to realize that reading has personal relevance and meaning for them and that various reading strategies have value and utility.

CHILDREN WITH DEFICITS IN SPEECH

For the purpose of differentiating from children with deficits in written language comprehension, in this chapter, *children with deficits in speech* refers to children with childhood speech disorders that affect articulation and intelligibility of speech to varying degrees. Childhood speech disorders can occur alone or be accompanied by language impairments (e.g., vocabulary and grammar) (McGuinness, 2004, 2005; Snowling & Hulme, 2005). Children with speech disorders accompanied by language impairments might have a similar language and literacy development process as that of children with deficits in written language comprehension, as discussed previously, because of the close relationship between spoken language and written language.

What about children with only speech disorders? Plante and Beeson (2008) categorized childhood speech disorders into *disorders of speech sound production* (e.g., misarticulations), *disorders of fluency* (e.g., stuttering), and *disorders of voice and swallowing* (e.g., voice disorders). Disorders of fluency and of voice and swallowing are typically associated with deficits in peripheral aspects of articulation (e.g., use of speech mechanisms for producing sounds and words). Current available research evidence has suggested that peripheral speech difficulties might carry a low risk of reading problems (McGuinness, 2004, 2005; Snow et al., 1998; Stackhouse, 1982).

There have been some interesting findings from research on the relationship between disorders of the phonological system (e.g., disorders of speech sound production) and reading difficulties. For example, in one of the seminal studies, Catts (1993) followed children with speech-language impairments from kindergarten to second grade and found that, although children with widespread language impairments in kindergarten developed reading difficulties in later grades, children with pure speech disorders did not. Despite conflicting results in a few other studies (Raitano, Pennington, Tunick, Boada, & Shriberg, 2004), the majority of the longitudinal studies with various age groups have reported similar findings. Moreover, research has indicated that once phonemic awareness skill was statistically controlled, neither speech perception nor speech production predicted variation in reading accuracy or spelling skills (Bishop & Adams, 1990; Bishop & Edmundson, 1987; Catts, Fey, Tomblin, & Zhang, 2002; McGuinness, 2004, 2005; Nathan, Stackhouse, Goulandris, & Snowling, 2004; Stothard, Snowling, Bishop, Chipchase, & Kaplan, 1998).

The above discussion indicates that the ability to *hear* phonemes and articulate them properly is not critical in reading. Instead, the primary goal of acquiring phonological knowledge is to understand that phonemes are the building blocks of a language and to obtain the ability to manipulate them (Adams, 1990). Snowling and Hulme (2005) also proposed: "... children who have speech difficulties *that persist to the point at which they need to use phonological skills for learning to read* are at high risk of reading problems ... it appears to be critical that these children's speech difficulties are accompanied by poor phoneme awareness; persisting speech difficulties without deficits in phoneme awareness (which only occurred in 4/19 children) do not appear to impact on reading ... [Emphasis added in the original]" (p. 403).

It should be underscored that phonology is the scaffold of learning a language, particularly a phonemic-based language such as English. Whether children and adolescents are expected to engage with through-the-air or captured forms of information, they need to obtain a proficient level of language use on which these forms are based. Phonology facilitates the development of other components of English as well as the development of beginning and advanced English reading (and writing) skills. As discussed in Chapters 7 to 9, developing phonological knowledge remains one of the most challenging areas for theorists, researchers, and educators.

LITERATE THOUGHT AND LANGUAGE/LEARNING DISABILITIES

So far, we have discussed four major groups of children with language/learning disabilities: children with deficits 1) in word recognition and 2) in written language comprehension; 3) children who are less engaged and less intrinsically motivated in reading; and 4) children with speech disorders. Many children have deficits in more than one area. When a child persistently fails to construct meaning from printed texts, s/he might eventually lose interest and motivation in reading. Limited experiences with reading, in turn, lead to a deprived vocabulary bank, insensitive metalinguistic awareness, limited discourse knowledge, world knowledge, or domain specific knowledge in long-term memory, and inexperienced use of cognitive and metacognitive strategies.

It is a swamp that is difficult to escape. Unfortunately, for many children with language/learning disabilities, for example, children with dyslexia, the phonological difficulty is neurobiological in origin. The degree of reading impairment in older children with severe phonologically-based reading disabilities thus can only be largely stabilized instead of completely remediated by intense interventions. This seems to lend support to a corollary deficit hypothesis, rather than one (e.g., Developmental Lag or the Qualitative-Similarity Hypothesis; see Chapter 4) based on Stanovich's *Matthew effects*, mentioned previously.

How can children with language/learning disabilities escape the mire of reading difficulty? To answer this question, we first need to explore the purpose of reading. Is the ultimate goal of reading to acquire the skill of constructing meaning from print or is it to acquire and later utilize the information from print? As discussed in Chapters 1 and 2 of this book, the ability to obtain and utilize literate information (i.e., to exhibit literate thought) is or should be the goal of literacy education, and the ability to read and write is only one of the means of being literate instead of the ends of being literate.

The *New and Multiple Literacies* model reconceptualizes literacy to emphasize its inherent plurality and multimodality (Harste, 2009; Masny, 2009; see also Chapter 3). Consequently, literacy evolves from a set of technical skills (i.e., reading and writing) to the use of literate information in its broadest sense (e.g., oral, visual, written, digital, etc.) (Tafaghodtari, 2009). It should be remembered that providing children and adolescents with multiple access is only one part of the equation, they still need to develop and use their interpretation skills to construct meaning and to apply it to other situations.

To exemplify our points, we return to the excerpt from Street (1984) quoted at the beginning of the chapter: "Many students who had blamed themselves for their 'failure' to learn to read and write came to recognize that the system had failed them" (p. 15). Similarly, Olson (1994) argued that the current predominant focus on the reading and writing skills of students seriously underestimates the significance of understanding that students bring to school as well as the importance of oral discourse in turning that into consciousness, or in other words, in turning it into an object of knowledge. The amount of time students spend on remedial reading exercises might be more appropriately spent acquiring and debating philosophical and scientific information.

The subsequent section is divided into three parts to discuss the following questions: 1) Can children with language/learning disabilities obtain and utilize information in modalities other than print? 2) Can skills acquired in other modalities of literacy be used to improve print literacy skills (see also, Chapter 2)? And 3) What are the instructional applications of the New and Multiple Literacies?

Can Children with Language/Learning Disabilities Obtain and Utilize Information in Modalities Other Than Print?

Disagreeing with Goody's (1977) reference to writing as *the technology of the intellect*, Street (1984) maintained: "No one material feature serves to define literacy itself" (p. 97). He insisted that although writing and speech are different, it does not necessarily mean that one is superior to the other. Snow, Griffin, and Burns (2005) summarized 15 different features between spoken language and written language. The decontextualization feature of written language is one of the most researched features (e.g., Nagy & Scott, 2000; Snow, 1991, 1994).

As discussed in Chapter 1, *decontextualization* asserts that communication success relies more heavily on the language itself, rather than shared knowledge or context. Contextualized language (also Chapter 1) such as spoken language can use gestures, intonations, and allusions to share knowledge or context. Decontextualized language such as written language has to be precise in choice of words and syntactical structures, which is the primary reason for the title of *the technology of the intellect* for written language.

The advance of technology makes it possible for speech (or sign) to be recorded in a CD, DVD, or MP3, and the captured information can be distributed on the Internet as a podcast (see Chapter 3). The author of the podcast can use decontextualized language in the speech-recorded mode in the audio/video file, and this is similar to writing the speech down. The emerging speech-to-text software further blurs the boundaries between the New and Multiple Literacies and traditional print literacy. If speech can be captured and utilized in a way similar to traditional script literacy, the *magic power* of script literacy disappears, and script literacy should only be considered as *one*, instead of *the*, particular vehicle to record or capture information (Paul, 2009; Paul & Wang, 2006a, 2006b; Wang, 2005).

Compared to written language, speech is easy because sounds are spontaneously produced, and speech progresses through simple play with sounds (Ong, 1967; Saljo, 1988). "Oral speech evolves naturally in the process of social interaction between children and adults" whereas "written speech emerges as the result of special learning" (Luria, 1982, p. 165). Olson (1994) also argued: "Writing is dependent in a fundamental way on speech. One's oral language, it is now recognized, is the fundamental possession and tool of mind; writing, though important, is always secondary" (p. 8). He further asserts:

> We don't want to say that we think in writing. Rather, writing offers us a set of options for cognition, options we choose among when we write. There is no magic about writing. It is not merely transcription, but neither is it a medium that operates independently of speech and thought. Writing, as Gombrich said of art, offers us a formulary into which we insert information. If there is no space on the formulary for a certain kind of information, it is just too bad for that information. Scholars have become increasingly attentive to what our formulary, our writing, leads us to overlook, but we also continue to believe that what it allows us to capture more than compensates for what is lost. Hence, we look forward to a long

literate tradition and with it increased interest in understanding just what all literacy involves. (p. 292)

Theoretically, it therefore is possible for children with language/learning disabilities (and others; see Chapters 7 to 9) to obtain and utilize literate information in modalities other than print. What about the practicality of this notion? As discussed previously in this chapter, word recognition accounted for the majority of variance in reading comprehension for beginning readers, especially children with language/learning disabilities. If the extra layer of decoding process is removed from the comprehension process, many children with language/learning disabilities without specific language impairments might be able to develop their literate thought in a mode that they are most comfortable with, most probably in speech.

As mentioned previously, this development is still pervasively contingent on a level of proficiency in the primary or through-the-air language form. In addition, these children do need to develop general language comprehension skills such as making inferences, drawing conclusion, synthesizing, and so on. This leads to our next question.

Can Skills Acquired in Other Modalities of Literacy Be Used to Improve Print Literacy Skills?

Instead of being modality-specific, early general comprehension skills range across a variety of media, which includes oral stories and televised narratives (Oakhill & Cain, 2007). These comprehension skills develop simultaneously with basic language skills. Children should not wait until being proficient in decoding print to begin receiving instruction in oral language comprehension skills (e.g., vocabulary, syntax, inference making, comprehension monitoring, etc.). Unfortunately, current early script literacy practice often focuses on the teaching of decoding skills to the omission of other general language and comprehension skills. Cain and Oakhill (2007) remarked:

> It is clear that we must be careful not to focus solely on word-reading skills in beginning reading instruction. Reading comprehension will not develop automatically and effortlessly once children have been taught to read words, and we need to consider how comprehension skills can be nurtured from an early age . . . children use the same skills to understand the causal structure of events in written, televised, and cartoon-based narratives. Work to engage children in the identification of causality, main events, and the extraction of the gist can be conducted with different media at differ-

ent ages. Many of the suggestions for skills-based teaching to remediate comprehension problems can be incorporated into the daily classroom for all children. (p. 292)

Cain and Oakhill further suggested that there is no distinction between *comprehension* of written text or spoken discourse in theories of comprehension: they both share the same general comprehension process (see also, Chapter 2). The outcome of skilled comprehension in either written text or spoken discourse is literate thought, rather than a particular technology to insert or retrieve information.

Many children with specific language impairments can recognize words in print fluently but lack the linguistic comprehension to construct meaning from what they have decoded. They have deficits in general comprehension processes, rather than the process of understanding information presented in a specific modality. For example, children fail to generate the necessary inferences to construct a coherent representation of meaning, which involves more than simply memorizing word and sentence meanings. They have difficulty in integrating ideas both within the text and from their background knowledge.

Children with specific language impairments typically do not use comprehension monitoring to alert them of the need to generate an inference. Specifically, they lack the explicit awareness of the discourse, syntax, or pragmatics to invoke relevant prior knowledge and schemas to facilitate the construction of meaning. Most components of the reading comprehension process discussed earlier in this chapter (i.e., metalinguistic awareness, prior knowledge, cognitive and metacognitive strategies) are involved in comprehending both spoken discourse and written text. Comprehension skills acquired in other modalities of literacy (e.g., speech or sign literacy) thus can be used to improve comprehension skills associated with print literacy.

We should end with a caveat: We do not mean to imply that general comprehension skills are sufficient for understanding printed texts for all (or even most) children with language and literacy difficulties or even for most children with other disabilities or conditions. Clearly, such skills are necessary, but for a number of children, there will be the need to address specific access challenges such as decoding and other identification areas. Nevertheless, decoding or other access skills should not impede the development of higher-level comprehension ability, particularly if the goal is literate thought.

What Are the Instructional Applications of the New and Multiple Literacies?

In our view, the New and Multiple Literacies (see also, Chapter 3) might offer the most viable option for developing literate thought in many children with language and literacy disabilities (and for other children with disabilities). One type, digital literacy such as hypertext, has received increasing attention due to its unique nonlinearity and multidimensionality (e.g., Spiro, 2006). "Digital hypertext affords multilayered and multimedia-based spaces to move across and within" (Tierney, 2009, p. 262). The *digitally-afforded multimodality* of hypertext integrates printed words with images, sound, music, and movements to assist reading (and general language) comprehension, which is an obvious advantage over printed words only.

Tierney (2009) concluded:

> Several literacy scholars have noted that access to multimedia tools (e.g., digital video) enhances youth's explorations, expression and expansion of their sense of identity. By affording students access to these multimedia environments spaces, Rogers and Winters (2006), Alvermann, Hagood, and Williams (2001), Hull and Nelson (2006), and Hudak, Hull, and James (in press) have argued that students are afforded the possibility of having their literacy practices travel across spaces, in and out of schools, blurring traditional boundaries and forms of literate practices. (p. 268)

Meanwhile, the *intertextual* and *multilayered* nature of hypertext requires the reader to plan within and across Web sites, to predict and follow leads, to monitor how and where to proceed, and to evaluate relevance and judging merits, all of which can be excellent practices for improving comprehension monitoring skills. Furthermore, because different readers might click on different links and proceed through the text in completely different sequences, hypertext is considered *nonlinear* and highly *interactive* (Kist, 2005; see also, Chapter 3).

A number of studies have demonstrated the advantages of using digital tools as scaffolding for learning (e.g., Kinzer & Leu, 1997). It should be emphasized that although multimodality and multilayered hypertext can provide a framework for the comprehension process; it also adds demands on the literacy skills of the reader. For example, the reader needs to be able to integrate the meaning of the multimedia document with the meaning of the printed text. The reader must decide whether or not to explore the links, and know how to navigate and return to the original page, both of which require a higher-level of cognitive and metacognitive skills (Kamil & Chou, 2009; see also, Chapter 3).

Kamil and Chou (2009) provided an example of how to use a podcast as an instructional tool in building students' vocabulary. For instance, the teacher can create a podcast of key vocabulary terms and concepts using a variety of audio and visual (e.g., slides) information on a weekly basis. Students can subscribe to the podcast and download the files onto their computers, MP3 players or CDs. They can be required to listen to the podcast before the lesson for pre-teaching difficult and key vocabulary words, which is an effective strategy for students, particularly those with language/learning disabilities. Students can also periodically revisit the archived podcasts to review learned vocabularies. Readers should refer to Kist (2010) for other tips on how to use Facebook, Twitter, blogs, and so forth to create a socially networked classroom.

It is worth emphasizing that the New and Multiple Literacies do not have to be completely dependent on technology; that is, *old fashioned* forms such as dance, music, and painting can be used as well. In addition, the mere presence of technology in a classroom does not necessarily transform the classroom into a New and Multiple Literacies classroom (Kist, 2005). Kist (2005) identified the following characteristics of New and Multiple Literacies classrooms: 1) classrooms feature daily work in multiple forms of representation; 2) there are explicit discussions of the merits of using particular symbol systems in particular situations; 3) there are metadialogues by the teacher who models working through problems using certain symbol systems; 4) students take part in a mix of individual and collaborative activities; and 5) classrooms are places of extensive student engagement activities.

Kist (2005) reported the findings of six case studies of New and Multiple Literacies classrooms in North America. One example, is an interdisciplinary Arts Seminar classroom at Parma High School in Parma, Ohio, where non-print media was used instead of the traditional lecture-based, paper-and-pencil assessed methods to cover the college preparatory content. The school was in a blue-collar neighborhood, and the classroom was not dominated by technology or news media at all. The class was team-taught by an art teacher, a music teacher, and an English teacher.

The elements of the Arts Seminar included project-based classroom work, student-led research, culminating presentations in multiple forms, and an assessment of product and process. For example, one of the class assignments was to design a monument for a person, event, or a phenomenon. One group of students had selected to pay tribute to Dr. Seuss. The challenge of the assignment was that the monument had to be designed in an entirely abstract fashion, and it could not be figurative in nature. That is, the students could not use a sculpture of Dr. Seuss or one of the characters from his books. Kist (2005) reported that the students used shapes such as spheres on the monument, and they were debating what each of the balls could represent of the life of Dr. Seuss.

Based on the interview transcripts from teachers and students, as well as the researcher's observation field notes, four major themes of students' achievements emerged from the data: 1) understanding of content; 2) understanding of symbol systems and forms of expression; 3) fluency; and 4) collaboration. "Overall, students appreciated that Arts Seminar centered around projects that required some application of knowledge and that it was empowering and gave them a sense of ownership. Students also appreciated that the class was interdisciplinary and that it was collaborative, both for students and teachers. Many students also cited that the course was fun and engaging as reasons for their learning more" (Kist, 2005, p. 41). In particular, students with language/learning disabilities or who were extremely shy and had great difficulty communicating reported that the class was enabling them to be free to communicate using alternative forms.

In sum, the research on the New and Multiple Literacies in classroom settings is still in its infancy, and much more is needed before we can fully evaluate its efficiency for children with language/learning disabilities (and for other children). The instructional value of the New and Multiple Literacies has great potential, however; in fact, we reiterate that this area might offer some of the best benefits for developing literate thought in these children. The success of this development is also contingent on what we have presented with respect to disciplinary structures (Chapter 4) and critico-creative thinking (Chapter 5). And, as discussed in the next set of chapters (Chapters 7 to 9), adjustments and modifications are necessary for children with other specific types of disabilities.

SUMMARY

The purpose of this chapter is to highlight the challenges of developing literate language in children with language/learning disabilities and to argue for the use of different types of literacy with this population; that is, literacies that do not depend on print. The chapter concluded with specific implications for developing literate thought using the New and Multiple Literacies.

A few of the major points expounded in this chapter are as follows.

- *Learning disability* is a general term typically used to refer to a collection of different types of learning problems, such as in reading, in mathematics, or in social/behavioral learning. *Language/learning disability* is used to specifically describe spoken and written language deficits. *Reading disability* is an even narrower term for different kinds of deficits in learning to read.
- Children with language/learning disabilities can be categorized as: 1) children with deficits in word recognition; 2) children with deficits in written language comprehension; 3) children who are less engaged and less intrinsically motivated in reading; and 4) children with deficits in spoken language (i.e., speech). The boundaries of these categories can be blurred in cases where an individual might have difficulties in multiple areas.
- Fluency in word recognition is a prerequisite for adequate reading comprehension.
- Children with deficits in written language comprehension typically have impoverished vocabulary knowledge and show a range of deficits during reading comprehension processes, which include impairments in metalinguistic awareness and prior knowledge as well as the use of cognitive and metacognitive strategies.
- It is not enough to simply possess knowledge on the various reading strategies (i.e., *declarative knowledge*), knowledge on how to employ reading strategies (i.e., *procedural knowledge*), or knowledge on when and why to apply certain strategies (i.e., *conditional knowledge*). Readers must have the willingness or motivation to actually use the various strategies.
- Once phonemic awareness skill is statistically controlled, neither speech perception nor speech production predicts variation in reading accuracy or spelling skills. Children with pure speech disorders therefore generally do not develop reading difficulties.
- The ability to obtain and utilize literate information (i.e., to exhibit literate thought) is or should be the goal of literacy education, and

the ability to read and write is only one of the many means of being literate instead of the ends of being literate.

- Children with language/learning disabilities can obtain and utilize information in modalities other than print. Skills acquired in other modalities of literacy can be used to improve general language comprehension skills associated with print literacy. The instructional applications of the New and Multiple Literacies represent one potential for developing literate thought in these children.

QUESTIONS FOR REFLECTION AND DISCUSSION

1. Describe the concept of an *ideological model of literacy*. What are the implications for the development of literate thought?

2. Discuss a few major highlights in the sections on the development of language and literacy for the *four* groups of children with language/learning disabilities.

3. How do the issues for each of the four groups (in question 2) relate to the three broad areas for reading difficulties as mentioned by the National Reading Panel?

4. What are the authors' responses (i.e., describe their major points) to the following questions discussed during the last part of the chapter?
    a. Can children with language/learning disabilities obtain and utilize information in modalities other than print?
    b. Can skills acquired in other modalities of literacy be used to improve print literacy skills?
    c. What are the instructional applications of the New and Multiple Literacies?

REFERENCES

Adams, M. (1990). *Beginning to read: Thinking and learning about print.* Cambridge, MA: The MIT Press.

Anderson, R. (1984). Role of the reader's schema in comprehension, learning, and memory. In R. C. Anderson, J. Osborn, & R. J. Tierney (Eds.), *Learning to read in American schools* (pp. 243-258). Hillsdale, NJ: Erlbaum.

Armbruster, B. B., Lehr, F., & Osborn, J. (2001). *Put reading first: The research building blocks for teaching children to read kindergarten through grade three.* Jessup, MD: National Institute for Literacy.

Baddeley, A. (1986). *Working memory.* Oxford, UK: Clarendon Press.

Baddeley, A. (1990). *Human memory: Theory and practice.* Hillsdale, NJ: Lawrence Erlbaum.

Baker, L., & Brown, A. (1984). Metacognition skills and reading. In P. D. Pearson, R. Barr, M. Kamil, & P. Mosenthal (Eds.), *Handbook of reading research* (pp. 353-394). White Plains, NY: Longman.

Bishop, D. V. M., & Adams, C. (1990). A prospective study of the relationship between specific language impairment, phonological disorders and reading retardation. *Journal of Child Psychology and Psychiatry, 31,* 1027-1050.

Bishop, D. V. M., & Edmundson, A. (1987). Language-impaired 4-year-olds: Distinguishing transient from persistent impairment. *Journal of Speech and Hearing Disorders, 52,* 156-173.

Cain, K., & Oakhill, J. (2007). Cognitive bases of children's language comprehension difficulties: Where do we go from here? In K. Cain & J. Oakhill (Eds.), *Children's comprehension problems in oral and written language: A cognitive perspective* (pp. 283-295). New York: The Guilford Press.

Catts, H. W. (1993). The relationship between speech-language and reading disabilities. *Journal of Speech and Hearing Research, 36,* 948-958.

Catts, H. W., Fey, M. E., Tomblin, J. B., & Zhang, X. (2002). A longitudinal investigation of reading outcomes in children with language impairments. *Journal of Speech, Hearing, and Language Research, 45,* 1142-1157.

Catts, H. W., Hogan, T. P., & Adlof, A. M. (2005). Developmental changes in reading and reading disabilities. In H. W. Catts & A. G. Kamhi (Eds.), *Connections between language and reading disabilities* (pp. 25-40). Mahwah, NJ: Erlbaum.

Catts, H. W., & Kamhi, A. G. (2005). Defining reading disabilities. In H. W. Catts & A. G. Kamhi (Eds.), *Language and reading disabilities* (pp. 50-71). Boston, MA: Pearson Education, Inc.

Dewitz, P., Carr, T., & Patberg, J. (1987). Effects of inference training on comprehension and comprehension monitoring. *Reading Research Quarterly, 22,* 99-121.

Dole, J. A., Nokes, J. D., & Drits, D. (2009). Cognitive strategy instruction. In S. E. Israel & G. G. Duffy (Eds.), *Handbook of research on reading comprehension* (pp. 347-372). New York: Routledge.

Ehri, L. (2002). Phases of acquisition in learning to read words and implications for teaching. In R. Stainthorp & P. Tomlinson (Eds.), *Learning and teaching reading* (pp. 7-28). London: British Journal of Educational Psychology Monograph Series II.

Ehri, L., & Robbins, C. (1992). Beginners need some decoding skill to read words by analogy. *Reading Research Quarterly, 27,* 12-26.

Goody, J. (1977). *The domestication of the savage mind.* New York: Cambridge University Press.

Gough, P., & Walsh, S. (1991). Chinese, Phoenicians, and the orthographic cipher of English. In S. Brady & D. Shankweiler (Eds.), *Phonological processes in literacy: A tribute to Isabelle Y. Liberman* (pp. 199-209). Hillsdale, NJ: Erlbaum.

Harste, J. C. (2009). Multimodality in perspective. In J. V. Hoffman & Y. Goodman (Eds.), *Changing literacies for changing times: An historical perspective on the future of reading research, public policy, and classroom practices* (pp. 34-48). New York: Routledge.

Hart, B., & Risley, T. R. (1999). *The social world of children learning to talk.* Baltimore, MD: Brookes.

Hoover, W., & Gough, P. B. (1990). The simple view of reading. *Reading and Writing: An Interdisciplinary Journal, 2,* 127-160.

Israel, S. E. (2008). Flexible use of comprehension monitoring strategies: Investigating what a complex reading framework might look like. In K. B. Cartwright (Ed.), *Literacy processes: Cognitive flexibility in learning and teaching* (pp. 188-207). New York: Guilford Press.

Kamil, M. L., & Chou, H. K. (2009). Comprehension and computer technology: Past results, current knowledge, and future promises. In S. E. Israel & G. G. Duffy (Eds.), *Handbook of research on reading comprehension* (pp. 289-304). New York: Routledge.

Kavale, K. A. (1988). The long-term consequences of learning disabilities. In M. C. Wang, H. J. Walburg, & M. C. Reynolds (Eds.), *The handbook of special education: Research and practice* (pp. 303-344). New York: Pergamon Press.

Kinzer, C., & Leu, D. (1997). The challenge of change: Exploring literacy and learning in electronic environments. *Language Arts, 74*(2), 126-136.

Kist, W. (2005). *New literacies in action: Teaching and learning in multiple media.* New York: Teachers College Press.

Kist, W. (2010). *The socially networked classroom: Teaching in the new media age.* Thousand Oaks, CA: Corwin.

Luria, A. R. (1982). *Language and cognition.* Washington, DC: V. H. Winston & Sons.

Lyon, G. R., Shaywitz, S. E., & Shaywitz, B. A. (2003). A definition of dyslexia. *Annals of Dyslexia, 53,* 1-14.

Masny, D. (2009). Literacies as becoming: A child's conceptualizations of writing systems. In D. Masny & D. R. Cole (Eds.), *Multiple literacies theory: A Deleuzian perspective* (pp. 13-30). Rotterdam, The Netherlands: Sense Publishers.

McAnally, P. L., Rose, S., & Quigley, S. P. (2007). *Reading practices with deaf learners.* Austin, Texas: PRO-ED.

McGuinness, D. (2004). *Early reading instruction: What science really tells us about how to teach reading.* Cambridge, MA: The MIT Press.

McGuinness, D. (2005). *Language development and learning to read: The scientific study of how language development affects reading skill.* Cambridge, MA: The MIT Press.

McKinney, J. D. (1990). Longitudinal research on the behavioral characteristics of children with learning disabilities. In J. Torgesen (Ed.), *Cognitive and behavioral characteristics of children with learning disabilities* (pp. 165-172). Austin, TX: PRO-ED.

Miller, S. D., & Faircloth, B. S. (2009). Motivation and reading comprehension. In S. E. Israel & G. G. Duffy (Eds.), *Handbook of research on reading comprehension* (pp. 307-322). New York: Routledge.

Nagy, W. E., & Scott, J. A. (2000). Vocabulary processes. In M. L. Kamil, P. B. Mosenthal, P. D. Pearson, & R. Barr (Eds.), *Handbook of reading research* (Volume III) (pp. 269-284), Mahwah, NJ: Lawrence Erlbaum Associates.

Nathan, L., Stackhouse, J., Goulandris, N., & Snowling, M. J. (2004). The development of early literacy skills among children with speech difficulties: A test of the "Critical Age Hypothesis". *Journal of Speech, Language and Hearing Research, 47*, 377-391.

National Reading Panel (NRP). (2000). *Report of the National Reading Panel: Teaching children to read – An evidence-based Assessment of the scientific research literature on reading and its implications for reading instruction.* Jessup, MD: National Institute for Literacy at EDPubs.

Oakhill, J., & Cain, K. (2007). Introduction to comprehension development. In K. Cain & J. Oakhill (Eds.), *Children's comprehension problems in oral and written language: A cognitive perspective* (pp. 3-40). New York: The Guilford Press.

Olson, D. (1994). *The world on paper.* New York, NY: Cambridge University Press.

Ong, W. (1967). *The presence of the word – Some prolegomena for cultural and religious history.* New Haven, CT and London: Yale University Press.

Palincsar, A. S., & Brown, A. L. (1984). Reciprocal teaching of comprehension-fostering and comprehension-monitoring activities. *Cognition and Instruction, 1*, 117-175.

Paul, P. (2009). *Language and deafness* (4th ed.). Sudbury, MA: Jones & Bartlett.

Paul, P., & Wang, Y. (2006a). Multiliteracies and literate thought. *Theory into Practice, 45*(4), 304-310.

Paul, P., & Wang, Y. (2006b). Literate thought and deafness: A call for a new perspective and line of research on literacy. *Punjab University Journal of Special Education* (Pakistan), *2*(1), 28-37.

Pearson, P. D., & Fielding, L. (1991). Comprehension instruction. In R. Barr, M. Kamil, P. Mosenthal, & P. D. Pearson (Eds.), *Handbook of reading research* (2nd ed., pp. 815-860). New York: Longman.

Perfetti, C. A. (1985). *Reading ability.* New York: Oxford University Press.

Perfetti, C. A., Landi, N., & Oakhill, J. (2005). The acquisition of reading comprehension skill. In M. J. Snowling & C. Hulme (Eds.), *The science of reading: A handbook* (pp. 227-247). Malden, MA: Blackwell Publishing.

Plante, E., & Beeson, P. M. (2008). *Communication and communication disorders: A clinical introduction* (3rd ed.). Boston, MA: Pearson Education.

Pressley, M. (2000). What should comprehension instruction be the instruction of? In M. L. Kamil, P. B. Mosenthal, P. D. Pearson, & R. Barr (Eds.), *Handbook of reading research* (Vol. III, pp. 545-560). Mahwah, NJ: Erlbaum.

Raitano, N. A., Pennington, B. F., Tunick, R. A., Boada, R., & Shriberg, L. D. (2004). Preliteracy skills of subgroup of children with speech sound disorder. *Journal of Child Psychology and Psychiatry, 45*, 821-835.

Saljo, R. (Ed.). (1988). *The written world – Studies in literate thought and action.* Berlin, Germany: Springer-Verlag.

Schumaker, J. B., Deshler, D. D., & Ellis, E. S. (1986). Intervention issues related to the education of learning disabled adolescents. In J. K. Torgesen & B. Y. L.

Wong (Eds.), *Psychological and educational perspectives on learning disabilities* (pp. 329-365). New York: Academic Press.

Snow, C. E. (1991). The theoretical basis for relationships between language and literacy development. *Journal of Research in Childhood Education, 6,* 5-10.

Snow, C. E. (1994). What is so hard about learning to read? A pragmatic analysis. In J. Duchan, L. Hewitt, & R. Sonnenmeier (Eds.), *Pragmatics: Form theory to practice* (pp. 164-184). Englewood Cliffs, NJ: Prentice Hall.

Snow, C. E., Burns, M. S., & Griffin, P. (1998). *Preventing reading difficulties in young children.* Washington, DC: National Academy Press.

Snow, C. E., Griffin, P., & Burns, M. S. (2005). *Knowledge to support the teaching of reading: Preparing teachers for a changing world.* San Francisco, CA: John Wiley & Sons, Inc.

Snowling, M., & Hulme, C. (Eds.). (2005). *The science of reading: A handbook.* Malden, MA: Blackwell.

Spear-Swerling, L., & Sternberg, R. J. (1994). The road not taken: An integrative theoretical model of reading disability. *Journal of Learning Disabilities, 27,* 91-103.

Spiro, R. J. (2006). The "New Gutenberg Revolution": Radical new learning, thinking, teaching, and training with technology. *Educational Technology, 46*(1), 3-4.

Stackhouse, J. (1982). An investigation of reading and spelling performance in speech disordered children. *British Journal of Disorders of Communication, 17,* 53-60.

Stahl, S., & Nagy, W. (2006). *Teaching word meanings.* Mahwah, NJ: Erlbaum.

Stanovich, K. E. (1986). Matthew effects in reading: Some consequences of individual differences in the acquisition of literacy. *Reading Research Quarterly, 86,* 360-406.

Stanovich, K. E. (1988). *Children's reading and the development of phonological awareness.* Detroit, MI: Wayne State University Press.

Stothard, S. E., Snowling, M. J., Bishop, D. V. M., Chipchase, B., & Kaplan, C. (1998). Language impaired pre-schoolers: A follow-up in adolescence. *Journal of Speech, Language and Hearing Research, 41,* 407-418.

Street, B. (1984). *Literacy in theory and practice.* New York: Cambridge University Press.

Tafaghodtari, M. H. (2009). Experimenting with multiple-literacies theory. In D. Masny & D. R. Cole (Eds.), *Multiple literacies theory: A Deleuzian perspective* (pp. 151-166). Rotterdam, The Netherlands: Sense Publishers.

Tierney, R. J. (2009). The agency and artistry of meaning makers within and across digital spaces. In S. E. Israel & G. G. Duffy (Eds.), *Handbook of research on reading comprehension* (pp. 261-288). New York: Routledge.

Torgesen, J. K. (2005). Recent discoveries on remedial interventions for children with dyslexia. In M. J. Snowling & C. Hulme (Eds.), *The science of reading: A handbook* (pp. 521-537). Malden, MA: Blackwell Publishing.

Torgesen, J. K., Otaiba, S. A., & Grek, M. L. (2005). Assessment and instruction for phonemic awareness and word recognition skills. In H. W. Catts & A. G. Kamhi (Eds.), *Language and reading disabilities* (pp. 127-156). Boston, MA: Pearson Education, Inc.

Torgesen, J. K., Rashotte, C. A., & Alexander, A. (2001). Principles of fluency instruction in reading: Relationships with established empirical outcomes. In M. Wolf (Ed.), *Dyslexia, fluency, and the brain* (pp. 333-355). Parkton, MD: York Press.

Trezek, B., Wang, Y., & Paul, P. (2010). *Reading and deafness: Theory, research and practice.* Clifton Park, NY: Cengage Learning.

Vellutino, F. R. (2003). Individual differences as sources of variability in reading comprehension in elementary school children. In A. P. Sweet & C. E. Snow (Eds.), *Rethinking reading comprehension* (pp. 51-81). New York: The Guilford Press.

Wang, Y. (2005). *Literate thought: Metatheorizing in literacy and deafness.* Unpublished doctoral dissertation, Ohio State University, Columbus.

FURTHER READING

Gee, J. (1996). *Social linguistics and literacy: Ideology in discourse* (2nd ed.). New York: Taylor & Francis.

Goody, J. (1987). *The interface between the written and the oral.* New York: Cambridge University Press.

Hoffman, J. V., & Goodman, Y. M. (2009). *Changing literacies for changing times: An historical perspective on the future of reading research, public policy, and classroom practices.* New York: Routledge.

Ong, W. (2002). *Orality and literacy.* New York: Routledge.

Street, B. (2001). *Literacy and development: ethnographic perspectives.* New York: Routledge.

CHAPTER 7

Children with Sensory Disabilities

To completely analyze what we do when we read would almost be the acme of a psychologist's dream for it would be to describe very many of the most intricate workings of the human mind as well as to unravel the tangled story of the most remarkable specific performance that civilization has learned in all of its history.

Huey, 1908/1968, p. 8

The question "Why do we use language?" seems hardly to require an answer. But, as is often the way with linguistic questions, our everyday familiarity with speech and writing can make it difficult to appreciate the complexity of the skills, we have learned. This is particularly so when we try to define the range of functions to which language can be put.

Crystal, 1997, p. 10

The juxtaposition of the two passages above is deliberate. On the one hand, one can imagine the possible connections among speech, language, reading, and writing. On the other hand, like it or not, much of the current focus in early literacy development is on the development of reading (and writing) via the use of print or Braille (National Early Literacy Panel [NELP], 2008). Whether the *wonders* of the human mind can be revealed by understanding the manner in which one learns and uses the conventions of language or those of literacy—print, Braille, and so on—is certainly open to question.

Nevertheless, understanding children with sensory disabilities complicates the above scenario and, at the least, adds to our contention that literate thought is or should be the main goal of education. The contributions of vision or hearing or both to the development of language and literacy have certainly captured the attention of researchers and schol-ars (Crystal, 1997; Paul & Whitelaw, 2011; Wang, Kretschmer, & Hart-man, 2008; Wormsley, 2008). Given the fact that some—perhaps, many—children who are blind or visually impaired can develop a high level of auditory or listening comprehension and that some deaf (i.e., severely-to-profoundly hearing impaired) children can develop strong sign comprehension skills, it may be that the predominant focus on print liter-acy or even Braille is misplaced in light of our model of literate thought.

Although it is difficult to define reading (see Chapter 4), we highlight a few aspects of the Adams (1990) model as a broad backdrop for some of our ensuing points. Adams argued that the reading process involves a circular connection of four processors—orthographic, phonological, meaning, and context—which are operating concurrently during reading after a sensory modality acquires encoded information from the outside. For example, during skillful visual reading, when light from the printed page is reflected onto the retinas, it is transferred to the brain for direct visual processing (i.e., orthographic processing). The brain applies higher cognitive functions that stimulate the orthographic processing and phonological translation simultaneously in word recognition. Meanwhile, meanings are attached to the arbitrary symbols to make sense of the word. In tandem, information from the context speeds up the reader's ability to comprehend the word. Orthographic, phonological, meaning, and con-textual processing thus occur harmoniously at the same time during read-ing of print information.

Figure 7-1 provides an illustration of the four processors for reading.

By creating an effective medium for sharing information, reading (and writing) has become an important *cultural invention* (Steinman, LeJeune, & Kimbrough, 2006). When vision is not available for script or print lit-eracy, as in the case of individuals with visual impairment, will there be an alternative sensory modality for orthographic processing? If so, then what is the impact of this alternative orthographic processing on developing reading? Similarly, when hearing is not available to readers, as in the case of individuals with hearing impairment, will there be an alternative sen-sory modality for phonological processing? If so, then what is the impact of this alternative phonological processing on the development of reading?

Orthographic processing obtains input from outside. Can ortho-graphic processing bypass phonological processing and be directly con-nected with meaning and context processing? If sensory impairments

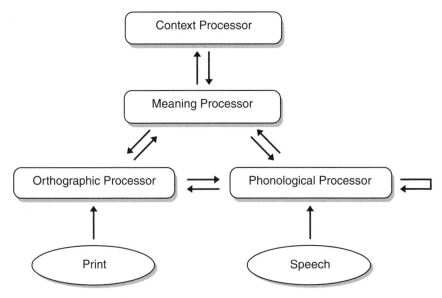

Figure 7-1. The four processors for reading.
Source: Adapted from Adams (1990).

prevent children from reading (print, Braille, etc.) as well as their peers without sensory disabilities, can they benefit equally from other effective media, particularly in the non-print modes, for sharing information?

This chapter provides tentative answers to the above questions. Before proceeding, we should emphasize again the challenges of categorizing children's abilities or disabilities in reading. There is no *typical* profile that fits all children who are blind or have low vision or those who are d/Deaf or hard of hearing. In short, we are dealing with heterogeneous populations—even though one could argue for fundamentals via the Qualitative-Similarity Hypothesis (QSH; see Chapter 4; see also, Paul, 2008; Paul & Lee, 2010).

This chapter uses a parallel structure to explore the challenges of developing language and literacy for children with visual or hearing impairment. For each group, we start with a general introduction of reading achievement and development and compare this to that of typical sighted or hearing readers. Then we investigate the application of the New and Multiple Literacies and conclude with specific implications for developing literate thought.

READING ACHIEVEMENT OF CHILDREN WITH VISUAL IMPAIRMENT

In every 1,000 school-aged children, there is approximately one child with visual impairment in the United States. Most children with visual impairment have low vision and use vision for reading along with tactile and auditory adaptations. Roughly 10% of children with visual impairment are legally blind and use primarily tactile and/or auditory methods of reading and information access (Council for Exceptional Children, n.d.).

Legally blind refers to people who have a central visual acuity of 20/200 or less in the better eye with the best possible correction, or a visual field of 20 degrees or less (American Printing House for the Blind, 2007). In general, children with visual impairment use one or more of the following media for literacy development: 1) standard print (often with decreased viewing distance, increased contrast, and color highlighting; lighting adaptations; or by optical devices such as a hand magnifier); 2) enlarged print; 3) Braille (an alphabet of raised dots read by touch; discussed later in this chapter); and 4) auditory materials (Council for Exceptional Children, n.d.).

Research on the reading achievement of children with visual impairment has mainly focused on Braille readers and has provided a mixed picture (e.g., see review in Wormsley, 2008). Some studies reported no difference or even slightly better reading achievement levels of children with visual impairment compared with those of sighted children (van Bon, Adriaansen, Gompel, & Kouwenberg, 2000; Williams, 1971), whereas others described approximately one year or less delays for children with visual impairment in reading achievement (Daugherty & Moran, 1982; Dodd & Conn, 2000; Douglas, Grimley, McLinden, & Watson, 2004; Fellenius, 1999; Lorimer, 1992; Nolan & Kederis, 1969; Tobin, 1985).

The differences between sighted children and children with visual impairment were not apparent in tasks such as making inference, comprehension, or spelling (Clark & Stoner, 2008; Edmonds & Pring, 2006; Gompel, van Bon, & Schreuder, 2004; Lowenfeld, Abel, & Hatlen, 1968), but differences tended to be found in phonological-related decoding skills (Dodd & Conn, 2000; Gillon & Young, 2002; Gompel, van Bon, Schreuder, & Adriaansen, 2002; Pring, 1982, 1984), which, as discussed later in this chapter, might be related to the orthography (i.e., contractions) of Braille. Furthermore, the phonological-related decoding skills of children with and without visual impairment are qualitatively similar but quantitatively different. For example, poor Braille readers had similar levels of phoneme awareness as those of sighted children who were three years younger but who demonstrated the same level of word-recognition ability (Gillon & Young, 2002). Finally, among children with visual impairment, there were strong relationships between phonological awareness and Braille reading accuracy and reading comprehension (Gillon & Young).

With respect to reading development, it seems that Braille users acquired literacy skills well from kindergarten to about second grade or age 7, when they began to show deficiencies. This is about the same time that many children with visual impairment start to learn contractions and encounter more demanding literacy tasks involving advanced decoding skills (Douglas et al., 2004; Emerson, Holbrook, & D'Andrea, 2009). Interestingly, by the time children with visual impairment reach a reading age of approximately 10 years, the differences between the efficiency of Braille and of print reading are few (Nolan & Kederis, 1969; Pring, 1982, 1984; 1994). It is possible that the mild reading delay of beginning Braille readers could be compensated by extensive literacy practice.

When the medium of testing is taken into consideration, the oral test scores of groups of students who were blind, sighted, or had low vision were not significantly different from each other. Students who were blind scored significantly higher on multiple-choice items on Braille tests compared with the other two groups (Erin, Hong, Schoch, & Kuo, 2006). Furthermore, compared with their sighted peers, children with visual impairment showed an advantage for literal questions under auditory presentation (Edmonds & Pring, 2006).

Overall, the pattern of research findings suggests that children with visual impairment experience mild, if any at all, delay in reading (Braille), and have a generally lower level of phonological awareness than their sighted peers. Nevertheless, the difference is not significant and may be related to the nature of contractions in Braille orthography and the limited literacy experience of Braille learners.

Interestingly, children with visual impairment perform equally well or even better than their sighted peers when their literacy skills are measured in the oral mode. Research on oral literacy skills of children with visual impairment is rare, however. With respect to our model of literate thought, this is an important area for future research.

READING DEVELOPMENT OF CHILDREN WITH VISUAL IMPAIRMENT

Traditionally, for parents and teachers of young children with visual impairment, one of the major challenges is to determine the most effective literacy medium or media for the individual child: Braille, print, or both (i.e., *dual media*) (Holbrook, 2009; Wormsley, 2008). Such a decision typically is made based on a series of data-driven and ongoing *Learning Media Assessment* (LMA) as required by *The Individuals with Disabilities Education Act of 2004.*

Nevertheless, a recent survey of 29 students with visual impairment, aged 3 to 21 years (McKenzie, 2009), revealed an alarming finding that only 13.8% of these students had a completed LMA. Another survey study of 108 students with visual impairment and 95 teachers (Lusk & Corn, 2006) found that the decision regarding a student's literacy medium or media was affected by the teachers' philosophies, the students' reading speed and stamina, as well as the teachers' subjective judgments in conducting an informal LMA. Based on a survey of 33 students with visual impairment, aged 9 to 18 years, and 24 teachers of students with visual impairment, Argyropoulos, Sideridis, and Katsoulis (2008) found that the more experienced the teachers were in terms of years of teaching and knowledge of Braille, the less the students preferred to study aurally.

In short, Braille is considered the *default* medium for the literacy development of children with vision impairment, and the decision on the literacy medium or media is heavily dependent on the teachers, instead of the individual needs of the child. Although Braille is the forefront mandated medium for literacy development of children with visual impairment, many of them are not Braille readers because their teachers are not proficient due to lack of training in university preparation programs, or because the Individualized Education Program (IEP) decision favors what is available in the school district instead of the needs of the child (Koenig & Holbrook, 2000).

A heavy reliance on teachers is also observed in the use of technology for children with visual impairment in their literacy development. For example, a survey of 410 teachers of students with visual impairment from 44 U.S. states and 4 Canadian provinces (Corn & Wall, 2002) revealed that the respondents preferred to use general technology (e.g., word processors, computers, CD-ROMs, or DVDs) in their classrooms, simply because they felt more at ease with them, not because it was more pertinent to the needs of their students. Additionally, in a survey study of 72 teachers, Abner and Lahn (2002) found that although teachers had access to and used computer-based technologies, they did not have the appropriate pre- and in-service training and support for teaching these technologies to their students; therefore, only half of their students used computer technologies.

Many assistive technologies (e.g., optical scanners, optical magnifiers, closed-circuit television systems (CCTVs), note-taking devices, and technology that produce large print, Braille, or speech) are rarely used in the classroom. Argyropoulos and colleagues (2008) found that teachers' involvement with technology was superficial and influenced only the usage of audiotapes. Furthermore, it appeared that the more the teachers used technology, the less their students were likely to select audiotapes for their schoolwork. In general, the use of technology by teachers in the classroom was not systematic with regard to instructional practices or curricula.

In terms of parental involvement, research studies suggest that parents who learn to read and write Braille have a positive influence on the literacy development of children with visual impairment (Argyropoulos et al., 2008); however, only a small proportion of parents know Braille (Lusk & Corn, 2006; Trent & Truan, 1997). Parents of children who are Braille readers might consider learning Braille as difficult as learning a foreign language. Without professional support, parents might not encourage their children to write with a Braillewriter or identify Braille letters (Brennan, Luze, & Peterson, 2009).

Braille Literacy

Braille is a tactile reading and writing system invented in 1824 by Louis Braille for individuals who are functionally blind and cannot use other media for reading and writing effectively. In Braille, each letter of the alphabet is represented by a character or cell with six embossed dots in two vertical columns of three dots each (for the orthography of Braille, see for example, Dodd & Conn, 2000).

Figure 7-2 illustrates a full numbered Braille cell.

There are 63 possible configurations. Braille cells are also used for punctuation, numbers, mathematical signs, and music notes. In Grade I Braille, each letter of a word is represented by a single configuration. In order to increase reading speed, many words and clusters of letters are

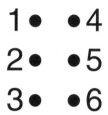

Figure 7-2.   A full numbered Braille cell.

represented by one or two tactile symbol(s) (i.e., contractions) in Grade II Braille.

Contractions do not correspond to the phonological units provided by the alphabetic orthography of English, that is, there is no symbol–sound correspondence between the contraction and the sound. For instance, the contraction for *the* is used for the words: *the*n, *The*lma, *the*ory, *the*ir, fur-*the*r and ca*the*dral. Additionally, approximately a quarter of the contractions found in Grade II Braille are seldom used in the general literature (Tobin, Douce, Lorimer, & Gill, 1980). These contractions might interfere with the ability of beginning Braille learners to detect phonemes in words, which consequently affects their reading and spelling ability. For example, research found that words with Braille contractions were less well segmented by children with visual impairment, although their phonological awareness skills on reading Grade 1 Braille were comparable to those of sighted peers matched for chronological age (Dodd & Conn, 2000).

It can be implied from the above discussion that the nature of the orthography learned (i.e., Braille contractions) affects the development of phonological awareness, although it is still unclear whether phonological awareness is a precursor of reading (Bradley & Bryant, 1983) or a result of learning to read (Morais, Cary, Alegria, & Bertelson, 1979). It might also be possible that there is a two-way relationship between phonological awareness and reading. Nevertheless, studies comparing the phonological awareness skills of Braille readers found that less skilled Braille readers were also delayed in their ability to understand the sound structure of spoken language at the phonemic level and to use phonological knowledge during reading (Barlow-Brown & Connelly, 2002; Gillon & Young, 2002). Furthermore, an advantage was found for both phoneme and onset-rime instruction (onset is the initial consonant sound and rime is the vowel and the rest of the syllable that follows) in learning Braille letters (Crawford, Elliott, & Hoekman, 2006).

Another challenge for Braille learners is that the Braille letter shapes are less distinctive than those in the Roman alphabet (Dodd & Conn, 2000), which leads to the fact that tactual acuity of Braille is significantly lower than that of vision and can resemble *blurred vision* (Apkarian-Stielau & Loomis, 1974; Pring, 1994). For example, as indicated in **Figure 7-3**, the letters *d, f, h* and *j* have the same triangular shape rotated in four different positions.

To obtain Braille reading readiness, children with visual impairment need to engage in tactual discrimination and fine motor activities, which may take them longer to reach readiness for formal reading instruction, particularly compared with their sighted peers (Lorimer, 1992).

The third challenge for Braille learners is that the different encoding strategies and redundancy characteristics in Braille and print result in a slower reading speed of Braille compared to print reading (Pring, 1994). For example, the tactual input of Braille tends to be successive whereas visual encoding of print may process several letters almost simultaneously because the *perceptual span* (i.e., the amount of information that can be acquired in one eye fixation) is estimated to be between 10 and 20 characters in reading print (Rayner & Pollatsek, 1989). Furthermore, whereas print can be read even with parts of letters missing, there is little redundancy in Braille orthography, which makes it harder to read and requires more attention to the letter recognition processes than does print reading (Pring, 1984; Wormsley, 2008).

Other than the tactical component of Braille, reading Braille is similar to reading print in terms of the similar factors affecting the reading time,

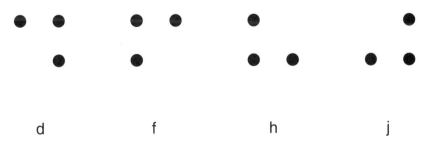

Figure 7-3. The letters *d, f, h,* and *j* in Braille.

for example, word length, word frequency, repetition, and semantic priming (Edmonds & Pring, 2006; Pring, 1984). Even with the use of contractions, however, experienced Braille readers read Braille for an average of 70 to 100 words per minute, which is significantly slower than sighted readers who generally read print at just under 300 words per minute (Edmonds & Pring, 2006; Nolan & Kederis, 1969). Generally speaking, a skilled Braille reader reads at approximately one-third or one-half of the speed of a sighted peer reading print (Nolan, 1966, discussed in Steinman et al., 2006). Furthermore, a study of 30 adolescent Braille readers (Trent & Truan, 1997) found that the most significant factor in Braille reading speed was age at first exposure to Braille, which highlights the importance of learning Braille early.

Last but not the least, in addition to the unique characteristics of Braille orthography, many other obstacles exist regarding the literacy experience of children with visual impairment: fewer Braille materials are available to Braille learners; many children with visual impairment do not have any literacy experience until school age; due to lack of incidental learning, they tend to have less contact with written words; and because of slow reading speed, they read less extensively (Dodd & Conn, 2000). All of these difficulties inherent in acquiring literacy through the medium of Braille can be potential risk factors for reading delays of children with visual impairment.

Braille and Print Literacy

In a nutshell, no matter whether the input stimulus is visual or tactile, the main information-processing tasks in reading are essentially the same (Gillon & Young, 2002; Pring, 1982). It appears that a level of phonological processing occurs between the child's tactical orthographic processing and meaning processing. That is, the spoken representation of a word helps to make a connection between the tactile stimulus for a word and its represented meaning. Once the input of orthographic information is connected with the meaning processor, there appears to be no difference in how the information is processed internally.

Similar to what we discussed in Chapter 6, the phonological and orthographic processing is essentially similar to the decoding process, and the meaning and context processing is fundamentally analogous to language comprehension. The input stimuli in Braille decoding are different from the ones used in print decoding, but once the stimuli are registered with meaning, it is language comprehension skills that distinguish good readers from poor readers. Examples are vocabulary knowledge, metalinguistic awareness, prior knowledge, and the use of cognitive and metacognitive strategies (see the discussions in Chapters 4 and 6).

Although there might be early language delays ranging from minor to major for some children (e.g., children with multiple disabilities), children with visual impairment generally have intact spoken language comprehension skills. As suggested by many researchers (e.g., Snow, Burns, & Griffin, 1998), visual impairment per se is generally not a risk factor for reading (i.e., Braille) delays. With disadvantaged phonological awareness skills and impoverished literacy experiences, a few children with visual impairment can fall into the category of delayed readers; but, compared with sighted children, the incidence is not significantly increased.

CONCLUSION: READING AND CHILDREN WITH VISUAL IMPAIRMENT

Children with visual impairment should have access to all choices of literacy media; however, in practice, the decision on the medium/media of literacy development is associated with teachers' personal experiences and subjective judgments. Similarly, the use of technology by children with visual impairment is heavily dependent on teachers, many of whom are not trained to use assistive technology themselves.

Because Braille is the default medium mandated for literacy development of children with visual impairment, most of the research on reading and blindness has been with Braille readers. The overall pattern of research findings suggests that children with visual impairment generally read at or less than one grade level below their sighted peers, although their delay on phonological decoding is more severe. Such a difference may be associated with the nature of contractions in Braille orthography and the reduced literacy experience of Braille learners. In addition, there is a positive relationship between the phonological awareness skills and reading comprehension. This confirms the hypothesis that regardless of the input stimulus of the orthographic processing (i.e., visual or tactile), phonological processing facilitates the connection between orthographic processing and meaning processing to make sense of the printed or Braille text.

A careful investigation on the reading development of children with visual impairment reveals that there are no categorical differences when compared to that of their sighted peers, although there might be some mild delays in the initial stages of development. For example, while sighted children see many vocabulary words in informal, incidental ways from an early age, children with visual impairment typically are not exposed to these instances in everyday life and must wait until entering school to learn them formally. In addition, vocabulary is usually not reinforced at home by parents reading Braille to their children and using it themselves. The lack of grapheme–phoneme correspondence between the contraction and the phoneme may prevent many beginning Braille readers from successful phonological decoding. Fortunately, eventually, Braille readers may read the same vocabulary words as do print readers, and after years of literacy experience, their delay in phonological decoding may be resolved automatically.

There is a dearth of research on oral literacy skills of children with visual impairment, although studies have found that they performed equally well or even better than their sighted peers when the oral method was used to measure their literacy skills. If children with visual impairment cannot fully benefit from the visual medium (i.e., standard or enlarged print) and there is inherent disadvantage of the tactile medium (i.e., Braille), why not take advantage of the auditory medium?

READING ACHIEVEMENT OF CHILDREN WHO ARE DEAF OR HARD OF HEARING

Hearing impairment is a generic term involving all causes, types, and degrees of hearing loss. Based on audiometric characteristics, individuals who are *hard of hearing* refer to those with slight, mild, or moderate hearing loss (up to about 70 decibels [dB] for a pure tone average in the better unaided ear; see Trezek, Wang, & Paul, 2010a) whereas individuals with severe or profound hearing loss (70 dB or greater) are typically labeled as *deaf* (Trezek et al., 2010a). In the United States, less than 1 of every 1,000 public school children is a d/Deaf child receiving special education while about 1 of every 1,000 is a hard of hearing child in special education (Mitchell, 2005).

It is well documented that the script reading achievement level of students with severe to profound hearing loss is not commensurate with that of their typical hearing peers. Children with severe-to-profound hearing loss leave the educational system in the United States reading at the beginning of the fourth grade level, and more than 90% of these individuals are reading at the sixth grade level or less. Furthermore, the annual growth rate of reading for many of them is approximately 0.3 grade level per year compared to roughly 1.0 grade level for their hearing peers (Allen, 1986; Luckner, Sebald, Cooney, Young, & Goodwin Muir, 2005/2006; Moores, 2006; Paul, 2003, 2009; Schirmer & McGough, 2005; Traxler, 2000; Trezek et al., 2010a).

Several explanations have been offered for the reading level: the artifacts associated with the types of assessments used to measure reading achievement; the inferential and language demands of reading materials, which increase dramatically after the third-grade level; the marked difficulty of many students with severe-to-profound hearing loss in developing or acquiring the language of written English; and the unpreparedness of teachers to teach reading and writing (Paul, 2001, 2009; Trezek et al., 2010a). Furthermore, Trezek, Wang, and Paul (2010b) suggested that the proliferation of reading theories provides numerous, sometimes conflicting, views, and there seem to be misinterpretations of these theories that are associated with the ongoing debates of whether the reading development of students who are d/Deaf or hard of hearing is similar to that of their hearing peers, thereby validating the use of mainstream literacy models for understanding and improving reading.

Fundamentally, the question is this: Is reading different for d/Deaf individuals when compared to hearing children? Rather than an either–or (yes or no) answer to the question, Hanson (1989) provided a dual (yes and no) response, which reflects the different language experiences that d/Deaf and hard-of-hearing individuals bring to the task of reading as well as the similarities among better d/Deaf and hard-of-hearing readers and better hearing readers in their perception of the structure of English, particularly the abstract phonology of English.

Hanson's answer concurs with the *Qualitative-Similarity Hypothesis* (QSH) (Paul, 2008, 2009; Paul & Lee, 2010), which claims that the reading development of students who are d/Deaf or hard of hearing is similar to that of students with typical hearing learning to read English as a first or second language (Hayes & Arnold, 1992; Paul, 1998, 2001, 2003; Paul , Wang, Trezek, & Luckner, 2009; Rose, McAnally & Quigley, 2004; Schirmer & McGough, 2005; Trezek et al., 2010a; Wang , Trezek, Luckner, & Paul, 2008). The essence of the QSH is that there are certain fundamental skills that apply to all children in learning to read and write (e.g., McGuinness, 2004, 2005), and the processes and components of reading development are qualitatively similar. That is, students who are d/Deaf or hard of hearing proceed through the same developmental stages, make the same errors, and use roughly the same reading strategies as their hearing counterparts, although progression through the developmental stages tends to be quantitatively delayed. These children therefore may require special instructional enhancements and an enriched intensity of instruction to achieve developmental milestones, but mainstream theories and recommendations for literacy practice should be applicable for this population (Trezek et al., 2010b; Wang et al., 2008).

It is also critical to recognize the different language experiences of children who are d/Deaf or hard of hearing, which is responsible for most of the reading delay. ASL is widely misunderstood as the primary language for children who are d/Deaf or hard of hearing. Actually, based on the 2007–2008 survey of 36,710 children in the United States (Gallaudet Research Institute, 2008), only 3.8% of these children use ASL at home and 11% use signing only as the communication mode, primarily used in the classrooms. Sign systems include not only visual-manual languages such as ASL but also many artificially developed *Manually Coded English (MCE)* systems (e.g., *Rochester Method, Signed English, Seeing Essential English (SEE I), Signing Exact English (SEE II), Conceptually Accurate Sign English (CASE), Pidgin Sign English, contact signing,* etc.), which use ASL-based signs and created grammar makers to represent the structure of English (e.g., see the discussion in Paul, 2009).

Table 7-1 offers an example of how the word *undecided* is represented by a few MCE systems.

As discussed later in this chapter, there is an inherent difficulty for d/Deaf students to use the skills acquired in a through-the-air language such as ASL to learn to read and write in a second language such as English without manipulation of the primary form (speech or sign) of English. But MCE systems are not the magic bullets either. Several degraded input hypotheses and structural limitation hypotheses have been offered to explain the limited success of MCE systems for improving d/Deaf children's script reading abilities (see the review in LaSasso & Crain, 2010). *Degraded input hypotheses* suggest that MCE systems represent English at the morphological level—albeit incompletely—rather than at the phonemic level. These systems therefore might not be effective in assisting chil-

---

Table 7-1. Representation of the Word *Undecided* by Four Manually Coded English Systems

---

English Sentence: *That is undecided.*
Rochester Method (fingerspelling): Each letter is represented by a fingerspelled handshape.

U-N-D-E-C-I-D-E-D

Signing Exact English (SEE 2): Two sign markers (*un-* and *–ed*) and an initialized ASL sign meaning *decide* are used to convey the message.

U̲N-D̲ECIDE-ED

Signed English (SE): The ASL sign for negation (not) is used along with the initialized sign for *decide* (same as SEE 2).

NOT D̲ECIDE

English Sign: There are several different ways to express this word. One common way is to use two ASL signs together to indicate what the signer means.

CAN'T DECIDE

Note: Underlined letters in SEE 2 and SE indicate that the fingerspelled handshape is used for that sign.

Source: Adapted from Paul (2009).

dren in acquiring the beginning awareness of the sound structures of words (Trezek et al., 2010a). Even speechreading and MCE systems combined cannot provide a complete picture of spoken English (Paul, 2001, 2009).

Only Cued Speech/Language has the potential to represent spoken English sufficiently at the phonemic level (see the details of Cued Speech/Language later in this chapter). 0.2% of school age children who are d/Deaf or hard of hearing in the United States are currently using Cued Speech/Language as their primary communication mode in the classrooms, however (Gallaudet Research Institute, 2008).

At present, the majority (i.e., 52%) of school age children who are d/Deaf or hard of hearing have speech only as their main mode of communication at school (Gallaudet Research Institute, 2008)—particularly in auditory oral programs. Children in the auditory oral programs are in a range of educational settings such as special or center schools, regular school settings with hearing students, self-contained classrooms in regular education settings, recourse rooms, and so on. The collection of oral methods focuses on the use of residual hearing with the development of oral speech and language as a goal. Many children with severe-to-profound hearing loss, however, cannot fully benefit from oral methods to develop their oral speech and spoken language skills. Their incomplete spoken language development might relate to their delay in reading print (see also the reviews in Paul, 2001, 2009).

In short, the average reading achievement level of children who are d/Deaf or hard of hearing is significantly lower than that of their hearing peers. Furthermore, children who are d/Deaf or hard of hearing are even more heterogeneous than children with visual impairment, given that, for example, they use different modes of communication and are in various educational placements.

Paul (2001, 2003; see also, Trezek et al., 2010b) proffered a *Process-and-Knowledge View* to describe the reading difficulties of children and adolescents who are d/Deaf or hard of hearing, which is used as the framework to discuss reading and deafness in the following section.

READING DEVELOPMENT AND CHILDREN WHO ARE DEAF OR HARD OF HEARING

The Process-and-Knowledge View (Paul, 2001, 2003; Trezek, et al., 2010b) suggests a reciprocal relationship between the processing of text and an understanding/interpretation of the information in the text. That is, the process domain facilitates the better use of the knowledge domain, and the knowledge domain assists the use of the process domain.

Trezek, Wang, and Paul (2010b) categorize the reading deficits of students who are d/Deaf or hard of hearing as difficulties with both process (i.e., text) and knowledge (i.e., reader) factors. Text factors are necessary for decoding (e.g., pronouncing, signing) linguistic information from print whereas reader factors are related to the mental representations needed for comprehending/interpreting decoded items. Both reader and text skills are essential during reading because it is possible for a reader to know the meaning of a word (knowledge) without identifying its written counterpart (process); whereas it is equally possible for a reader to pronounce or sign a word (process) without knowing its meaning (knowledge).

Apparently, the process and knowledge factors of reading difficulties for students who are d/Deaf or hard of hearing are very similar to the word recognition and written language comprehension deficits of children with language/learning disabilities. Processing print involves *word identification* and larger discourse processes as well as converting print to construct meaning in the head. The goal of processing is to have the process become automatic so that much of the reader's energy and resources can be allocated to understand/interpret the text. The knowledge domain is a broad entity, which includes mainly language comprehension skills such as *metalinguistic awareness* (i.e., syntactic awareness and pragmatic awareness), *prior knowledge* (i.e., passage-specific prior knowledge or discourse knowledge and topic-specific prior knowledge including world knowledge and domain specific knowledge), and the use of *cognitive strategies* such as critical analysis, inference, reasoning, problem solving and comprehension, specific *metacognitive strategies* including monitoring and evaluating comprehension (see the discussion on language comprehension skills in Chapter 6; see also Chapters 4 and 5).

As we discussed in Chapter 6, when poor readers constantly experience difficulties in reading, they might be less engaged and less intrinsically motivated to read. These readers thus might have less reading practice, which will further extend their deficits in reading. Such a *Matthew effect* (see the discussion in Chapter 6) is not only applicable for children with language/learning disabilities, but also for children who are d/Deaf or hard of hearing.

Because several factors contributing to reading difficulties for children who are d/Deaf or hard of hearing are essentially parallel to those for children with language/learning disabilities, here we address mainly a few outstanding differences between children who are d/Deaf or hard of hearing and children with language/learning disabilities. Our focus is on phonology, morphology, and syntax, which serve as our exemplars.

Access to Phonology of English

One of the most controversial lines of reading research in deafness is whether readers can bypass phonological processing and connect orthographic processing directly with meaning processing during reading (Allen et al., 2009; Paul et al., 2009; Wang et al., 2008). Those who believe reading is different for d/Deaf individuals maintain that they are visual learners and their reading acquisition process is so fundamentally different from that of hearing individuals that they can bypass phonological coding by using orthography via signs or fingerspelling or by going straight from print to meaning (Allen et al.).

In this view, phonological coding is unrealistic, and effective reading instructional strategies on phonemic awareness and phonics skills founded on the research of hearing children (e.g., National Reading Panel [NRP], 2000) are meaningless and inappropriate for them. Proponents believe that d/Deaf readers can use their knowledge of ASL to acquire adequate independent English literacy skills without ever manipulating or having exposure to the through-the-air (i.e., speech or signing) form of English print. This is the predominate basis for using ASL to teach English as a second language or for ASL/English bilingualism/biculturalism programs (Paul, 1998, 2001, 2009; Paul et al., 2009; Trezek et al., 2010a; Wang et al., 2008). Although some educational programs, particularly many state schools for d/DHH children adhere to this philosophical approach for literacy instruction, thus far, a paucity of research exists to support its efficacy (Luckner & Handley, 2008; Luckner et al., 2005/2006; Moores, 2008; Schirmer & McGough, 2005).

Leybaert, Colin, and LaSasso (2010) illustrate the difficulty in using signed languages to teach an alphabetic orthography:

> Indeed, the phonological units of signs, including: hand configuration, hand placement, hand movement, and hand location (Stokoe, 1971) do not have any systematic correspondence with graphemes. The link between a written word and a sign could only be arbitrary, as in the logographic stage. Important consequences for children who cannot make associations between the phonemes and graphemes of a language include the following: (1) they cannot be "autonomous readers" (in Jorm & Share's 1983 terminology) meaning that they cannot independently access the meaning of "new" written words that they have not encountered in print before; (2) they will not develop "redundancy" in Perfetti's terms; (3) they will be at risk of not developing orthographic representations of high quality. Such children must either *guess* the meaning of novel print words, via contextual analysis, for example; use a dictionary; or ask the help of a more skilled reader. The way that reading is taught in some classes in which a signed language is the instructional language well illustrates this possibility: the teacher first translates the written text into the signed language, which is understood by the children; and then, the children try to *read* the written text by associating the written words with the corresponding signs. It should be noted that although the signing children in this scenario may be experiencing pleasure in learning to read when they are provided a signed translation, they are *not* presenting as autonomous readers. (p. 253)

On the other hand, proponents who believe that reading is *not* different for d/Deaf or hard of hearing individuals argue not only that the use of a phonological code via a development of phonemic awareness and phonic skills is important for any beginning reader of English as a first or second language, but also that it is feasible for children who are d/Deaf or hard of hearing to acquire these skills (Paul et al., 2009; Wang et al., 2008). Although a few studies have documented limited phonological processing (Allen et al., 2009), substantial research over the last 30 years has reached a growing consensus that phonology plays a critical role in reading comprehension, and the ability to process phonological information during reading distinguishes skilled readers from average or poor readers (see reviews in Alegria, 1998; Hanson, 1991; Marschark & Harris, 1996; Perfetti & Sandak, 2000; Wang et al., 2008).

Several alternative techniques can be used, with varying levels of success, to facilitate the acquisition of phonology in d/Deaf or hard of hearing children (**Table 7-2**).

Two of the most promising techniques for developing phonology are Cued Speech/Language and Visual Phonics.

Cornett (1967) created *Cued Speech* (or *Cued Speech/Language*) as a sound-based, visual communication system that uses eight handshapes in four different locations in combination with the natural mouth movements of speech. Sets of consonants are represented by handshapes whereas sets of vowels are represented by hand positions and sometimes hand positions plus movements. During cuing, the speaker keeps his or her hand near the mouth while speaking (for further details, see Shull & Crain, 2010). The underlying hypothesis of Cued Speech/Language is that a prelingually d/Deaf child can acquire spoken language in a way that is similar to that of a hearing child through a visual channel rather than an auditory channel (Cornett).

As a reading instructional tool specifically designed for delivering the phonological information of English, *Visual Phonics* is the abbreviated title for *See The Sound/Visual Phonics* (STS/VP), a multisensory system of hand cues and corresponding written symbols that represents aspects of the phonemes of a language and grapheme–phoneme relationships. Similar to Cued Speech/Language, it incorporates speechreading (visual information), articulatory feedback (tactile information), and hand motions (kinesthetic information). Different from Cued Speech/Language, however, the hand cues of Visual Phonics mirror the articulatory features of the sound, and the written symbols reflect the gestures used in the cues (Trezek et al., 2010a). Also, because it is an instructional tool

---

Table 7-2. Four Alternative Means of Acquiring Phonology

Method	Details
Speechreading	
Definition	Also *lipreading*, is the process of understanding a spoken message through observation of the speaker's face
Advantages	• Direct and easy access
Disadvantages	• Incomplete or ambiguous representation of phonology
Articulatory Feedback	
Definition	Also *tactile-kinesthetic feedback system*, involves mouth movements and vocal sensations produced for each phoneme
Advantages	• Direct and easy access
Disadvantages	• Incomplete or ambiguous representation of phonology
Cued Speech/Language	
Definition	A sound-based, visual communication system that uses eight handshapes in four different locations in combination with the natural mouth movements of speech
Advantages	• Represents the cued language at the syllable level, and for reading instructional purposes, also at the phoneme level • Can be used for language acquisition • Has been adapted to 56 languages • Can be learned in a relatively short period of time • Can be produced in real time
Disadvantages	• The hand cues do not contain articulatory features of the sounds
Visual Phonics	
Definition	The abbreviated title for *See The Sound/Visual Phonics* (STS/VP), a multisensory system of hand cues and corresponding written symbols that represents aspects of the phonemes of a language and the grapheme-phoneme relationships
Advantages	• Represents English at the phoneme level • The hand cues contain articulatory features of the sounds • The written symbols reflect the gestures used in the cues • Can be learned in a relatively short period of time • Can be used with any communication philosophy
Disadvantages	• A reading instructional tool, not a language acquisition device • Cannot be produced in real time

---

Sources: Adapted from Shull & Crain (2010) and Trezek et al. (2010a).

instead of a communication system, Visual Phonics can be used with any communication methodology, and once students gain information about phonemes, the use of Visual Phonics is likely to fade. Visual Phonics can only be used as a tool to gain access to phonology of English, not as a phonological or even a language acquisition device.

Although relatively little research is available, Cued Speech/Language and Visual Phonics can be effective methods for delivering phonological information. For example, there is ample evidence that French-speaking d/Deaf children who use Cued Speech/Language at home and at school make significant improvements in spoken language and print literacy development (Marschark & Spencer, 2006; see also the reviews in Leybaert et al., 2010; Trezek et al., 2010a). In addition, evidence supports a relationship between phonological awareness and exposure to Cued Speech/Language for English-speaking d/Deaf children as well (e.g., Crain & LaSasso, 2010).

In conjunction with a phonics-based reading curriculum, Visual Phonics has been used in several classroom-based intervention studies for students with various degrees of hearing loss in preschool (Smith & Wang, 2010), kindergarten and first grade (Syverud, Guardino, & Selznick, 2009; Trezek & Wang, 2006; Trezek, Wang, Woods, Gampp, & Paul, 2007) to adolescents in high school (Trezek & Malmgren, 2005). The collective results indicate a significant improvement in participants' reading achievement as well as in aspects of phonology.

In sum, traditional reading instructional practices for students who are d/Deaf or hard of hearing have attempted to circumvent or substitute the role of the phonological processor (e.g., see Adams, 1990), which might directly relate to the disappointing general reading achievement level. Phonological processing does not necessarily have to be based on hearing (i.e., the use of audition), and children who are d/Deaf or hard of hearing can and should use alternative means such as Cued Speech/Language or Visual Phonics to acquire and develop their phonological knowledge, which might be the key to ultimately improving their English reading skills.

It should be emphasized that a growing number of d/Deaf and hard-of-hearing children are obtaining access to the phonology of English through assistive listening devices such as cochlear implants or digital hearing aids (for a detailed description of the devices, see Paul &

Whitelaw, 2011). Currently, research on the literacy skills of cochlear implant users is emerging (Marschark, Rhoten, & Fabich, 2007; Spencer & Tomblin, 2009; Trezek et al., 2010a). Empirical evidence on the positive effects of cochlear implantation on reading and academic achievement of young d/Deaf children has been inconsistent or equivocal to some degree, although some promising results, particularly on their phonological processing skills, are apparent. Further research is needed to control potentially confounding variables such as age at implantation, language and reading skills prior to implantation, and consistency of implant use (Marschark et al., 2007).

Access to Morphology

Morphology and syntax are two aspects of the indirect connection between spoken and written languages (Nunes & Bryant, 2006, 2009). Children use their morphological and syntactical awareness to infer the meaning of new words. For example, when a child encounters *pictography* for the first time in the following sentence: "It is a *pictograph* of a bird," s/he can, first, use his/her syntactical awareness to figure out that *pictography* might be a noun due to its position in the sentence. The child then uses his/her morphological awareness to identify the two morphemes (i.e., *picto, graphy*) and guess that it might related to *picture graph*.

Morphemes are the smallest meaningful units of language. Morphological awareness refers to individuals' "conscious awareness of the morphemic structure of words and their ability to reflect on and manipulate that structure" (Carlisle, 1995, p. 194). It includes knowledge of both inflectional morphemes and derivational morphemes (see descriptions in Paul, 2009). A typical English-speaking child begins to produce two-morpheme words (e.g., *Sara's* cat, I *singing*, *Birds* fly) during Stage 2 of Brown's Stage of Language Development in his/her late second year or beginning third year, and the growth in the use of affixes (mainly inflections) is rapid and exceptionally impressive during early childhood (Brown, 1973). Their morphological awareness in writing mirrors that in their speech: inflectional morphology is largely mastered by the time s/he reaches age 9 or 10, and the skills with derivational morphology continue to develop in middle childhood (Green et al., 2003).

Table 7-3 illustrates Brown's Stages of Language Development.

Table 7-3. **Brown's Stages of Language Development with Comparable Mean Lengths of Utterances (MLUs) and Ages**

Stage	MLU	Approximate age (months)	Characteristics
I	1.0–1.99	12–26	Linear semantic rules, e.g., "actor + action"
II	2.0–2.49	27–30	Morphological development
III	2.5–2.99	31–34	Sentence-form development
IV	3.0–3.99	35–40	Embedding sentences
V	4.0	41+	Coordination of simple sentences and propositional relations

Source: Adapted from Brown (1973).

Children who are d/Deaf or hard of hearing and use ASL or other sign systems as their mode of communication from an early age proceed through Brown's Stage 1 comparable with their hearing peers. That is, they produce first signs and sign combinations that express the same functional relationship as first words and two word utterances of hearing children (Rose et al., 2004). The sign language development of children who are d/Deaf or hard of hearing seems to parallel the spoken language development of hearing children.

The subsequent development of English is another story, particularly for the morphological development of English. For example, many English morphemes do not exist in ASL and, as shown in Table 7-1, although many MCE systems represent English at the morphological level, their representation is incomplete. For children who communicate orally, many morphemes (e.g., *-s, -ed, 's*) are difficult to hear because they are unstressed in speech. With respect to the Morphological Development Stage, therefore, many children who are d/Deaf or hard of hearing exhibit delays in English language development, which contributes to their reading difficulties at school.

English orthography is *morphophonemic*, which means that the spelling system of English is based on both representation of sounds (phonemes) and units of meaning (morphemes). That is, grapheme–phoneme mappings do not offer a complete account of English orthography; therefore, meaning relations across words are also required in reading and spelling, particularly, the so-called *irregular* spelling patterns (Carlise & Stone, 2005; Deacon & Kirby, 2004; Green et al., 2003).

Similar to the *chicken-and-egg* relationship between phonological awareness and reading, it is unclear if morphological awareness is a predictor of reading or vice versa. It might also be possible that morphological awareness and reading are connected through a third underlying factor, most likely phonological awareness (Arnbak & Elbro, 2000).

Access to Syntax

On the other hand, *syntax* refers to the rules that govern the order or arrangement of words. Syntactic knowledge is often required during reading to integrate information across connected linguistic units such as phases, sentences and paragraphs (Paul, 2003). Syntax has been one of the most researched components in reading and deafness (Paul, 2003) whereas it seldom appears to be a focus for studying reading difficulties in hearing students, except for some studies on second language learners.

Typical hearing children acquire syntactical knowledge of English through daily communication with adults and peers in the spoken form of the language. For d/Deaf children who use ASL as their primary mode of communication, without ever manipulating or having exposure to the performance (i.e., speech or signing) form of English print, they are learning the English language and the artifacts associated with reading print simultaneously at the beginning reading stage. It is a double-burden for them. MCE systems were designed for children who are d/Deaf or hard of hearing to be exposed to the syntactic structures of English through exposure to signing from teachers and significant others. As discussed previously, however, putting ASL signs into English order is not equivalent to teaching English syntax.

Quigley and his team (see the review in Paul, 2009) studied the English syntactic knowledge of d/Deaf children (i.e., with profound hearing impairment) and found that d/Deaf children have difficulties with most sentences that did not adhere to a subject-verb-object (SVO) structure, particularly the ones with verb inflectional processes and auxiliaries (e.g., *The cat was bitten by a dog*) or the ones with embedded structures such as relative clauses (e.g., *The boy who kissed the girl ran away*). Quigley and colleagues further demonstrated that, despite the quantitative delays, d/Deaf children acquired syntactic structures in a developmental manner similar to that of younger hearing children. That is, they went through stages, produced errors, and employed strategies that appeared to be developmentally similar to those of younger hearing students who are native speakers of English, providing further support for the Qualitative-Similarity Hypothesis (Paul, 2008, 2009; Paul & Lee, 2010).

CONCLUSION: READING AND DEAFNESS

Most d/Deaf and many hard-of-hearing children experience challenges in reading print English, although the reasons for the difficulties vary. One problematic area is the lack of access to the phonology of English. In addition, many children also have problems in two other critical forms of English, namely, morphology and syntax. These three forms are language-specific; that is, it is almost impossible to develop knowledge of the forms of English via the use of another language such as ASL. The content (i.e., semantics) and use (i.e., pragmatics) of English may be acquired via explanations in another language but not the forms.

Research in reading and deafness over the past century has confirmed the basic tenets of the Qualitative-Similarity Hypothesis (Paul, 2008, 2009; Paul & Lee, 2010). That is, despite their unique language experiences, students who are d/Deaf or hard of hearing progress through parallel developmental stages, make matching errors, and use roughly the same reading strategies as their hearing peers to read English as a first or second language—albeit, the rate of acquisition is quantitatively slower.

Let's revisit the questions posed at the beginning of the chapter. *When vision is not available to readers, as in the case of individuals with visual impairment, will there be an alternative sensory modality for orthographic processing?* The answer is: *Yes*. Many children with visual impairment use the tactile sense for orthographic processing (in Braille).

If so, then what is the impact of alternative orthographic processing on reading? We asserted that the tactile orthographic processing is roughly similar to the visual orthographic processing and that the reading achievement of Braille readers is generally at or slightly below that of sighed peers.

Similarly, when hearing is not available to readers, as in the case of individuals with hearing impairment, will there be an alternative sensory modality for phonological processing? The answer is: *Yes.* There are alternative means of phonological processing that use visual and/or tactile-kinesthetic senses.

If so, then what is the impact of alternative phonological processing on reading? Two techniques (e.g., Cued Speech/Language or Visual Phonics) have demonstrated promising empirical results on improving d/Deaf and hard-of-hearing children's reading achievement, but more research is needed to establish a firm cause–effect relationship.

Or, can reading be successful without phonological processing? Orthographic processing obtains input from outside. Can orthographic processing bypass phonological processing and be directly connected with meaning and context processing? Our response is: *Probably not.* Traditional reading instruction for d/Deaf and hard-of-hearing children has attempted to bypass phonological processing, and the reading achievement of many d/Deaf and some hard-of-hearing high school graduates seems to plateau at the third or fourth grade level.

LITERATE THOUGHT AND CHILDREN WITH SENSORY DISABILITIES

Let's consider the last question, which is related to our proposal of literate thought as the main goal: *If sensory impairments prevent children with sensory disabilities from reading as well as their peers without disabilities, can they benefit equally from other effective media for sharing information?*

The use of media in addition to print seems to be necessary for a large number of d/Deaf or hard of hearing children—particularly those who have difficulty accessing phonology with or without amplification. The use of performance literacy (see Chapter 2) is under-researched as well as other aspects of the New and Multiple Literacies,especially for children with sensory disabilities and other disabilities (see Chapters 6 and 8). As is discussed later, there is some research on caption literacy.

Approximately 90% of children with visual impairment have low vision and benefit from standard or enlarged print. The risk of having reading difficulties is not higher than that of their sighted peers. Although the majority of reading research is on children who use Braille as their literacy medium, the American Printing House for the Blind (2007) reported that only about 9.5% of children with visual impairment are Braille readers. 26.9% are visual (print) readers, 7.5% are auditory readers, 21.7% are pre-readers, and the highest percentage (34.4%) is non-readers. The *pre-reader* label refers to children who are working on or toward a reading readiness level (or are in the emergent literacy stage), including infants, preschoolers, or older students with reading potential. *Non-readers* are children who show *no reading (Braille or otherwise) potential* and do not fall in any of the other categories.

The purported low risk factor of reading difficulties for children with visual impairment is misleading. The available research data concern only a small percentage (i.e., Braille readers) with the majority in the *non-reader* category.

Braille is not practical for everyone with visual impairment, particularly those who are legally blind. Children with visual impairment often have delayed development in their fine motor and object manipulation skills (Ferrell et al., 1990). In addition, approximately 60% of these children have multiple disabilities, including physical disabilities with motor control (Wormsley, 2008), which might lead to their difficulties and frustrations with tactile processing in Braille.

In Chapter 6, we suggest that children with language/learning disabilities can obtain and utilize information in modalities other than print. The skills that they acquired in other modalities of literacy can be used to improve aspects of their print literacy skills as well. This assertion is also applicable to children with sensory impairments. Particularly, for children with sensory impairments, technology plays a key role in their development of literate thought.

Use of Technology

Hasselbring (2001) suggested that often "students with disabilities have a greater need for accessing technology than do their non-disabled peers. This may be especially true for those students who need technology just to function within the school environment such as students with sensory and physical impairments" (p. 16). Technology is particularly important for children with sensory impairments because their sensory impairments might create barriers for them to retrieve or consume information presented in only the print mode.

As discussed in Chapter 6 and elsewhere, the advances in technology make it feasible for literate information to be stored in a CD, DVD, or MP3. For instance, the *Scholastic Storybook Treasures* series includes hundreds of award-winning and classic children literature stories (e.g., *Click, Clack, Moo, Where the Wild Things Are, Why Mosquitoes Buzz in People's Ears*) on DVD, featuring celebrity narrations (e.g., Sarah Jessica Parker, James Earl Jones). Paul (2009) has suggested:

> You can listen to or watch this DVD version of *Moby-Dick* in the same manner as you would read the book or print version. For example, you can replay it (i.e., relisten and rewatch) jump ahead, stop it, and reflect about what you have heard and seen, and so on. In essence, this is similar (without the pictures) to today's audiobooks – however, with advanced technology, you can maneuver back and forth in a faster manner and with greater ease with the DVD. (pp. 361-362)

If children with visual impairment can reflect upon captured information in an oral form on a DVD similar to the way sighted people analyze information in print, then we ask: What is the magical or talismanic power of print? In general, children with visual impairment have an intact spoken language development, although some of them might experience a late start during their early age. These children should be able to understand and/or produce oral information that is equivalent to, or might even be richer than, the print information their sighted peers comprehend and/or generate. Similarly, for children who are d/Deaf or hard of hearing who cannot access print, they should be able to access and/or utilize the captured information—assuming a level of competence in either a sign language or a form of signed English (Paul, 2009; Paul & Wang, 2006a; Paul & Wang, 2006b; Wang, 2005).

Little empirical research is available to test this hypothesis, and almost all available studies focus on the effectiveness of improving print literacy skills through assistive technology such as multimedia presentations that include print. This approach and the findings should be interpreted with caution: The sheer use of assistive technology does not necessarily ensure the development of literate thought in the New and Multiple Literacies. Many assistive technologies (e.g., *Computer Aided Realtime Translation* or *CART, C-Print*) are only translation services and rely heavily on print literacy skills.

Interactive multimedia is assumed to be useful for d/Deaf or hard of hearing students to connect information presented in graphics, sign language animation, and written text (Gentry, Chinn, & Moulton, 2004/

2005). Few studies, however, have explored the effectiveness of multimedia on improving reading comprehension of print, and most studies are descriptive. For example, Hanson and Padden (1990) developed a system, *HandsOn*, to simultaneously present ASL video and English print. Theoretically, this system allows the child's proficiency in ASL to transfer to literacy skills in English. Unfortunately, there are no empirical data to date on the efficacy of this system. Similarly, *Project UTERACY-HI* (Horney, Anderson-Inman, & Chen, 1994) created electronic versions of textbooks and included multimedia resources designed to support reading comprehension. Again, no data are available regarding any improvement of reading comprehension.

Wang and Paul (in press) conducted one of the first intervention studies on the effectiveness of educational technology in the classroom for literacy instruction of children who are d/Deaf or hard of hearing, aged 7 to 11 years. The *Cornerstones* instructional units were story-based and included materials that were visually rich, engaged students in content, and incorporated signing or cuing (e.g., ASL, signed English and Cued Speech/Language). Each Cornerstones unit was built around an animated story taken from Public Television's literacy series, *Between the Lions.*

Other technology materials supported comprehension and vocabulary objectives and enabled teachers to spend considerable time on literacy lessons. Except for the television program, all Cornerstones materials included lesson guides, lesson plans, and digitized videos. Supportive interactive computer games and materials were freely available on the PBSKIDS Web site (http://pbskids.org/lions/cornerstones/) and could be accessed in the classroom or the home. Research results revealed positive teacher feedback and provided evidence for the effectiveness of this literature-based technology-infused literacy program.

Another technology-enhanced literacy program was designed by Mueller and Hurtig (2010). Four children with prelingual hearing loss, aged 2 to 4 years, 10 months, participated. The researchers examined the effectiveness of the *Iowa Signing E-book*, a multimedia tool that created e-books with or without a video of a narrator signing the story in ASL, fingerspelling, Signed English, or contact sign. Children could make comments on the story or ask comprehension questions of different levels of structure/complexity and were provided feedback.

Results indicated that a greater time was spent in shared reading activities, and the sign vocabulary level improved for both the parents and children. Although these results are promising, large-scale intervention studies are needed to investigate further the effectiveness of technology-enhanced literacy practices for children who are d/Deaf or hard of hearing.

Caption Literacy

Television is one of the most important media that hearing children use to further their learning and understanding of culture. As a medium, however, television is designed to be heard and seen—and *entertaining*. Captioning has been used to make television more accessible for individuals who are d/Deaf or hard of hearing as well as for others such as those who are English language learners (Chapter 9) or who are young viewers. For example, in a study of 76 typically developing children who had just completed second grade, Linebarger (2001) found that these beginning readers recognized more words when they watched television that used captions, and appeared to focus more on central story elements and away from distracting information such as sound effects and visual glitz.

One accommodation that has been used to address the reading difficulty of individuals who are d/Deaf or hard of hearing is *edited captioning*. Edited captions present less information with less complex vocabulary and syntax, and the edited text remains on the screen longer than that of verbatim or near verbatim captions. An example of a near verbatim caption is, "Safety is everyone's responsibility," and an example of an edited caption is "Everyone must be safe." Research on the efficiency of using caption (i.e., edited or verbatim) literacy for developing the literate thought of children who are d/Deaf or hard of hearing is still in its infancy, however (see the discussion in Ward, Wang, Paul, & Loeterman, 2007).

A common misunderstanding of this medium is to "focus on technical surface features at the expense of more meaningful generic qualities" (Leander, 2009, p. 163). For example, there are several underlying skills associated with using captions that make this medium somewhat different than that of print literacy (e.g., books, etc.):

> In a captioned program, the video provides a portion of the narrative so children need to switch their gaze from text to picture and back again. To read captions, children need, at least, a large sight vocabulary, knowledge of syntax and other language variables, and to be able to recognize words and sentences quickly. They also need to be able to switch their gaze from picture to text and back again integrating the two sources of information quickly. (Ward et al., 2007, p. 21)

Nevertheless, there are some similarities between print and caption literacy. For example, Lewis and Jackson (2001) found that although the comprehension of the captioned video was significantly better than that of print for students who are d/Deaf or hard of hearing, caption comprehension test scores were highly associated with print reading grade level. In addition, the students' caption comprehension test scores were significantly lower than those of hearing students with equivalent reading abilities.

Finally, for many students who are d/Deaf or hard of hearing, as linguistic complexity increases in caption literacy, the comprehension of the captions decreases (Berman & Jorgensen, 1980). To proceed to higher levels of understanding in caption literacy, children thus need to have some generic print literacy skills.

Role of Language

As mentioned throughout this book, a bona fide language is one major prerequisite for literacy development (and literate thought), regardless of the mode of literacy or form of captured information (see also, the discussion in Chapter 2). This assertion becomes evident in other recent studies using various forms of multimedia.

For example, Gentry et al. (2004/2005) investigated the effectiveness of multimedia compared to print-only presentation in d/Deaf students, aged 9 to 18 years, to test story retelling skills in four treatments: 1) print alone; 2) print plus pictures; 3) print and digital video of sign language; and 4) print, pictures and digital video of sign language. Comprehension was strongest in Treatment 2 and weakest in Treatment 1. No significant differences were found between Treatment 2 and Treatment 4, nor were there significant differences between Treatment 1 and Treatment 3.

The authors concluded that the multimedia presentation of reading materials is significantly more effective for reading comprehension than is the use of print only. It is not significantly better than the use of print plus pictures alone, however. Most interesting was that the integration of sign language with print but without pictures did not appear to enhance reading comprehension.

From another perspective, Marschark and colleagues (Marschark, Sapere, Convertino, Mayer, Waters, & Sarchet, 2009) investigated college students' learning of materials. Science texts were presented to d/Deaf students in print or ASL and to hearing students in print or auditorially.

Immediately following each passage, the participants were first asked to write down, in one or two sentences, the main idea of the passage, and then answer eight-questions on a post-test.

Results showed that d/Deaf students learned as much or more from print as they did from ASL, but less than hearing students in both cases (i.e., print and auditorially). The authors concluded that challenges to d/Deaf students' reading comprehension are not specific to print, but are related to the students' difficulties or development in language comprehension, particularly—in this case—in the language of signs (e.g., ASL). In other words, d/Deaf students' did not possess higher-level language and cognitive processes in *any mode* as did their hearing peers.

Instructional Applications of the New and Multiple Literacies

Leander (2009) categorized the current teaching and research stances on the relationship between the New and Multiple Literacies and more conventional print-based literacy into four groups: resistance, replacement, return, and remediation. People with the *resistance* stance believe firmly in traditional print literacy practices, which may be a practical response to the increased pressure from standardized assessments that emphasize conventional literacy skills. The New and Multiple Literacies are considered as interfering with the development of traditional print literacy skills.

Contrary to the resistance stance, the *replacement* stance underscores the *outdatedness* and *irrelevance* of traditional print literacy. For example, "Film analysis might replace novel interpretation, multimedia persuasion through websites may be a more appropriate set of skills for the future work place than the academic argument, and the aesthetics of poetry writing and analysis may be better updated by engaging the aesthetics of weblogs" (Leander, 2009, p. 148). Educators with a replacement stance are often *technophilic* counterparts to their *technophobia* foils with the resistance stance.

A common stance between resistance and replacement is *return*, which values the New and Multiple Literacies but validates and defends them with respect to print literacy. Skills in the New and Multiple Literacies are primarily measured by how they are a foundation to print literacy skills. For example, in the Iowa E-book project discussed previously (Mueller & Hurtig, 2010), the e-books were designed to "provide a form of scaffolding support for reading growth. Initially, the e-book may provide the sign and picture support for the child who is just beginning the reading process. As the child becomes a more efficient reader, the sign and picture support can be systematically removed until the child is able to read the text alone" (p. 78). The stance of return is essentially *printcentric*.

Leander (2009) remarked that the *remediation* stance is an imperfect label to describe the belief that the meaning of familiar, conventional print literacy is mediated once again through the less familiar New and Multiple Literacies. The new is never completely apart from the old; that is, skills developed in the New and Multiple Literacies include and embed those in print literacy instead of abandoning them. The remediation stance is agnostic regarding the existence of any supreme media.

In essence, Leander (2009) asserts the need for a *parallel pedagogy* in which old and new literacy practices, including print, performance, or multimedia literacies, are effectively taught equally in the classroom, instead of the old being a precursor to the new or being replaced by it. Access to information captured in the New and Multiple Literacies is only part of literacy development. Equally as important, children need to be able to interpret the information, that is, to discuss and analyze the captured information as well as to produce new information.

Consider the following as an example: After children watch an ASL-based *Click, Clack, Moo*, they can engage in group or class discussions on the content of the e-book, answer comprehension questions, and provide alternative endings for the story, all in ASL. Children's answers can be videotaped and used as the basis for grading. If children have the required ASL skills to participate in these activities, they are developing their literate thought in an equally, if not more, efficient manner as in print, and the skills that they acquired can be transferred into their skills in print literacy (see also the discussion in Chapters 2, 3, and 5). Similarly, children with visual impairment can listen to an audio book, contribute to class/group discussions, and they can be assessed based upon the recorded oral performance of their understanding and application of the text.

Most important, teachers of children with sensory disabilities should update their knowledge of literacy development for both typical children and children with sensory disabilities (Barlow-Brown & Connelly, 2002; Paul, 2001, 2009; Wang et al., 2008). The decision on the literacy medium or media should be based on the individual needs of the child. Regardless of the mode, an effective literacy instruction should be research-based, systematic, and consistent.

SUMMARY

This chapter emphasizes the challenges of developing literate language in children with sensory disabilities and promotes the use of alternative media. Specific implications are provided for developing literate thought.

The major points are as follows.

- Many children with visual impairment experience mild, if any, delay in reading (Braille), and the delay may be related to the nature of contractions in Braille orthography as well as limited literacy experiences.

- Many children with visual impairment perform equally well or even better than their sighted peers when their literacy skills are measured in the oral mode. Research on oral literacy skills of children with visual impairment is rare, however.

- Whether the input stimulus is visual as in print or tactile as in Braille, the main information-processing tasks in *reading* are essentially the same.

- The reading development of Braille readers is qualitatively similar to that of print readers.

- Many children with severe to profound hearing loss leave the educational system in the United States reading at the beginning of the fourth grade level, and more than 90% are reading at the sixth grade level or less.

- To understand reading and deafness, we need to recognize the different language experiences that d/Deaf or hard-of-hearing individuals bring to the task of reading as well as the similarities among better d/Deaf or hard-of-hearing readers and better hearing readers in their perception of the structure of English, for example, phonology, morphology, and syntax.

- The reading development of children who are d/Deaf or hard of hearing is qualitatively similar to that of hearing peers; however, many children have limited access to the sound structures of words and experience delays. Children who acquire the ability to process phonological and other information during early reading distinguish themselves from the average or struggling readers.

- Children with sensory impairments can use alternative media for developing literate thought, particularly with the assistance of technology.

- It is suggested that the literacy development of children with sensory disabilities be based on a parallel pedagogy that is research-based, systematic, consistent, and one that considers the individual needs of the child.

QUESTIONS FOR REFLECTION AND DISCUSSION

1. Describe the reading achievement level and development of students who are blind or have low vision.

2. Compare Braille literacy to print literacy. Discuss similarities and differences.

3. Describe the reading achievement level and development of students who are d/Deaf or hard of hearing.

4. Do the general findings of reading achievement and development support the basic tenets of the Qualitative-Similarity Hypothesis? Why or why not?

5. With respect to the use of technology, what are the implications for developing literate thought?

REFERENCES

Abner, G. H., & Lahm, E. A. (2002). Implementation of assistive technology with students who are visually impaired: Teachers' readiness. *Journal of Visual Impairment & Blindness, 96,* 98-105.

Adams, M. (1990). *Beginning to read: Thinking and learning about print.* Cambridge, MA: The MIT Press.

Alegria, J. (1998). The origin and functions of phonological representations in deaf people. In C. Hulme & R. M. Joshi (Eds.), *Reading and spelling: Development and disorders* (pp. 263-286). Mahwah, NJ: Erlbaum.

Allen, T. (1986). Patterns of academic achievement among hearing impaired students: 1974 and 1983. In A. Schildroth & M. Karchmer (Eds.), *Deaf children in America* (pp. 161-206). San Diego, CA: Little, Brown.

Allen, T., Clark, M. D., del Giudice, A., Koo, D., Lieberman, A., Mayberry, R., & Miller, P. (2009). Phonology and reading: A response to Wang, Trezek, Luckner, and Paul. *American Annals of the Deaf, 154*(4)*, 338-345.

American Printing House for the Blind (2007). *2007 annual report: American Printing House for the Blind.* New York: American Printing House for the Blind, Inc.

Apkarian-Stielau, P., & Loomis, J. M. A. (1974). A comparison of tactile and blurred visual form perception. *Perception and Psychophysics, 18,* 362-368.

Argyropoulos, V. S., Sideridis, G. D., & Katsoulis, P. (2008). The impact of the perspectives of teachers and parents on the literacy media selections for independent study of students who are visually impaired. *Journal of Visual Impairment & Blindness, 102,* 221-231.

Arnbak, E., & Elbro, C. (2000). The effects of morphological awareness training on the reading and spelling of young dyslexics. *Scandinavian Journal of Educational Research, 44,* 229-251.

Barlow-Brown, F., & Connelly, V. (2002). The role of letter knowledge and phonological awareness in young Braille readers. *Journal of Research in Reading, 25*(3), 259-270.

Berman, V., & Jorgensen, J. (1980). Evaluation of a multilevel linguistic approach to captioning television for hearing-impaired children. *American Annals of the Deaf, 125,* 1072-1081.

Bradley, L., & Bryant, P. (1983). Categorizing sounds and learning to read – a causal connection. *Nature, 301,* 419-421.

Brennan, S. A., Luze, G. J., & Peterson, C. (2009). Parents' perceptions of professional support for the emergent literacy of young children with visual impairments. *Journal of Visual Impairment & Blindness, 103*(10), 694-704.

Brown, R. (1973). *A first language.* Cambridge, MA: Harvard University Press.

Carlisle, J. (1995). Morphological awareness and early reading achievement. In L. B. Feldman (Ed.), *Morphological aspects of language processing* (pp. 189-209). Hillsdale, NJ: Erlbaum.

Carlisle, J., & Stone, C. A. (2005). Exploring the role of morphemes in word reading. *Reading Research Quarterly, 40,* 428-449.

Clark, C., & Stoner, J. B. (2008). An investigation of the spelling skills of braille readers. *Journal of Visual Impairment and Blindness, 102,* 553-563.

Corn, A. L., & Wall, R. S. (2002). Access to multimedia presentations for students with visual impairments. *Journal of Visual Impairment & Blindness, 96,* 197-211.

Cornett, R. O. (1967). Cued Speech. *American Annals of the Deaf, 112,* 3-13.

Council for Exceptional Children. (n.d.). *Blindness and visual impairment.* Retrieved January 12, 2011 from http://www.cec.sped.org/AM/Template.cfm?Section=Home&CONTENTID=7568&TEMPLATE=/CM/ContentDisplay.cfm

Crain, K. L., & LaSasso, C. J. (2010). Generative rhyming ability of 10- to 14- year-old readers who are deaf from oral and cued speech backgrounds. In C. J. LaSasso, K. L. Crain, & J. Leybaert (Eds.), *Cued Speech and Cued Language for deaf and hard of hearing children* (pp. 345-358). San Diego, CA: Plural Publishing.

Crawford, S., Elliott, R. T., & Hoekman, K. (2006). Phoneme, grapheme, onset-rime and word analysis in braille with young children. *The British Journal of Visual Impairment, 24*(3), 108-116.

Crystal, D. (1997). *The Cambridge encyclopedia of language (2nd ed).* New York: Cambridge University Press.

Daugherty, K. M., & Moran, M. F. (1982). Neuropsychological, learning, and developmental characteristics of the low vision child. *Visual Impairment & Blindness, 76,* 398-406.

Deacon, S. H., & Kirby, J. R. (2004). Morphological awareness: just "more phonological"? The roles of morphological and phonological awareness in reading development. *Applied Psycholinguistics, 25,* 223-238.

Dodd, B., & Conn, L. (2000). The effect of braille orthography on blind children's phonological awareness. *Journal of Research in Reading, 23,* 1-11.

Douglas, G., Grimley, M. McLinden, M., & Watson, L. (2004). Reading errors made by children with low vision. *Ophthalmic and Physiological Optics, 24*(4), 319-322.

Edmonds, C. J., & Pring, L. (2006). Generating inferences from written and spoken language: A comparison of children with visual impairment and children with sight. *British Journal of Developmental Psychology, 24,* 337-351.

Emerson, R. W., Holbrook, M. C., & D'Andrea, F. M. (2009). Acquisition of literacy skills by young children who are blind: Results of the ABC Braille study. *Journal of Visual Impairment and Blindness, 103,* 610-624.

Erin, J. N., Hong, S., Schoch, C., & Kuo, Y. (2006). Relationships among testing medium, test performance, and testing time of high school students who are visually impaired. *Journal of Visual Impairment & Blindness, 100,* 523-532.

Fellenius, K. (1999). Reading environment at home and at school of Swedish students with visual impairments. *Journal of Visual Impairment & Blindness, 93,* 211-224.

Ferrell, K. A., Trief, E., Dietz, S. J., Bonner, M. A., Cruz, D., Ford, E., & Stratton, J. M. (1990). Visually impaired infants research consortium (VIIRC): First-year results. *Journal of Visual Impairment & Blindness, 84*(8), 404-410.

Gallaudet Research Institute (2008). *Regional and national summary report of data from the 2007-2008 annual survey of deaf and hard of hearing children and youth.* Washington, D.C.: GRI, Gallaudet University.

Gentry, M. M., Chinn, K. M., & Moulton, R. D. (2004/2005). Effectiveness of multimedia reading materials when used with children who are deaf. *American Annals of the Deaf, 149*(5), 394-403.

Gillon, G., & Young, A. (2002). The phonological awareness skills of children who are blind. *Journal of Visual Impairment & Blindness, 96,* 38-49.

Gompel, M., van Bon, W. H. J., & Schreuder, R. (2004). Reading by children with low vision. *Journal of Visual Impairment & Blindness, 98,* 77-89.

Gompel, M., van Bon, W. H. J., Schreuder, R., & Adriaansen, J. J, M. (2002). Reading and spelling competence of Dutch children with low vision. *Journal of Visual Impairment & Blindness, 96,* 435-447.

Green, L., McCutchen, D., Schwiebert, C., Quinlan, T., Eva-Wood, A., & Juelis, J. (2003). Morphological development in children's writing. *Journal of Educational Psychology, 95,* 752-761.

Hanson, V. L. (1989). Phonology and reading: Evidence from profoundly deaf readers. In D. Shankweiler & I. Liberman (Eds.), *Phonology and reading disability: Solving the reading puzzle* (pp. 69-89). Ann Arbor: University of Michigan Press.

Hanson, V. L. (1991). Phonological processing without sound. In S. A. Brady & D. P. Shankweiler (Eds.), *Phonological processes in literacy: A tribute to Isabelle Y. Liberman* (pp. 153-162). Hillsdale, NJ: Erlbaum.

Hanson, V L., & Padden, C. A. (1990). Computers and videodisc technology for bilingual ASL/English instruction for deaf children. In D. Nix & R. Spiro (Eds.), *Cognition, education, and multimedia: Exploring ideas in high technology* (pp. 49-63). Hillsdale, NJ: Erlbaum.

Hasselbring, T. A. (2001). A possible future of special education technology. *Journal of Special Education Technology, 16*(4), 15-21.

Hayes, P., & Arnold, P. (1992). Is hearing-impaired children's reading delayed or different? *Journal of Research in Reading, 15,* 104-116.

Holbrook, M. C. (2009). Supporting students' literacy through data-driven decision making and ongoing assessment of achievement. *Journal of Visual Impairment & Blindness, 103,* 133-136.

Horney, M., Anderson-Inman, L., & Chen, D. (1994). Project LITERACY-HI: Hypermedia for readers with hearing impairments. *The Oregon Conference Monograph, 7,* 195-208.

Huey, E. (1908/1968). *The psychology and pedagogy of reading.* New York: Macmillan. (Reprint: Cambridge, MA: The MIT Press).

Koenig, A. J., & Holbrook, M. C. (Eds.). (2000). *Foundations of education: Instructional strategies for teaching children and youths with visual impairments* (2nd ed.). New York, NY: American Foundation for the Blind.

LaSasso, C. J., & Crain, K. L. (2010). Cued language for the development of deaf students' reading comprehension and measured reading comprehension. In C. J. LaSasso, K. L. Crain, & J. Leybaert (Eds.), *Cued Speech and Cued Language for deaf and hard of hearing children* (pp. 285-321). San Diego, CA: Plural Publishing.

Leander, K. (2009). Composing with old and new media: Toward a parallel pedagogy. In V. Carrington & M. Robinson (Eds.), *Digital literacies: Social learning and classroom practices* (pp. 147-163). London: SAGE.

Lewis, M., & Jackson, D. (2001). Television literacy: Comprehension of program content using closed captions for the Deaf. *Journal of Deaf Studies and Deaf Education, 6*(1), 43-53.

Leybaert, J., Colin, S., & LaSasso, C. J. (2010). Cued Speech for the deaf students' mastery of the alphabetic principle. In C. J. LaSasso, K. L. Crain, & J. Leybaert (Eds.), *Cued Speech and Cued Language for deaf and hard of hearing children* (pp. 245-283). San Diego, CA: Plural Publishing.

Linebarger, D. (2001). Learning to read from television: The effects of using captions and narration. *Journal of Educational Psychology, 93*(2), 288-298.

Lorimer, J. (1992). *Braille teaching and learning.* Birmingham: University of Birmingham.

Lowenfeid, B., Abel, G. L., & Hatlen, P. H. (1968). *Blind children learn to read.* Springfield, IL: Charles C Thomas.

Luckner, J. L., & Handley, C. M. (2008). A summary of the reading comprehension research undertaken with students who are deaf or hard of hearing. *American Annals of the Deaf, 153*(1), 6-36.

Luckner, J. L., Sebald, A. N., Cooney, J., Young, J., & Goodwin Muir, S. (2005/2006). An examination of the evidence-based literacy research in deaf education. *American Annals of the Deaf, 150*(5), 443-456.

Lusk, K. E., & Corn, A. L. (2006). Learning and using print and braille: A study of dual-media learners, Part 1. *Journal of Visual Impairment & Blindness, 100,* 606-619.

Marschark, M., & Harris, M. (1996). Success and failure in learning to read: The special case (?) of deaf children. In C. Cornoldi & J. Oakhill (Eds.), *Reading comprehension difficulties: Processes and intervention* (pp. 279-300). Mahwah, NJ: Erlbaum.

Marschark, M., Rhoten, C., & Fabich, M. (2007). Effects of cochlear implants on children's reading and academic achievement. *Journal of Deaf Studies and Deaf Education, 12*(3), 269-282.

Marschark, M., Sapere, P., Convertino, C., Mayer, C., Waters, L., & Sarchet, T. (2009). Are deaf students' reading challenges really about reading. *American Annuals of the Deaf, 154*(4), 357-370.

Marschark, M., & Spencer, P. E. (2006). Spoken language development of deaf and hard-of-hearing children: Historical and theoretical perspectives. In P. E. Spencer & M. Marschark (Eds.), *Advances in the spoken language development of deaf and hard-of-hearing children* (pp. 3-21). New York: Oxford University Press.

McGuinness, D. (2004). *Early reading instruction: What science really tells us about how to teach reading.* Cambridge, MA: The MIT Press.

McGuinness, D. (2005). *Language development and learning to read: The scientific study of how language development affects reading skill.* Cambridge, MA: The MIT Press.

McKenzie, A. R. (2009). Emergent literacy supports for students who are deaf-blind or have visual and multiple impairments: A multiple-case study. *Journal of Visual Impairment & Blindness, 103,* 291-302.

Mitchell, R. E. (2005, February). *A brief summary of estimates for the size of the deaf population in the USA based on available federal data and published research.* Retrieved June 1, 2010 from http://research.gallaudet.edu/Demographics/deaf-US.php

Moores, D. (2006). Print literacy: The acquisition of reading and writing skills. In D. Moores & D. Martin (Eds.), *Deaf learners: Development in curriculum and instruction* (pp. 41-55). Washington, DC: Gallaudet University Press.

Moores, D. (2008). Research on Bi-Bi instruction. *American Annals of the Deaf, 153*(1), 3-4.

Morais, J., Cary, L., Alegria, J., & Bertelson, P. (1979). Does awareness of speech as a sequence of phones arise spontaneously? *Cognition, 7,* 323-331.

Mueller, V., & Hurtig, R. (2010). Technology-enhanced shared reading with deaf and hard-of-hearing children: The role of a fluent signing narrator. *Journal of Deaf Studies and Deaf Education, 15*(1), 72-101.

National Early Literacy Panel (NELP). (2008). *Developing early literacy: Report of the National Early Literacy Panel.* Washington, DC: National Institute for Literacy. Available at http://www.alabamaschoolreadiness.org/uploadedFiles/File/NELPReport09.pdf.

National Reading Panel (NRP). (2000). *Report of the National Reading Panel: Teaching children to read – An evidence-based assessment of the scientific research literature on reading and its implications for reading instruction.* Jessup, MD: National Institute for Literacy at EDPubs.

Nolan, C. (1967). A 1966 reappraisal of the relationship between visual acuity and mode of reading for blind children. *New Outlook for the Blind, 61*(8), 255-261.

Nolan, C., & Kederis, C. (1969). Perceptual factors in braille word Recognition. *Research series, No.20.* New York: American Foundation for the Blind.

Nunes, T., & Bryant, P. (2006). *Improving literacy by teaching morphemes.* New York: Routledge.

Nunes, T., & Bryant, P. (2009). *Children's reading and spelling: Beyond the first steps.* West Sussex, UK: Wiley-Blackwell.

Paul, P. (1998). *Literacy and deafness: The development of reading, writing, and literate thought.* Needham Heights, MA: Allyn & Bacon.

Paul, P. (2001). *Language and deafness* (3rd ed.). San Diego, CA: Singular Publishing Group.

Paul, P. (2003). Processes and components of reading. In M. Marschark & P. Spencer (Eds.), *Handbook of deaf studies, language, and education* (pp. 97-109). New York: Oxford University Press.

Paul, P. (2008). Introduction: Reading and children with disabilities. *Balanced Reading Instruction, 15*(2), 1-12.

Paul, P. (2009). *Language and deafness* (4th ed.). Sudbury, MA: Jones & Bartlett.

Paul, P., & Lee. C. (2010). The qualitative similarity hypothesis. *American Annals of the Deaf, 154*(5), 456-462.

Paul, P., & Wang, Y. (2006a). Multiliteracies and literate thought. *Theory into Practice, 45*(4), 304-310.

Paul, P., & Wang, Y. (2006b). Literate thought and deafness: A call for a new perspective and line of research on literacy. *Punjab University Journal of Special Education* (Pakistan), *2*(1), 28-37.

Paul, P., Wang, Y., Trezek, B., & Luckner, J. (2009). Phonology is necessary, but not sufficient: A rejoinder. *American Annals of the Deaf, 154*(4), 346-356.

Paul, P,. & Whitelaw, G. (2011). *Hearing and deafness: An introduction for health and educational professionals.* Sudbury, MA: Jones & Bartlett Learning.

Perfetti, C. A., & Sandak, R. (2000). Reading optimally builds on spoken language: Implications for deaf readers. *Journal of Deaf Studies and Deaf Education, 5*(1), 32-50.

Pring, L. (1982). Phonological and tactual coding of Braille by blind children. *British Journal of Psychology. 73,* 351-359.

Pring, L. (1984). A comparison of the word recognition processes of blind and sighted children. *Child Development, 55,* 1865-1877.

Pring, L. (1994). Touch and go: Learning to read Braille. *Reading Research Quarterly, 29,* 67-74.

Rayner, K., & Pollatsek. A. (1989). *The psychology of reading.* Hillsdale, NJ: Lawrence Erlbaum.

Rose, S., McAnally, P., & Quigley, S. (2004). *Language learning practices with deaf children* (3rd ed.). Austin, TX: PRO-ED, Inc.

Schirmer, B. R., & McGough, S. M. (2005). Teaching reading to children who are deaf: Do the conclusions of the National Reading Panel apply? *Review of Educational Research, 75*(1), 83-117.

Shull, T. F., & Crain, K. L. (2010). Fundamental principles of Cued Speech and Cued Language. In C. J. LaSasso, K. L. Crain, & J. Leybaert (Eds.), *Cued Speech and Cued Language for deaf and hard of hearing children* (pp. 28-51). San Diego, CA: Plural Publishing.

Smith, A., & Wang, Y. (2010). The impact of Visual Phonics on the phonological awareness and speech production of a student who is deaf: A case study. *American Annals of the Deaf, 155*(2), 124-130.

Snow, C., Burns, S., & Griffin, P. (Eds.). (1998). *Preventing reading difficulties in young children*. Washington, DC: National Academy Press.

Spencer, L. J., & Tomblin, J. B. (2009). Evaluating phonological processing skills in children with prelingual deafness who use cochlear implants. *Journal of Deaf Studies and Deaf Education, 14*(1), 1-21.

Steinman, B., LeJeune, B. J., & Kimbrough, B. T. (2006). Developmental stages of reading processes in children who are blind and sighted. *Journal of Visual Impairment & Blindness, 100,* 36-46.

Syverud, S. M., Guardino, C., & Selznick, D. N. (2009). Teaching phonological skills to a deaf first grader: A promising strategy. *American Annals of the Deaf, 154*(4), 382-388.

Tobin, M. (1985). The reading skills of the partially sighted: Their implications for integrated education. *International Journal of Rehabilitation Research, 8,* 467-472.

Tobin, M., Douce, J., Lorimer, J., & Gill, J. (1980). *A study of Braille contractions*. Report to the DHSS: Birmingham and Warwick Universities.

Traxler, C. (2000). The Stanford Achievement Test, 9th edition: National norming and performance standards for deaf and hard-of-hearing students. *Journal of Deaf Studies and Deaf Education, 5,* 337-348.

Trent, S. D., & Truan, M. B. (1997). Speed, accuracy, and comprehension of adolescent Braille readers in a specialized school. *Journal of Visual Impairment & Blindness, 91,* 494-500.

Trezek, B. J., & Malmgren, K. W. (2005). The efficacy of utilizing a phonics treatment package with middle school deaf and hard of hearing students. *Journal of Deaf Studies and Deaf Education, 10*(3), 256-271.

Trezek, B. J., & Wang, Y. (2006). Implications of utilizing a phonics-based reading curriculum with children who are deaf or hard of hearing. *Journal of Deaf Studies and Deaf Education, 11*(2), 202-213.

Trezek, B., Wang, Y., & Paul, P. (2010a). *Reading and deafness: Theory, research and practice*. Clifton Park, NY: Cengage Learning.

Trezek, B., Wang, Y., & Paul, P. (2010b). Processes and components of reading. In M. Marschark & P. Spencer (Eds.), *Handbook of deaf studies, language, and education* (Vol. 1, Part II; pp. 99-114). New York: Oxford University Press.

Trezek, B. J., Wang, Y., Woods, D. G., Gampp, T. L., & Paul, P. V. (2007). Using Visual Phonics to supplement beginning reading instruction for students who are deaf/hard of hearing. *Journal of Deaf Studies and Deaf Education, 12*(3), 373-384.

van Bon, W. H. J., Adriaansen, L., Gompel, M., & Kouwenberg, I. (2000). The reading and spelling performance of visually impaired Dutch elementary school-children. *Visual Impairment Research, 2*(1), 17-31.

Wang, Y. (2005). *Literate thought: Metatheorizing in literacy and deafness.* Unpublished doctoral dissertation, Ohio State University, Columbus.

Wang, Y., Kretschmer, R., & Hartman, M. (2008). Reading and students who are d/Deaf or hard of hearing. *Journal of Balanced Reading Instruction, 15*(2), 53-68.

Wang, Y., & Paul, P. (2011). Integrating technology and reading instruction with children who are deaf or hard of hearing – The effectiveness of the Cornerstones Project. *American Annals of the Deaf, 156*(1), 56-68.

Wang, Y., Trezek, B. J., Luckner, J. L., & Paul, P. V. (2008). The role of phonology and phonological-related skills in reading instruction for students who are deaf or hard of hearing. *American Annals of the Deaf, 153*(4), 396-407.

Ward, P., Wang, Y., Paul, P., & Loeterman, M. (2007). Near verbatim versus edited captioning for students who are deaf or hard of hearing: A preliminary investigation of effects on comprehension. *American Annals of the Deaf, 152*(1), 20-28.

Williams, M. (1971). Braille reading. *Teacher of the Blind, 59*, 103-116.

Wormsley, D. P. (2008). Literacy instruction for children who are blind or visually impaired. *Journal of Balanced Reading Instruction, 15*(2), 69-87.

FURTHER READING

Brueggemann, B.J. (Ed). (2004). *Literacy and Deaf people: Cultural and contextual perspectives.* Washington, DC: Gallaudet University Press.

Harley, R. K., Truan, M. B., & Sanford, L. D. (1997). *Communication skills for visually impaired learners.* Springfield, IL: Charles C Thomas.

Koenig, A. J., & Farrenkopf, C. (1995). *Assessment of Braille literacy skills.* Houston, TX: Region IV Education Service Center.

Marschark, M., & Clark, M. D. (Eds.). (1992). *Psychological perspectives on deafness.* Hillsdale, NJ: Lawrence Erlbaum Associates.

Marschark, M., & Spencer, P. (Eds.). (2011). *Handbook of deaf studies, language, and education.* New York: Oxford University Press.

Troughton, M. (1992). *One is fun: Guidelines for better Braille literacy.* Brantford. Ontario, Canada: Dialatype.

CHAPTER 8

Children with Developmental Disabilities

Racial segregation, with its manifest restrictions on literacy, was ultimately realized in the Brown decision to represent an arbitrary and thus unconstitutional denial of equal protection. In contrast, the presumption of intellectual disabilities continues to provide what is commonly considered to be an objective, intrinsic rationale for the educational separation of labeled from nonlabeled individuals. Restricted literacy among people with disabilities has become institutionalized as a presumably natural manifestation of organic defects thought to objectively exist well beyond the reach of social, cultural, or historical consideration.

Kliewer, Biklen, & Kasa-Hendrickson, 2006, p. 164

The goal of education for students with moderate and severe disabilities is to provide skills that will enable them to live, work, and participate in an integrated community. Active integration requires the ability to access goods and services and to engage in purposeful and safe mobility around the community. Such engagement requires the ability to discern information in multiple ways. Definitions of literacy that focus solely on reading words provide too narrow a framework and are functionally insufficient for many students with moderate and severe intellectual disabilities as they engage in natural community settings. . . . A more inclusive definition of functional literacy is the ability to obtain information—from the environment, through a variety of modes—with which to make decisions and choices, alter the environment, and gain pleasure.

Alberto, Fredrick, Hughes, McIntosh, & Cihak, 2007, p. 234

As advocated by Kliewer et al. (2006) in the first cited passage above, many scholars have criticized society's constant denial of literate citizenship for people with developmental disabilities. Associated with the experiences of other devalued and marginalized groups such as minority racial groups, who were historically segregated from the educational privilege, a number of scholars challenge the common perception that citizenship in the literate community is impossible for people with developmental disabilities. Kliewer et al. called for "a science of literacy for all" (p. 163) to provide every child with opportunities to develop as literate citizens, particularly the labeled children, who are still legally segregated from "valued access to the citizenship tools of literacy" (p. 164).

From another perspective, scholars such as Alberto et al. (2007) in the second cited passage above questioned the value or relevance of traditional literacy skills (i.e., reading and writing) for individuals with moderate or severe developmental disabilities. Yes, these individuals deserve a seat within the circle of educational privilege, but do they want the same *citizenship tools of literacy* as their typically developing peers or are these tools even practical for them? In this *No Child Left Behind* era, schools are required to document adequate yearly progress (AYP) in reading as well as math and science for all children, including those with disabilities, with the exception of up to 1% of children with significant developmental disabilities who can use alternative achievement standards.

Is this realistic? If we allow some children to be left behind (i.e., becoming the exception), who should make the decision and what should be the criteria? Most importantly, what should be the appropriate alternative achievement standards? Or, maybe we should ask the question: *No child left behind of what?* Citizenship tools of print literacy or citizenship tools of the New and Multiple Literacies that allow individuals to acquire and utilize information in the community through multiple pathways?

In an attempt to answer these questions and highlight the need for the focus on literate thought, this chapter starts with a general introduction of the reading skills of children with developmental disabilities. Then it is divided into several sections to cover reading and subgroups of children, that is, children with Down syndrome, Williams syndrome, or autism spectrum disorders. Word recognition and language comprehension skills of each subgroup are discussed in detail. Finally, with an eye on the development of literate thought, the application of concepts of the New and Multiple Literacies and its specific implications are examined.

Similar to children with reading (i.e., language and literacy) disabilities (discussed in Chapter 6), sensory disabilities (discussed in Chapter 7) or those who learn English as a second language (discussed in Chapter 9), children with developmental disabilities comprised a widely varied group with heterogeneous language and reading skills. Most of the available research studies on the reading skills of children with developmental disabilities are on those with mild or moderate disabilities who were reading at a reasonably advanced level or who had some minimal measurable language skills. Readers should interpret the research results with caution to avoid overestimating the language and reading achievements of children with developmental disabilities.

GENERAL READING SKILLS OF CHILDREN WITH DEVELOPMENTAL DISABILITIES

Developmental disabilities are a diverse group of severe chronic conditions that are linked to mental and/or physical impairments (Centers for Disease Control and Prevention, 2010). In this chapter, we mainly focus on mental impairments such as intellectual disabilities and autism spectrum disorders. Although some scholars use intellectual disability and developmental disability interchangeably, in this text, we purposefully distinguish between these two terms.

Intellectual disability, also known as *cognitive disability* or sometimes *mental retardation*, is the most common developmental disorder. Intellectual disability is more prevalent in boys than in girls and more common in African-American children than in white children. Mild intellectual disability is three times more prevalent than severe intellectual disability (Centers for Disease Control and Prevention, 2010). The cause of intellectual disability for many children is unknown. The primary focus of this chapter is on reading research and children with *Down syndrome* or *Williams syndrome*—two of the most commonly known or widely researched causes of cognitive disability.

Autism Spectrum Disorders (ASD) is a broad category of psychological conditions that typically feature abnormalities of social interactions and communication along with severely restricted interests and highly repetitive behavior (Snowling & Hulme, 2007). There are three types of ASD: *autism*, *Asperger syndrome*, and *Pervasive Developmental Disorder not Otherwise Specified* (PDD-NOS), or *atypical autism*. In this chapter, we discuss the reading ability of children and adolescents with ASD in general, and then we focus on those with Asperger syndrome specifically. **Figure 8-1** provides a structure of the different developmental disability groups introduced in this chapter.

Reading Instruction: Sight Word Versus Phonics

In a comprehensive review of 128 studies on reading instruction for children with developmental disabilities, considered in light of the National Reading Panel's components of effective reading instruction (i.e., phonemic awareness, phonics, fluency, vocabulary and text comprehension), Browder and colleagues (Browder, Wakeman, Spooner, Ahlgrim-Delzell, & Algozzine, 2006) found a few high quality (i.e., peer-reviewed scientific) studies with positive results for vocabulary, specifically, sight word instruction, fluency, and text comprehension. Browder et al. documented only three studies that focus on phonics instruction with positive findings associated with one high-quality study.

For many children with developmental disabilities, reading instruction is often exclusively focused on sight word reading (see also the reviews in Browder & Xin, 1998; Conners, 1992). Teaching sight words, using systematic prompting and fading such as constant time delay (CTD), has the strongest research evidence for effectiveness (Browder, Ahlgrim-Delzell, Spooner, Mims, & Baker, 2009). As Browder and Xin reported, however, sight word studies might offer strong demonstrations of teaching children to name words, but these studies have not established that children understand the words or apply them to their daily routine.

As a non-transparent language, English has many irregular words that do not lend themselves to decoding and must be acquired as sight words. Sight word reading can build vocabulary as part of a reading program, but without appropriate phonemic awareness and phonics skills, children cannot generalize to decode untaught words (see also the discussion in Chapter 6). Phonics decoding skills are the means of adding new words to the body of words that individuals can recognize promptly by sight as

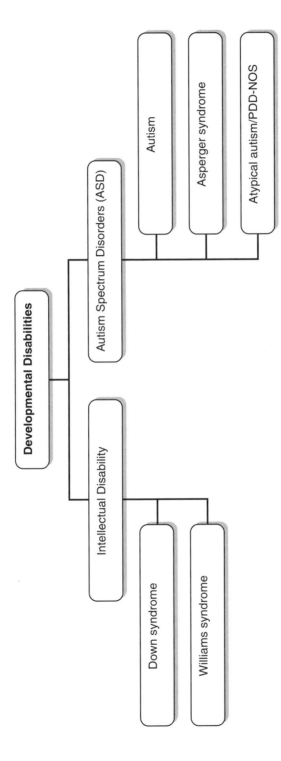

Figure 8-1. Structure of Developmental Disability Groups

a whole. That is, new words that are initially recognized by phonics decoding skills eventually should be read quickly by sight.

There remains a dearth of research on phonemic awareness and phonics instruction for children with developmental disabilities (see the review in Conners, 1992, and the updated review since 1992 in Joseph & Seery, 2004). Saunders (2007) provided two possible reasons: 1) developmental disability is a low-incidence, heterogeneous population, making it difficult to produce statistically significant effects; 2) historically, the research community is slow in applying findings from the mainstream reading literature to this population.

Role of Phonological-Related Skills in Decoding

The role of phonological-related skills in decoding for children with developmental disabilities, especially an intellectual disability such as Down syndrome, is not without controversy. Two of the most cited and debated studies were conducted by Cossu and colleagues (Cossu & Marshall, 1990; Cossu, Rossini, & Marshall, 1993). In a case study of an Italian boy with a severe intellectual disability, Cossu and Marshall (1990) reported that the boy obtained a perfect score for reading both words and nonwords, but exhibited poor phonological and phonemic awareness skills. For example, he was not able to understand the task for rhyming and phoneme blending. Although his performance was better on phoneme segmentation and deletion, it was still well below that of a group of typically developing control subjects matched on chronological age.

In a second study (Cossu et al., 1993), 10 Italian children with Down syndrome were matched with 10 younger, normally developing children on their ability to read aloud both regular and irregular words and nonwords. The children with Down syndrome performed significantly poorer than the comparison group on all four phonological and phonemic awareness tasks (i.e., phoneme segmentation, deletion, blending, and oral spelling). Cossu et al. concluded that children with Down syndrome were able to learn to read "despite signal failure on tests of 'phonological awareness'" (p. 133).

The Cossu studies have been criticized for various reasons. For example, several researchers (Byrne, 1993; Cupples & Iacono, 2000) argued that the children with Down syndrome did not achieve a score of *zero* on the phonological and phonemic awareness tasks, although they performed significantly poorer when compared with normally developing children. It might be possible that the minimal phonological-related skills that they had were sufficient for reading acquisition.

Second, the apparently poor performance of children with Down syndrome in these two studies on phonological-related skills might be a result of poor general cognitive ability rather than a lack of competence in phonological-related skills (Byrne, 1993; Cupples & Iacono, 2000). One of the phonemic awareness skills is phoneme blending, which requires a child to remember a string of phonemes to combine them in order to form a word. For example, when presented three separated phonemes: /d/, /o/, /g/, the child is expected to say them slowly /d/-/o/-/g/ and then fast /dog/.

Blending phonemes to form words appears to be difficult for many children with developmental disabilities due to their lack of experience with phonemes produced in isolation, memory difficulties, or failure to understand the given directions (Hoogeveen, Birkhoff, Smeets, Lancioni, & Boelens, 1989; Hoogeveen, Kouwenhoven, & Smeets, 1989). In the Cossu et al. (1993) study, although 7 out of 10 participating children with Down syndrome had digit spans of 3 or lower, they were presented with either 4 or 6 individual phonemes for blending, whereas all children in the comparison group achieved digit span scores of 4 or above. It might be possible that the participating children with Down syndrome in the study had the targeted phonemic awareness skills but were not able to demonstrate these skills in the tasks.

One of the most outstanding features of children with intellectual disabilities is memory difficulties, which appear to affect phonological working memory, especially in the rehearsal process (Cohen, Heller, Alberto, & Fredrick, 2008; Coleman-Martin, Heller, Cihak, & Irvine, 2005; Conners, Atwell, Rosenquist, & Sligh, 2001). As discussed in detail in Chapter 6, an adequate phonological working memory is necessary for holding phonological information to allow remembering meanings of words within the sentence, retrieving information from preceding text, parsing the sentence, and so on. Many researchers have warned that the metacognitive demands of some assessments on phonological related skills might be too great for children with intellectual disabilities (see the review in Saunders, 2007).

Conners and colleagues (2001) found that a phonological rehearsal process was the strongest predictor of decoding ability for children with mild/moderate intellectual disabilities. Other factors involved in the decoding abilities of these children included age (with older children being better decoders), language skills, and phonemic awareness skills. It should be noted that Intelligence Quotient (IQ) was not found to be a significant factor for decoding ability (Siegel, 1993; Stanovich, Cunningham, & Freeman, 1984).

In response to the Cossu studies, Cupples and Iacono (2000) investigated the relationship between phonological awareness and early oral reading development of 22 children with Down syndrome between the ages of 6 and 10 years, inclusive. Participants were initially assessed on receptive language, cognitive function, oral reading, and phonological awareness. Then oral reading and phonological awareness were assessed again approximately nine months later. The researchers reported better oral reading associated with superior phoneme segmentation skills on reassessment, and early segmentation ability as a predictor for later nonword reading, even after controlling for the effects of age, digit span, receptive vocabulary, and early reading ability.

In light of the finding that phoneme segmentation ability was positively associated with early oral reading skill, Cupples and Iacono (2000) concluded that these children learned to read in a manner that was qualitatively similar to that of children developing typically—a conclusion that is similar to ours in Chapter 4 (i.e., Qualitative-Similarity Hypothesis). The fact that segmentation, rather than blending, was positively associated with reading seems to support Stuart and Coltheart's (1988) account of the role of phonological awareness in reading development. As described earlier, they argued that children with good segmentation skills were at an advantage when it came to establishing lexical representations for printed words because they could use their segmentation skills along with their knowledge of letter–sound correspondences to predict how newly encountered spoken words should look in print.

Additional evidence can be found in the literature on young, typically developing children. That is, it seems to be clear that phoneme segmentation skills are more strongly associated with early reading than phoneme blending skills (Wagner, Torgeson, & Rashotte, 1994; Yopp, 1988). Finally, it is also reported that the onset-rime distinction (assessed in rhyme and alliteration tasks) is not crucially important in early reading (Duncan, Seymour, & Hill, 1997).

Overall, the general consensus is that although children with intellectual disabilities have poor phonological-related skills, similar to their typically developing peers, their phonological-related skills are associated with their decoding skills. Furthermore, children with intellectual disabilities are able to perform phonological-related tasks after adequate training is provided (Hoogeveen & Smeets, 1988; Hoogeveen, Smeets, & Lanconi, 1989). In fact, research has found that, with or without instruction, children with mild/moderate intellectual disabilities demonstrated the ability to: 1) produce letter–sound correspondences; 2) segment phonemes; 3) blend phonemes to form words; and most importantly, 4) decode unknown words of similar phonetic structure (Browder et al., 2006; Cohen, et al., 2008). In a review of the literature on the use of phonetic analysis for children with intellectual disabilities, Joseph and Serry (2004) concluded that children with intellectual disabilities not only have the potential to benefit from phonics instruction but also could make progress in their decoding skills.

Reading Interventions on Word Recognition and Language Comprehension

A variety of phonics instructional methods have been used with children with mild/moderate developmental disabilities with varying degrees of success. For example, using the *Corrective Reading Program* (Engelmann, Becker, Hanner, & Johnson, 1980), Bradford, Shippen, Alberto, Houchins, and Flores (2006) were successful in teaching decoding to middle school children with moderate intellectual disabilities. In another study conducted by Cohen et al. (2008), a three-step decoding explicit phonics instruction with CTD was used with five students with mild/moderate intellectual disabilities, aged 9 to 14. The three steps consisted of a) attention-getting, b) decoding, and c) reading-the-word. All participants were able to learn words although only one student was able to read unknown words of phonetically similar structures. These results further confirmed that phonological memory, instead of IQ, was associated with the acquisition rate of learning words.

What about children with severe developmental disabilities, who are either nonverbal or who utilize augmentative communication systems? These children typically do not have adequate verbal skills to respond to instruction in the typical phonics instruction format, and the language deficits for many of them are so severe that they cannot derive meaning from printed text. Coleman-Martin et al. (2005) investigated the effectiveness of computer-assisted instruction to promote word identification using the Nonverbal Reading Approach (NRA), a metacognitive strategy for decoding words. Results from three students with severe speech impairments and concomitant physical disabilities or autism showed that the NRA could be effectively delivered through computer-assisted instruction to free up teacher time and provide students with the independent ability to practice decoding and word identification.

Evaluating the effectiveness of an adapted early literacy curriculum (i.e., *Early Literacy Skills Builder*) for children with severe developmental disabilities, Browder, Ahlgrim-Delzell, Courtade, Gibbs, and Flowers (2008), found significant differences between the intervention group and the control group on two research team-designed measures of early literacy and two standardized language measurements by using finger pointing responses and an eye gazing system. The authors concluded (providing more evidence for the Qualitative-Similarity Hypothesis, discussed in Chapter 4):

> What will be important is to build on the science of reading that is already available. Until research indicates otherwise, the best starting point will be in adapting interventions proven effective for typically developing students. This requires gaining deeper knowledge of this literature as well as knowing what has been effective in teaching reading to students with significant disabilities. Research is especially needed on comprehensive and longitudinal curricula that school systems can adapt and modify for this population. It will be difficult for teachers to piece together a reading program from studies that focus on only one component of reading. Research also is needed on measures that show gains relevant to reading, but that are not biased against students who are nonverbal or have sensory or physical impairments. Through such research more students with significant disabilities may gain the skills needed to become readers. (p. 50)

Reading Interventions on Self-Confidence and Motivation

Other than the difficulties on word recognition and language comprehension, many children with developmental disabilities also suffer from lack of self-confidence and motivation in reading due to the impact of limited instruction, poor skills, and failure at academic tasks (Basil & Reyes, 2003; see also the risk factor of less engaged and less intrinsically motivated readers in Chapter 6). One critical reason for the failure of children with developmental disabilities to acquire literacy skills might be that they do not have sufficient understanding of the required instructional tasks to be fully interested in reading and writing activities.

Many children might not benefit from traditional instruction in which teachers lead or direct. Instead, they need more active and self-directed learning to make the tasks more meaningful for them. A *scaffolding* approach that emphasizes spontaneous dialogues and co-construction of language should support these children and encourage active involvement in solving meaningful tasks.

Basil and Reyes (2003) examined the performance of three boys and three girls with severe developmental disabilities, between 8 and 16 years old, to evaluate the effectiveness of a multimedia software *Delta Messages* and a scaffolding approach. During the intervention, the participants were able to follow their own course and speed, and were offered feedback on their self-directed productions. The participants showed significant gains not only in targeted skills such as sentence production through a whole-word selection strategy, but also in non-targeted skills such as the ability to synthesize and spell words. The observed gains were maintained and even improved in the two follow-up periods. The authors concluded that substantial practice of self-initiated and meaningful literacy activities promotes the literacy acquisition of children with severe developmental disabilities.

Conclusion

Historically, the reading instruction of children with developmental disabilities overwhelmingly has been focused on sight word reading, despite mounting evidence that, similar to their typically developing peers, these children can and should be taught to use phonemic awareness and phonics skills in decoding. It is possible that children with significant developmental disabilities "may not have learned to read in the past because they were either not taught to read or were not taught with methods that promote literacy" (Browder et al., 2006, p. 404). Furthermore, in addition to word recognition and language comprehension difficulties, many children with developmental disabilities also suffer from low self-confidence and lack of motivation. In essence, an effective, comprehensive reading intervention for children with developmental disabilities should include components to address all three above areas.

In the next section, the focus is on specific groups within the population of children with developmental disabilities.

READING AND CHILDREN WITH DOWN SYNDROME

As the most frequent human chromosomal abnormality (i.e., trisomy of Chromosome 21), Down syndrome occurs in approximately 1.5 per 1,000 live births (Snowling & Hulme, 2007). Children with Down syndrome typically have full-scale IQ between 50 and 70 and often have language acquisition difficulties including phonological problems.

The delayed language development of children with Down syndrome, particularly, their expressive language deficits (e.g., expressive grammatical difficulties), have been reported as greater than expected on the basis of nonverbal cognitive impairments. Although their lexical knowledge is relatively strong, children with Down syndrome are reported to have language problems in speech production, phonological memory, and syntactic, conversational, and narrative difficulties (Chapman, Seung, Schwartz, & Kay-Raining Bird, 1998; Snowling & Hulme, 2007).

Chapman et al. (1998) investigated the validity of four popular hypotheses regarding children and adolescents with Down syndrome: 1) a specific expressive language impairment; 2) a critical period for language acquisition; 3) a simple sentence syntactic ceiling in language production; and 4) a deficit in grammatical morphology. Based on their analyses of conversational and narrative language samples from children and adolescents aged 5 to 20 years, and those from typically developing comparison children aged 2 to 6 years, matched for nonverbal mental age, the authors concluded that children and adolescents with Down syndrome: 1) appeared to have a specific language impairment in terms of the number of different words, total words, and mean length of utterance (MLU) and, particularly, their intelligibility of narratives was significantly poorer; 2) showed no evidence of a critical period for language development ending at adolescence; 3) demonstrated no proof of a syntactic ceiling corresponding to simple sentences; and 4) omissions of grammatical morphology were more frequent in the older participants than in the younger comparison sample matched on MLU. Overall, the study reported that children and adolescents with Down syndrome had specific expressive language deficits across measures of syntax, lexicon, amount and rate of speaking, and intelligibility, in contrast to mental-age matched typically developing children.

Although there is no longer a debate on the ability of children with Down syndrome to learn to read, many individuals with Down syndrome still have never been offered the opportunity to learn to read (Moni & Jobling, 2001). Studies reporting the reading abilities of individuals with Down syndrome have been limited. A group of Australian scholars (Bochner, Outhred, & Pieterse, 2001) measured the literacy skills of 29 young adults with Down syndrome aged 18 to 36 years, and found that all but one of them had learned to read, although the levels of reading skills varied. The mean age-equivalent score for receptive language skills was 7 years, 2 months; and the mean reading age of the participants as a group was 8 years, 1 month. In addition, the highest scores on the reading achievement assessments were recorded by the same three participants who had scored highest on the receptive language measurements; the lowest scores were attained by the same two participants who performed poorly on the receptive language measurements. Overall, the reading achievement scores of the participants were highly correlated with their receptive language scores.

Similarly, Fowler, Doherty, and Boynton (1995) measured the reading skills of 33 young adults with Down syndrome, aged 17 to 25 years, using a variety of formal assessments and concluded that their reading abilities varied greatly. Nevertheless, phonological skills and verbal memory were the strongest predictors of reading achievements. Interestingly, one of the participants was able to read without possessing phonemic awareness (see also the previous discussion on the Cossu et al. studies).

Some of the reading difficulties of children with Down syndrome can be traced to constitutional, genetic, and neurological abnormalities, which lead to delayed, albeit highly variable language development. For example, many children with Down syndrome might make more rapid progress in comprehension and vocabulary acquisition than in formation of syntactical utterances and production of speech sounds, which is related to their low muscle tone and abnormalities of the speech canal (Bochner et al., 2001). Other reading difficulties of children with Down syndrome might be related to the fact that their "deficiencies in the central nervous system include difficulties with attention (increased distractibility), short- and long-term memory (in processing, storing, and retrieving visual and, more particularly, auditory information), and completion of more complex cognitive tasks" (Bochner et al., p. 67).

Overall, children with Down syndrome often have language deficits that exceed what is expected from their nonverbal cognitive impairments. Along with cognitive challenges, their language difficulties in speech production, phonological memory, syntax, morphology, conversational and narrative pragmatics contribute to their reading difficulties. With appropriate reading instruction methods and sufficient reading practices, however, many children with Down syndrome are able to read, albeit at significantly varying levels. Most important, the predictors of reading achievement for children with Down syndrome are similar to those for typically developing children, for example, phonological skills, verbal memory, and language skills. This suggests that the Qualitative-Similarity Hypothesis (QSH) (see Chapters 4 and 7) might be applicable to children with Down syndrome as well.

READING AND CHILDREN WITH WILLIAMS SYNDROME

Although Williams syndrome is a rare genetic disorder affecting only 1 in 20,000 live births (Greenberg, 1990), there has been interest in studying these children because of their atypical reading development. Children with Williams syndrome are generally reported as having an IQ range between 50 and 65 (Snowling & Hulme, 2007). Many have severe impairments in nonlinguistic functions, for example, spatial cognition, planning, and problem solving.

The language profile of children with Williams syndrome is highly uneven. Individuals often have good oral language skills, normal auditory short-term memory and verbal working memory, and typical vocabulary skills (Levy, Smith, & Tager-Flusberg, 2003). Compared with their unexpectedly good vocabulary skills, their morphosyntax and semantics skills are often disproportionately poor (see the review in Laing, Hulme, Grant, & Karmiloff-Smith, 2001). These children may acquire letter–sound correspondences fairly effortlessly and utilize phonological processing during reading; however, their reading comprehension skills are impaired (Laing, et al., 2001; Snowling & Hulme, 2007).

Children with Williams syndrome have been reported to be overdependent on phonological decoding and may not process semantic information in the typical way (Laing, et al., 2001). They generally perform well on phonological short-term memory tasks but poorly on visuospatial short-term memory, which is the opposite pattern to what is found in children with Down syndrome (Snowling & Hulme, 2007). Furthermore, for many individuals with Williams syndrome, such a persistent reliance on phonological short-term memory to support word reading continues beyond what is typically expected for normal development and many times into adulthood (Grant et al., 1997).

Laing and colleagues (2001) measured the reading, general cognitive, and phonological skills of individuals with Williams syndrome, aged 9 to 27 years, and those of a group of typically developing children matched on reading age and verbal mental age. The researchers confirmed that individuals with Williams syndrome had better phonological decoding skills than reading comprehension skills. They further found that phonological skills were associated with individual differences in reading comprehension in both groups, although more poorly for individuals with Williams syndrome.

These researchers concluded that, although the reading levels of children with Williams syndrome depended on phonological skills, their full development of reading comprehension was compromised by poor semantics. That is, learning to read appeared only to involve the creation of mappings between orthography and phonology. Mappings between orthography and semantics, which happens in typical reading, had failed to be created (see related discussion in Chapter 7 for the processors in reading).

In short, whereas the word recognition scores of children with Williams syndrome are often reported to be surprisingly higher than what would be expected by their level of general intelligence, the morphosyntactic levels have been reported closer to their nonverbal mental age. Although they may acquire phonics decoding skills fairly easily and utilize phonological processing during reading, these children thus cannot comprehend what they have read. Their reading profiles are analogous to children with hyperlexia, which is discussed in the next section on children with ASD.

READING AND CHILDREN WITH AUTISM SPECTRUM DISORDERS (ASD)

Centers for Disease Control and Prevention (2010) estimates that an average of 1 in 110 children in the United States has an ASD. Boys are three to four times more likely than girls to be identified as having ASD (Griffin, Griffin, Fitch, Albera, & Gingras, 2006).

Many children with ASD have general language comprehension difficulties despite fairly good reading accuracy (i.e., single word reading; see the review in Nation, Clarke, Wright & Williams, 2006). The comprehension difficulties of children with ASD might include delays in pragmatics development, overall deficits of integrating information (i.e., text cohesion), struggles with understanding and problem solving, difficulties with incorporating prior knowledge and context during reading, and lack of comprehension monitoring (O'Connor & Klein, 2004; Snowling & Hulme, 2007; Wahlberg, & Magliano, 2004).

Many children with ASD have been reported to have well-developed word recognition skills and reading behaviors similar to *hyperlexia*, which, albeit controversial, refers to children who demonstrate remarkably advanced word recognition skills incommensurable with their cognitive and linguistic deficits. That is, they develop superior reading accuracy but have severely impaired reading comprehension skills (Nation et al., 2006; Snowling & Hulme, 2007; Walberg, 2008). For example, Frith and Snowling (1983) demonstrated that the phonological-based reading levels of children with ASD were commensurate with typically developing children of equivalent reading level. Children with ASD, however, performed less well than the control group on a test of reading comprehension albeit the two groups were matched in reading accuracy.

A nonautistic child can also have a hyperlexic reading profile; nevertheless, a strong association between autism and hyperlexia has been documented (Nation, Clarke, & Snowling, 2002; Snowling & Frith, 1986). Nation (1999) offered several hypotheses for hyperlexia: special cognitive and linguistic strengths and weaknesses, a preoccupation with local features rather than global coherence, and an obsession with text and reading. Meanwhile, it should be highlighted that most studies only recruited participants who were reading at a reasonably advanced level. It is possible that the reported levels of reading skills of children with ASD have been overestimated (Nation et al., 2006).

Nation and colleagues (2006) investigated the patterns of reading ability in children with ASD, aged 6 to 15 years, on four measurements: word recognition, nonword decoding, text reading accuracy, and text comprehension. Children were included in the study as long as their language skills were sufficient enough to allow them to participate. In spite of considerable variability, the overall levels of word and nonword reading and text reading accuracy of the participants fell within the average range with a delayed reading comprehension. 65% of the children with measurable reading ability obtained reading comprehension scores below the norm, and approximately one-third of the sample exhibited significantly severe delays in reading comprehension. Within the sample, 20 had normal or above normal word-reading levels. Ten of these achieved reading comprehension levels in the normal range or above; the other 10 demonstrated delayed reading comprehension, which was accompanied by poor oral language skills and vocabulary.

Collectively, the hyperlexia feature of many children with ASD reiterates the importance of language comprehension in overall reading acquisition. That is, superb word recognition skill alone is not sufficient for adequate reading development. Furthermore, the available literature suggests that, although there might be some overestimation, children with ASD can and should be taught to read with evidence-based best practices.

In a review of the literature from 1986 to 2006 on reading instruction and children with ASD with a focus on text (i.e., academic reading) comprehension and sight word (i.e., functional) comprehension, Chiang and Lin (2007) reported that effective instructional strategies included picture-word matching, graphic cues, and computer-based multimedia programs. It should be noted that none of the studies that met criteria for inclusion in the review by Chiang and Lin involved children with Asperger syndrome—the topic of our next section.

Reading and Children with Asperger Syndrome

Children with Asperger syndrome are often considered as high-functioning ASD who demonstrate few or no significant cognitive delays or impaired language development, and speak and read as well as their typically developing peers (Griffin et al., 2006). Their problems are often associated with their motor or social skills, for example, being easily overstimulated by crowded rooms or overwhelming visual situations, and having problems with social interaction, communication, and thought flexibility, which is reflected by narrow interests, lack of imagination, and obsession with routine (Griffin et al., 2006; Kaufman, 2002). The impact of their disability on reading comprehension is mainly from their frustration with novel learning situations and difficulties with understanding complex social interactions. As reported by Asperger (1944), the academic performance of these children is uneven.

There are few research studies on the reading skills of children with Asperger syndrome. In one of the seminal studies, Church, Alisanski, and Amanullah (2000) reported that many children with Asperger syndrome enter elementary school with reading skills above grade level. These children had difficulties with comprehension, however, especially when the material was not factual. Similar reading comprehension problems were reported for students at the middle school level but, surprisingly, not at the high school level. One limitation of the study was that no distinctions were made between word recognition and reading comprehension (Myles et al., 2002).

Using an informal *Classroom Reading Inventory*, Myles and colleagues (2002) measured the word recognition and comprehension skills of children with Asperger syndrome (aged 6 to 16 years; IQ 66–133). The overall scores suggested that students with Asperger syndrome had grade-level-appropriate skills on *Instructional*, *Frustration*, and *Listening Capacity*, but below-grade-level skills on *Silent Reading* and *Independent Reading*. The fact that both their Instructional level and Frustration level occurred at grade level presents difficulties in selecting appropriate classroom texts for students with Asperger syndrome because they can easily go from effective word recognition and text comprehension to a point of frustration. The authors hypothesized the possibilities of other interference variables such as attention, motivation, time-on-task, and so on. Based on their below-grade-level Independent reading, the authors also underscored the possibility that typical classroom-based silent reading tasks could be difficult for students with Asperger syndrome because they might need additional auditory input to facilitate comprehension or need to read aloud to better focus their attention on the reading materials.

The word recognition skills of children with Asperger syndrome are often reported as strong. In fact, both oral expression and word recognition have been the strengths of many children with Asperger syndrome (Myles et al., 2002). This might be due to the fact that these children have above-average intelligence (Williams, 1995). Such an advance in vocabulary and word recognition skills conceals their deficits in critical thinking, problem solving, and reading comprehension, however. These children often have weak written expression skills, which is also reflective of their literal thinking styles (i.e., lack of abstract thinking), poor problem-solving and organizational skills, inflexibility, difficulty discriminating important information, and inability to handle complex social interactions (Griffin et al., 2006).

In sum, many children with Asperger syndrome have reading difficulties similar to those of other children with ASD; however, their average or above-average skills in oral expression, vocabulary, and word recognition cloak their deficits in critical thinking, problem solving, and reading comprehension. In addition, although most children with Asperger syndrome are currently educated with typically developing children in general education classrooms, many instructional practices, for example, silent reading, might not be appropriate for them. Adaptations or accommodations include: familiarizing students with academic materials before a lesson to establish predictability, decrease stress, and increase the chances of success (Griffin et al., 2006).

Interestingly, many adaptations/accommodations for children with Asperger syndrome might be beneficial for other children as well. For example, effective techniques such as using graphic organizers in organizing and sequencing writing, providing additional clarifications in simpler terms to discuss complex concepts in a lesson, and breaking information down into smaller chunks, may be effective for other children with disabilities (e.g., see discussions in Klingner, Vaughn, & Boardman, 2007; Trezek, Wang, & Paul, 2010).

Table 8-1 provides profiles of the different developmental disability groups discussed in this chapter. Readers should keep in mind that children with developmental disabilities are a heterogeneous group with varying levels of reading abilities. These profiles should be interpreted with caution.

Table 8-1. Profiles of Developmental Disability Groups

Developmental Disabilities	Prevalence Rate	Word Recognition Skills	Language Comprehension Skills
Down syndrome	1.5/1,000	• Poor phonological-related skills, but able to perform phonological-related tasks after adequate training is provided • Phonological skills and verbal memory are the strongest predictors of reading achievements	• Significant expressive language deficits (e.g., grammatical and speech production) • Relatively strong lexical knowledge
Williams syndrome	1/20,000	• Acquire letter–sound correspondences fairly effortlessly and utilize phonological processing during reading	• Good oral language skills • Normal auditory short-term memory and verbal working memory • Typical vocabulary skills • Poor morphosyntax and semantics skills • Poor overall text comprehension skills
Autism spectrum disorders (ASD)	1/110	• Good reading accuracy (i.e., single word reading)	• Delays in pragmatics development • Deficits of integrating information (i.e., text cohesion) • Struggles with understanding and problem solving • Difficulties with incorporating prior knowledge and context during reading • Lack of comprehension monitoring • Poor overall text comprehension skills

LITERATE THOUGHT AND CHILDREN WITH DEVELOPMENTAL DISABILITIES

There is no doubt that children with developmental disabilities encounter obstacles in learning to read (i.e., script or print) for diverse reasons. With the use of adequate reading instructional methods and practices, many of them can learn or have learned to read (albeit at varying levels). A number of individuals with developmental disabilities, however, never learn to read and write well due to the severity of the disability, existence of multiple disabilities, inappropriate instructional methods, and so on.

In traditional print literacy, the reading process involves the simultaneous processing of four processors: orthographic, phonological, meaning and context (see the discussion in Chapter 7). For children with visual impairment, the major obstacle is the orthographic processing. For children with hearing impairment, the primary difficulty comes from phonological processing (although meaning and context processing could be difficult for children with additional language impairment as well).

For children with developmental disabilities, the key problem is associated with meaning and context processing in which they need to comprehend what they have read. For some children with moderate-to-severe developmental disabilities, the cognitive demands for abstract meaning and context processing might be too great for them to handle. In an alphabetic language such as English, the relationships between the printed words and their associated meanings are arbitrarily assigned. An individual thus cannot associate the word *cat* with the furry animal by simply looking at the shape of the word.

Given these difficulties, it is critical to explore alternative routes to developing literacy or, rather, there is a need to reconceptualize literacy (see Chapters 1 and 2). As discussed at the beginning of the chapter, every individual, regardless of ability/disability, race, or gender, deserves to be in the circle of educational privilege and is entitled to the citizen tools of literacy. The definition of literacy needs to be expanded to include multiple pathways to meet the special needs of individual citizens of the community.

Consider this: When discussing the literacy skills of children with developmental disabilities, many researchers make the distinction between *academic literacy* and *functional literacy* (Note: The validity of the phrase, *functional literacy*—in the narrow sense—is discussed in Chapter 10). Alberto et al. (2007) remarked:

> Academic literacy refers to the ability to engage in and master academic material taught in school. It also includes word analysis, comprehension, and fluency skills for deriving information from adult reading materials in the general community. For example, a minimum of a fifth-grade reading level is needed for a person to be able to read newspapers and other materials encountered in adult life (Browder, 2001). Functional literacy refers to sight word reading and the communication abilities necessary to perform daily routines in various environments. For students with moderate and severe disabilities, the outcomes of a functional reading program include (a) comprehending words needed to manage activities at home (e.g., food preparation, medication directions), in the community (e.g., grocery words, menus), at work (e.g., job schedule), and at school (e.g., schedules, room names); (b) making safe responses when encountering warning words (e.g., "Do not enter"); (c) using printed words to make choices (e.g., music or TV selections); and (d) accessing new opportunities through increased skills in reading (e.g., taking up hobbies that involve some reading, participating more fully in general education lessons; Browder, 2001). (p. 234)

In addition to the various forms of literacies discussed in this book, the New and Multiple Literacies for children with developmental disabilities promote a broad view of *functional literacy*: the ability to obtain information via multiple pathways from the environment and use it to make decisions and choices, to modify the environment, and to acquire pleasure (Alberto et al., 2007). The most important feature of functional literacy is multimodal, which encourages children with developmental disabilities not only to discern information conveyed in multiple forms but also to use various modes of expression, such as verbal language and alternative and augmentative communication (AAC) devices.

One form of functional literacy, in the broad sense, is *visual literacy*, which is the ability to recognize and use meaning conveyed through images (e.g., photos, films, pictorial, and simple graphic symbols and signs) (Alberto et al., 2007; Considine & Haley, 1992; Dondis, 1973). Visual literacy is based on the system for "expressing, recognizing, understanding and learning visual messages that are negotiable by all people . . . each medium has meaning to an individual because of its historical uses, resulting in a seemingly fixed meaning" (Alberto et al., p. 234). There are three categories of signs with various degrees of abstraction: iconic signs, symbolic signs, and indexual signs (Alberto et al.).

Iconic signs are photographs that entail a perceptual relationship to experienced reality. For example, a photograph of a local community hospital reminds people of the place to go when they become sick. *Symbolic signs* are meaningful pictures of the entities that they depict, for example, a picture of a hospital that does not necessarily resemble the one to which people have visited. *Indexual signs* are signs in an abstract or conventional mode. For example, the sign for hospital may not necessarily look like a hospital, but it is accepted by the community/society due to repeated usage. The ability to read individual or sequences of signs/pictures allow children with developmental disabilities to perform classroom, community, and job-related tasks such as reading a picture cook book.

Various forms of the New and Multiple Literacies can be used to facilitate comprehension skills in ways similar to those used in print literacy. For example, through connected pictures, wordless books can be used to teach the skills in using context and picture cues to make interpretations and predictions similar to skills taught via the use of written text (Alberto & Fredrick, 2000; Alberto et al., 2007). Most importantly, by requiring active processing of comprehending the relationships among a series of pictures and orally composing a story that connects the meaning among events depicted and implied in the pictures, wordless books can be used to teach the skill of constructing meaning, which is a weakness for many children with developmental disabilities.

In a sense, as a symbol system, written languages are forms of visual literacy. The outstanding feature that distinguishes written languages from other media of visual literacy is that written languages are more complex and abstract, which poses obstacles for a number of children with moderate-to-severe developmental disabilities. If the same or similar messages carried by written languages can be delivered through other media of visual literacy, many children with developmental disabilities might be able to have equal access to the cultural capital that is enjoyed by others. *Cultural capital* refers to non-economic social assets (e.g., educational or intellectual) that might promote social mobility beyond financial means, for example, the attitudes, knowledge, skills, and education that a person needs to be successful in society such as finding a job (Bourdieu & Passeron, 1990).

Technology in the New and Multiple Literacies

To maintain or enhance the functional competence of individuals with disabilities, including those with developmental disabilities, assistive or adaptive technology is often used in the following ways:

- Provide access for participation in activities that otherwise would be closed to the individual
- Assists in expressive language
- Increases endurance or ability to persevere and complete tasks that otherwise are too laborious to be attempted on a routine basis
- Allows greater access to information
- Supports normal social interactions with peers and adults
- Helps individuals achieve greater independence in performing daily living tasks. (Smith, DeMarco, & Worley, 2009, p. 48)

In addition to the traditional low-tech assistive technology, multimedia computer programs with graphics, sounds, and animations are often used in literacy instruction for children with developmental disabilities to capture their attention, motivate their literacy learning, and assist with their literate language development (see the review of educational technology for literacy instruction of children with developmental disabilities in Chiang & Lin, 2007; see a list of vendors offering assistive technology devices in Smith et al., 2009). For example, Mechling, Gast, and Krupa (2007) documented the effectiveness of SMART Board along with a 3-second constant time delay (CTD) procedure for three adolescents with developmental disabilities (aged 19–20 years; IQ 52–54). Results indicated that all three participants showed competence in: 1) reading target grocery words; 2) matching grocery item pictures to target grocery words; 3) reading fellow students' target grocery words through observational learning; and 4) matching grocery item pictures to observational non-target grocery words.

Collectively, returning to the questions posted at the beginning of this chapter, we believe that with appropriate literacy instructional approaches and adequate literacy practices, most children and adolescents with developmental disabilities are capable of accessing and utilizing information from traditional reading and writing to various degrees. In essence, everyone, including children and adolescents with moderate or severe developmental disabilities for whom the cognitive and/or physical demands of traditional reading and writing are too great, should have the choice of using the New and Multiple Literacies as an avenue for the development of literate thought.

SUMMARY

This chapter highlights the challenges of developing literate language in children with developmental disabilities and promotes the use of the New and Multiple Literacies. The chapter concludes with specific implications for developing literate thought in multiple pathways.

Several major points are as follows:

- *Developmental disabilities* encompass a diverse group of severe chronic conditions that are linked to mental and/or physical impairments. The main focus is on mental impairments such as intellectual disabilities and autism spectrum disorders.
- *Intellectual disability* (also known as *cognitive disability* or *mental retardation*) is the most common developmental disorder.
- *Autism Spectrum Disorders* (ASD) is a spectrum of psychological conditions that typically feature abnormalities of social interactions and communication along with severely restricted interests and highly repetitive behavior. There are three types of ASD: *autism, Asperger syndrome*, and *Pervasive Developmental Disorder not Otherwise Specified* (PDD-NOS), or *atypical autism*.
- For many children with developmental disabilities, reading instruction is often exclusively sight word reading, and there remains a dearth of research on phonemic awareness and phonics instruction.
- In general, although children with intellectual disabilities have poor phonological-related skills similar to those of their typically developing peers, their phonological-related skills are associated with their decoding skills. Furthermore, these children are able to perform phonological-related tasks after adequate training is provided.
- A variety of newer phonics instructional methods, including computer-assisted instruction, have been developed for children with developmental disabilities. There are varying rates of success associated with the use of these methods.
- In addition to the difficulties on word recognition and language comprehension, many children with developmental disabilities also exhibit lack of self-confidence and motivation in reading due to the

impact of limited instruction, poor skills, and failure at academic tasks. A scaffolding approach that emphasizes spontaneous dialogues and co-constructions of language may facilitate the success and involvement of children with meaningful tasks.

- Children with Down syndrome often have language deficits exceeding what is expected from their nonverbal cognitive impairments. With appropriate reading instruction methods and practices, however, many children are able to read, albeit at significantly varying levels. The predictors of reading achievement for children with Down syndrome are similar to those for typically developing children.

- Although many children with Williams syndrome may acquire phonics decoding skills fairly easily and utilize phonological processing during reading, they cannot comprehend what they have read. Even though their vocabulary scores are often reported to be surprisingly higher than what would be expected by their level of general intelligence, the morphosyntactic levels of these children have been reported to be closer to their nonverbal mental age.

- The hyperlexia feature of many children with ASD reiterates the importance of language comprehension in overall reading skills; that is, superb word recognition skill alone is not sufficient for reading development. Furthermore, the available literature suggests that, although there might be some overestimation, children with ASD can and should be taught to read with evidence-based best practices.

- Many children with Asperger syndrome have reading difficulties that are similar to those of other children with ASD; however, their average or above-average abilities in oral expression, vocabulary, and word recognition cloak their deficits in critical thinking, problem solving, and reading comprehension. Teachers should be sensitive to the special needs of children with Asperger syndrome.

- The New and Multiple Literacies for children with developmental disabilities reflect a broad view of *functional literacy*—that is, the ability to obtain information through multiple pathways from the environment and use it to make decisions and choices, to modify the environment, and to acquire pleasure.

- Various forms of the New and Multiple Literacies can be used to facilitate comprehension skills in ways similar to those used in print literacy.

- If the same or similar messages carried by written languages can be delivered via other media of visual literacy, many children with developmental disabilities should be able to have equal access to the cultural capital that is enjoyed by others.
- In addition to traditional low-tech assistive technology, multimedia computer programs with graphics, sounds, and animations are often used in literacy instruction for children with developmental disabilities to capture their attention, motivate their literacy learning, and assist with their literate language development.

QUESTIONS FOR REFLECTION AND DISCUSSION

1. How do the authors of this book define children with developmental disabilities?

2. Discuss highlights regarding reading development and specific subgroups of children. What are the similarities and differences (if any)?
   a. Children with Down syndrome
   b. Williams syndrome
   c. Autism spectrum disorders

3. Is there evidence for the Qualitative-Similarity Hypothesis for *each specific group of children* with developmental disabilities (question 2)? Why or why not?

4. What are the authors' suggestions on the development of literate thought for children with developmental disabilities?

REFERENCES

Alberto, P., & Fredrick, L. (2000). Teaching picture reading as an enabling skill. *Teaching Exceptional Children, 33,* 60-64.

Alberto, P. A., Fredrick, L., Hughes, M., McIntosh, L., & Cihak, D. (2007). Components of visual literacy: Teaching logos. *Focus on Autism and Other Developmental Disabilities, 22*(4), 234-243.

Asperger, H. (1944). Die 'Autistichen Psychopathen' imkindesalter. *Archiv fur Psychiatrie und Nervenkrankheiten, 117,* 76-136.

Basil, C., & Reyes, S. (2003). Acquisition of literacy skills by children with severe disability. *Child Language Teaching and Therapy, 19*(1), 27-48.

Bochner, S., Outhred, L., & Pieterse, M. (2001). A study of functional literacy skills in young adults with Down syndrome. *International Journal of Disability, Development and Education, 48,* 67-88.

Bourdieu, P., & Passeron, J. (1990). *Reproduction in education, society, and culture* (2nd ed.). Thousand Oaks, CA: SAGE Publications Inc.

Bradford, S., Shippen, M., Alberto, P., Houchins, D., & Flores, M. (2006). Using systematic instruction to teach decoding skills to middle school students with moderate intellectual disabilities. *Education and Training in Developmental Disabilities, 41,* 333-343.

Browder, D., Ahlgrim-Delzell, L., Courtade, G., Gibbs, S. L., & Flowers, C. (2008). Evaluation of the effectiveness of an early literacy program for students with significant developmental disabilities. *Exceptional Children, 75*(1), 33-52.

Browder, D., Ahlgrim-Delzell, L., Spooner, F., Mims, P. J., & Baker, J. N. (2009). Using time delay to teach literacy to students with severe developmental disabilities. *Exceptional Children, 75*(3), 343-364.

Browder, D., Wakeman, S. Y., Spooner, F., Ahlgrim-Delzell, L., & Algozzine, B. (2006). Research on reading instruction for individuals with significant cognitive disabilities. *Exceptional Children, 72*(4), 392-408.

Browder, D. M., & Xin, Y. P. (1998). A meta-analysis and review of sight word research and its implications for teaching functional reading to individuals with moderate and severe disabilities. *Journal of Special Education, 32,* 130-154.

Byrne, B. (1993). Learning to read in the absence of phonemic awareness? A comment on Cossu, Rossini, and Marshall (1993). *Cognition, 48,* 285-288.

Centers for Disease Control and Prevention (2010). *Developmental disabilities.* Retrieved January 17, 2011 from http://www.cdc.gov/ncbddd/dd/dd1.htm

Chapman, S., Seung, H., Schwartz, S., & Kay-Raining Bird, E. (1998). Language skills of children and adolescents with Down syndrome II: Production deficits. *Journal of Speech, Language and Hearing Research, 42,* 861-873.

Chiang, H., & Lin, Y. (2007). Reading comprehension instruction for students with autism spectrum disorders: A review of the literature. *Focus on Autism and Other Developmental Disabilities, 22*(4), 259-267.

Church, C., Alisanski, S., & Amanullah, S. (2000). The social, behavioral, and academic experiences of children with Asperger syndrome. *Focus on Autism and Other Developmental Disabilities, 15,* 12-20.

Cohen, E. T., Heller, K. W., Alberto, P., & Fredrick, L. D. (2008). Using a three-step decoding strategy with constant time delay to teach word reading to students with mild and moderate mental retardation. *Focus on Autism and Other Developmental Disabilities, 23*(2), 67-78.

Coleman-Martin, M. B., Heller, K. W., Cihak, D. F., & Irvine, K. L. (2005). Using computer-assisted instruction and the nonverbal reading approach to teach word identification. *Focus on Autism and Other Developmental Disabilities, 20,* 80-89.

Conners, F. A. (1992). Reading instruction for students with moderate mental retardation: Review and analysis of research. *American Journal on Mental Retardation, 96,* 577-597.

Conners, F. A., Atwell, J. A., Rosenquist, C. J., & Sligh, A. C. (2001). Abilities underlying decoding differences in children with intellectual disability. *Journal of Disability Research*, *45*, 292-299.

Considine, D., & Haley, G. (1992). *Visual messages*. Englewood, CO: Teacher Ideas Press.

Cossu, G., & Marshall, J. C. (1990). Are cognitive skills a prerequisite for learning to read and write? *Cognitive Neuropsychology*, *7*, 21-40.

Cossu, G., Rossini, F., & Marshall, J. C. (1993). When reading is acquired but phonemic awareness is not: A study of literacy in Down syndrome. *Cognition*, *46*, 129-138.

Cupples, L., & Iacono, T. (2000). Phonological awareness and oral reading skills in children with Down's syndrome. *Journal of Speech, Language, and Hearing Research*, *43*, 595-608.

Dondis, D. (1973). *A primer of visual literacy*. Cambridge, MA: The MIT Press.

Duncan, L., Seymour, P., & Hill, S. (1997). How important are rhyme and analogy in beginning reading? *Cognition*, *63*, 171-208.

Engelmann, S., Becker, W. C., Hanner, S., & Johnson, G. (1980). *Corrective reading program*. Chicago: Science Research Associates.

Fowler, A. E., Doherty, B. J., & Boynton, L. (1995). Basis of reading skill in young adults with Down syndrome. In L. Nadel & D. Rosenthal (Eds.), *Down syndrome: Living and learning in the community* (pp. 182-196). New York: Wiley-Liss.

Frith, U., & Snowling, M. (1983). Reading for meaning and reading for sound in autistic and dyslexic children. *British Journal of Developmental Psychology*, *1*, 329-342.

Grant, J., Karmiloff-Smith, A., Gathercole, S., Paterson, S., Howlin, P., Davies, M., & Udwin, O. (1997). Phonological short-term memory and its relationship to language in Williams syndrome. *Cognitive Neuropsychiatry*, *2*, 81-99.

Greenberg, E. (1990). Introduction to special issue on Williams syndrome. *American Journal of Medical Genetics Supplement*, *6*, 85-88.

Griffin, H. C., Griffin, L. W., Fitch, C. W., Albera, V., & Gingras, H. (2006). Educational interventions for individuals with Asperger syndrome. *Intervention in School and Clinic*, *41*, 150-155.

Hoogeveen, F. R., Birkhoff, A. E., Smeets, P. M., Lancioni, G. E., & Boelens, H. H. (1989). Establishing phonemic segmentation in moderately retarded children. *Remedial and Special Education*, *10*(3), 47-53.

Hoogeveen, F. R., Kouwenhoven, J. A., & Smeets, P. M. (1989). Establishing sound blending in moderately retarded children: Implications of verbal instruction and pictorial prompting. *Research in Developmental Disabilities*, *10*, 333-348.

Hoogeveen, F. R., & Smeets, P. M. (1988). Establishing phoneme blending in trainable mentally retarded children. *Remedial and Special Education*, *9*(2), 46-53.

Hoogeveen, F. R., Smeets, P. M., & Lanconi, G. (1989). Teaching moderately mentally retarded children basic reading skills. *Research in Developmental Disabilities*, *10*, 1-18.

Joseph, L. M., & Seery, M. E. (2004). Where is the phonics? A review of the literature on the use of phonetic analysis with students with mental retardation. *Remedial and Special Education*, *25*, 88-94.

Kaufman, C. (2002). Asperger syndrome: Implications for educators (Expert speaks out). *The Brown University Child and Adolescent Behavior Letter, 18*, 1-4.

Kliewer, C., Biklen, D., & Kasa-Hendrickson, C. (2006). Who may be literate? Disability and resistance to the cultural denial of competence. *American Educational Research Journal, 43*(2), 163-192.

Klingner, J., Vaughn, S., & Boardman, A. (2007). *Teaching reading comprehension to students with learning difficulties.* New York: The Guilford Press.

Laing, E., Hulme, C., Grant, J., & Karmiloff-Smith, A. (2001). Learning to read in Williams syndrome; Looking beneath the surface of atypical reading development. *Journal of Child Psychology and Psychiatry, 42*(6), 729-739.

Levy, Y., Smith, J., & Tager-Flusberg, H. (2003). Word reading and reading-related skills in adolescents with Williams syndrome. *Journal of Child Psychology and Psychiatry, 44*(4), 576-587.

Mechling, L. C., Gast, D. L., & Krupa, K. (2007). Impact of SMART Board technology: An investigation of sight word reading and observational learning. *Journal of Autism & Developmental Disorder, 37*, 1869-1882.

Moni, K. B., & Jobling, A. (2001). Reading-related literacy learning of young adults with Down syndrome: Findings from a three year teaching and research program. *International Journal of Disability, Development and Education, 48*(4), 377-394.

Myles, B., Hilgenfeld, T., Barnhill, G., Griswold, D., Hagiwara, T., & Simpson, R. (2002). Analysis of reading skills in individuals with Asperger syndrome. *Focus on Autism and Other Developmental Disabilities, 17*, 44–47.

Nation, K. (1999). Reading skills in hyperlexia: a developmental perspective. *Psychological Bulletin, 125*(3), 338-355.

Nation, K., Clarke, P., & Snowling, M. J. (2002). General cognitive ability in children with poor reading comprehension. *British Journal of Educational Psychology, 72*, 549-560.

Nation, K., Clarke, P., Wright, B., & Williams, C. (2006). Patterns of reading ability in children with autism spectrum disorder. *Journal of Autism & Developmental Disorder, 36*, 911-919.

O'Connor, I. M., & Klein, P. D. (2004). Exploration of strategies for facilitating the reading comprehension of high-functioning students with autism spectrum disorders. *Journal of Autism and Developmental Disorders, 34*(2), 115-127.

Saunders, K. J. (2007). Word-attack skills in individuals with mental retardation. *Mental Retardation and Developmental Disabilities Research Reviews, 13*, 78-84.

Siegel, L. S. (1993). Phonological processing deficits as the basis of a reading disability. *Developmental Review, 13*, 246-257.

Smith, D. D., DeMarco, J. F., & Worley, M. (2009). *Literacy beyond picture books: Teaching secondary students with moderate to severe disabilities.* Thousand Oaks, CA: Corwin.

Snowling, M., & Frith, U. (1986). Comprehension in hyperlexic readers. *Journal of Experimental Child Psychology, 42*(3), 392–415.

Snowling, M., & Hulme, C. (2007). Learning to read with a language impairment. In M. Snowling & C. Hulme (Eds.), *The science of reading – A handbook* (pp. 397-412). Malden, MA: Blackwell Publishing.

Stanovich, K. E., Cunningham, A. E., & Freeman, D. J. (1984). Intelligence, cognitive skills and early reading progress. *Reading Research Quarterly, 19*, 278-303.

Stuart, M., & Coltheart, M. (1988). Does reading develop in a sequence of stages? *Cognition, 30*, 139-181.

Trezek, B., Wang, Y., & Paul, P. (2010). *Reading and deafness: Theory, research and practice.* Clifton Park, NY: Cengage Learning.

Wagner, R. K., Torgeson, J. K., & Rashotte, C. A. (1994). Development of reading-related phonological processing abilities: New evidence of bidirectional causality from a latent variable longitudinal study. *Developmental Psychology, 30*, 73-87.

Wahlberg, T., & Magliano, J. P. (2004). The ability of high function individuals with autism to comprehend written discourse. *Discourse Processes, 38*(1), 119-144.

Walberg, J. L. (2008). Reading and autism: Why is there a paucity of research? *Balanced Reading Instruction, 15*(2), 41-52.

Williams, K. (1995). Understanding the student with Asperger's syndrome: Guidelines for teachers. *Focus on Autistic Behavior, 10*, 1-8.

Yopp, H. (1988). The validity and reliability of phonemic awareness tests. *Reading Research Quarterly, 23*, 160-177.

FURTHER READING

Cohen, D. J., & Volkmar, F. R. (Eds.). (2005). *Handbook of autism and developmental disorders* (3rd ed). New York: Wiley.

Goswami, U., & Bryant, P. (1990). *Phonological skills and learning to read.* London: Lawrence Erlbaum.

Jacobson, J. W., Foxx, R. M., & Mulick, J. A. (Eds.). (2005). *Controversial therapies for developmental disabilities: Fad, fashion, and science in professional practice.* Mahweh, NJ: Lawrence Erlbaum.

Simpson, R. L. (2005). *Autism spectrum disorders: Interventions and treatments for children and youth.* Thousand Oaks, CA: Corwin.

CHAPTER 9

English Language Learners

The challenge of being, becoming, or remaining a bilingual has an entirely different character in the United States than in the highlands of Peru, in Stockholm, or in Riga; even within the United States, the challenge is quite different in National City, California, than it is in Des Moines, Iowa. We are failing to understand the phenomenon of biliteracy development if we do not integrate the sociocultural context with developmental and instructional data. Thus, it is important to connect the topic of sociocultural context to the treatment of language and literacy development, integrating data about the sociocultural context with developmental and instructional data.

Snow, 2006, pp. 647-648

The cited passage above is from the conclusion of the *Report of the National Literacy Panel on Language-Minority Children and Youth* (August & Shanahan, 2006), the most recent and comprehensive synthesis of research on the literacy skills of English language learners (ELLs). Because neither the National Reading Panel (NRP) (2000) nor the resulting Reading First or Early Reading First legislation (see also, the National Early Literacy Panel [NELP], 2008) examined or provided recommendations specifically on literacy instruction of ELLs, the Panel (i.e., *Report of the National Literacy Panel*) was formally charged to identify, evaluate, and synthesize research on the education of language-minority children and youth regarding their literacy achievement. Approximately 1,800 studies from 1980 to 2003 were initially identified through the literature, and 293 of those met the methodological criteria established by the Panel and included in the report. There were only a few high-quality intervention studies, however, and the majority of those studies were focused on ELLs in kindergarten through fifth grade. Based on the available data, the Panel identified five domains for investigation: 1) the development of literacy in language-minority children and youth; 2) cross-linguistic relationships; 3) sociocultural contexts and literacy development; 4) instruction and professional development; and 5) student assessment.

The Panel's comprehensive review concluded that multiple factors influence second-language English literacy development, which include: individual differences in the age at which literacy skills are acquired; second-language oral proficiency, first-language oral proficiency, and literacy skills as well as cognitive abilities; classroom and school factors; and sociocultural variables. Consequently, to understand the challenges of developing literate thought, including critico-creative skills, this chapter discusses the developmental, instructional, and sociocultural variables related to the language and literacy skills of ELLs. Special attention is given to cross-linguistic relationships because, based on Cummins' interdependence and threshold hypotheses (1978, 1979, 1980, 1981, 1984, 1989), the successful transfer of knowledge and expertise across languages is dependent on the development of cognitive proficiency in the involved languages, including the dominant language.

The structure of this chapter is as follows. First, an explanation of the various terms associated with English language learners is provided. Then the literacy development of ELLs is discussed, including their word recognition skills, written language comprehension skills, and motivational factors. The role of first-language literacy and oral proficiency in the literacy development of ELLs is also covered at the word-level and at the text-level. This chapter examines literacy instruction and assessment for ELLs, which entails literacy instructional strategies, programs, and assessments. Next, we explore the relationships between sociocultural contexts and literacy achievements of ELLs, incorporating the influences of the home environment/culture as well as community/culture on literacy achievements. We conclude with implications for developing literate thought in ELLs.

DIFFERENT TERMS ASSOCIATED WITH ENGLISH LANGUAGE LEARNERS

The *National Literacy Panel on Language-Minority Children and Youth*— known simply as the Panel—used the term *language minority* to refer to individuals from homes where a language other than a societal language is actively used (August & Shanahan, 2006). A language minority student may have limited second-language proficiency, be bilingual, or basically monolingual in the second-language. Language minority students whose second-language proficiency is not yet developed to benefit fully from instruction solely in the second-language are called *second-language learners*. Meanwhile, second-language learners who are acquiring English as a second-language are referred as *English language learners (ELLs)*—the focus of this chapter.

The most recent U.S. Department of Education report entitled, the *Condition of Education 2010* (Aud et al., 2010), estimates that, in 2008, approximately 21% (or 10.9 million) of school-age children (aged 5 to 17 years old) spoke a language other than English at home (i.e., language minority learners). Of the 5% (or 2.7 million) school-age children who spoke English with difficulty (i.e., ELLs), 75% of them spoke Spanish. ELLs are a heterogeneous group with a wide range of individual differences, however; in general, 71% of ELLs from 2004 to 2007 were performing below grade level, and they continue to be among the nation's lowest achieving students (Short & Fitzsimmons, 2007). Furthermore, although assessment tools and testing policies differ from state to state, even differing among districts within a state, only 18.7% of the ELLs assessed scored above the state-established norm on reading comprehension (Kindler, 2002). Improving the literacy skills of ELLs is critical, particularly considering the increasing prevalence of ELLs in U.S. school-age children.

Other terms are used interchangeably with English language learners, such as *Limited English Proficient (LEP)*, which is used in many federal legislation and other official documents. ELL is often preferred over LEP because it highlights accomplishments rather than deficits. *English as a Second Language (ESL)*, also known as *English Speakers of Other Languages (ESOL)*, is typically used to refer to students in traditional special education programs taught by teachers who have explicit training in teaching students in acquiring English as a second-language (Hill & Flynn, 2006).

In this chapter, one might expect to see LEP or ESL when we quote a source or cite legal requirements. Readers should be aware that findings from studies with ELLs who receive special education services (i.e., ESLs or ESOLs) need to be carefully considered before these findings can be applied to the general ELL population, however, because most ELLs do not need special education services (Prater, 2009).

Figure 9-1 summarizes the different terms associated with ELLs.

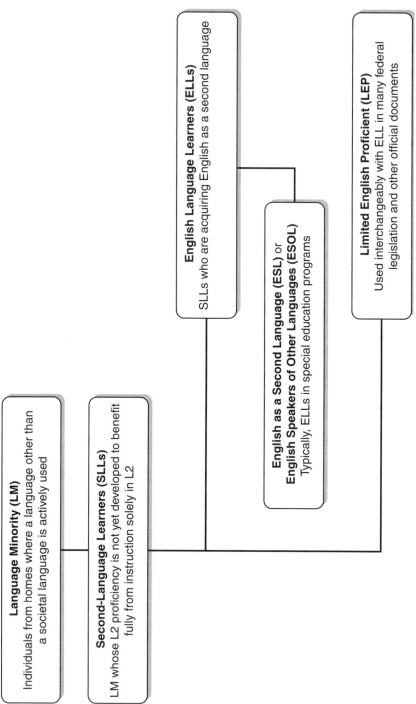

Figure 9-1.   Summary of different terms associated with English language learners.

LITERACY DEVELOPMENT OF ENGLISH LANGUAGE LEARNERS

The Panel (August & Shanahan, 2006) remarked: "Rapid increases in the numbers of language-minority children and youth, as well as their low levels of literacy attainment and its consequences—high dropout rates, poor job prospects, and poverty—create an imperative to attend to the literacy development of these students" (p. xiii). Unfortunately, as mentioned previously, the literature on literacy development of language-minority students, particularly ELLs, is limited. Readers should interpret the findings reported in this chapter with caution.

Consistent with the findings on literacy development of typical English monolingual students (Adams, 1990; Chall, 1983, 1996; McGuinness, 2004, 2005; NELP, 2008; NRP, 2000), the Panel (August & Shanahan, 2006) concluded that, for ELLs, certain components of literacy cannot fully develop until precursor skills are acquired. For example, good decoding and orthographic skills are prerequisites for subsequent efficient word recognition skills, and satisfactory levels of reading comprehension cannot be achieved without accurate and fast word recognition skills. We emphasize that efficient word recognition skills are necessary but not sufficient for proficient reading comprehension—general language proficiency also plays a critical role.

The Panel (August & Shanahan, 2006) also emphasized the dynamic nature of literacy development. That is, the relationships among the components of literacy are fluid and may change with the learners' age, levels of second-language oral proficiency, previous learning experiences, and underlying cognitive abilities (e.g., working memory, phonological short-term memory, phonological awareness, and phonological recoding such as Rapid Automatic Naming [RAN]). Many of these issues are similar to those for first-language literacy development for monolingual learners (e.g., NELP, 2008; NRP, 2000).

This section is divided into three parts to discuss the literacy development of ELLs: word recognition skills, written language comprehension skills, and motivational factors.

Word Recognition Skills

Consistent with decades of research on early reading development of English monolingual learners (Adams, 1990; Chall, 1983, 1996; McGuinness,

2004, 2005; NELP, 2008; NRP, 2000), the Panel (August & Shanahan, 2006) reported that the best predictors of English word-level literacy skills (i.e., word recognition and spelling) of language-minority students are phonological processing skills (e.g., phonological awareness, rapid letter naming, and phonological short-term memory) and concepts of print. It is possible that the similarities in factors influencing first- and second-language reading are due to the universality of the requirements for reading acquisition across languages, or the *universal grammar of reading* (Perfetti, 2003).

On the other hand, the effects of English oral proficiency (e.g., vocabulary or grammatical skills) on English word-level skills of ELLs are limited (August & Shanahan, 2006). Although measures of English oral proficiency correlate positively with English word and pseudoword reading, they are not strong predictors of these skills. In addition, measures of English oral proficiency are not strongly related to English spelling skills. In fact, Durgunoglu, Nagy, and Hancin-Bhatt (1993) reported that first-language word recognition was a better predictor of bilingual students' second-language performance on reading than was their second-language oral proficiency. Again, readers should interpret these findings with caution. It does not necessarily mean that English oral proficiency does not play a role in English reading performance of ELLs; instead, as suggested by Garcia (2000), the measures might not accurately reflect aspects of oral knowledge that are important for reading.

Figure 9-2 provides a summary on predictors of word recognition skills of ELLs.

In general, with adequate instruction, ELLs can acquire word recognition skills that either are or can be commensurate with those of their English monolingual peers. A similar proportion of ELLs have difficulties in word recognition that resemble the reading difficulties of English monolingual students with reading disabilities, however. English monolingual students and ELLs who are poor spellers also have similar cognitive profiles despite their different vocabulary and grammatical proficiency in English.

Interestingly, three studies reviewed by the Panel (August & Shanahan, 2006) suggested that ELLs with reading disabilities outperformed their English monolingual reading disabled peers on phonological measures. The Panel concluded with caution that the results might be possibly related to the cross-language transfer of phonological awareness skills.

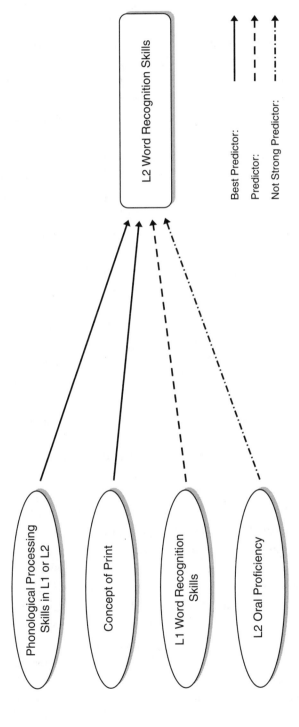

Figure 9-2.   Predictors of word recognition skills of ELLs.

Obviously, there is a great need for additional research on cross-language transfer.

The purported advanced phonological awareness skills of bilingual children are even more apparent when they are younger. Such a phonological advantage seems to fade after age 6, however, possibly because these children receive English-only instruction at school that impedes their bilingual development (August & Shanahan, 2006). Based on the limited available data, the Panel concluded that the cross-language effects in phonological awareness are more likely to occur among younger ELLs or during early—not later—stages of second-language development because phonological awareness might be less important once students have acquired higher levels of second-language proficiency.

In response to the need for further study of cross-language transfer, Cardenas-Hagan, Carlson, and Pollard-Durodola (2007) conducted a large-scale longitudinal investigation of the relationship between initial phonological awareness performance in Spanish and performance on a parallel English phonological awareness task a year later in a sample of over 1,000 Spanish–English bilingual kindergarten students in Texas and California. After controlling for initial English kindergarten performance on the same task, the researchers found that Spanish phonological awareness at the beginning of kindergarten predicted English phonological awareness at the beginning of first grade. This transfer effect across phonological awareness performance in Spanish and English only emerged for the Spanish-instructed students, however, not for English-instructed Spanish-English bilingual kindergarteners. In addition, after controlling for initial English performance on the same task, participants' performance on English letter name and letter-sound identification skills was predicted by Spanish performance on the letter name and letter-sound identification tasks measured a year earlier. Such a cross-language transfer of orthographic skills only emerged for students with poor performance on the initial measures of English orthographic knowledge. It appears that Spanish-speaking students may use their knowledge of Spanish orthography during the initial stages of learning English orthography, but it becomes less useful to them once they have developed a greater amount of knowledge about English orthography.

Whether or not the first-language of ELLs entails the use of an alphabetic script might have some impact on the subsequent development of phonological awareness in English. For example, Liow and Poon (1998) involved 9- to 10-year-old multilingual students (English-Bahasa Indonesian-Mandarin Chinese) in a study to investigate the impact of exposure to different types of script on phonological awareness in English. Results indicated that students whose dominant language was English or Bahasa Indonesian exhibited higher levels of phonological awareness than those whose dominant language was Mandarin Chinese. Because English and Bahasa Indonesian use an alphabetic script whereas Mandarin Chinese uses a logographic script, the researchers suggested that language minority students who had exposure to written forms of the first-language are likely to have better phonological awareness in English if their first-language uses an alphabetic script.

In sum, similar to the situation of their English monolingual peers, the English word recognition skills of ELLs are best predicted by their phonological processing skills (in either their first-language or English) and concept of print, whereas English oral proficiency as measured by vocabulary or grammatical skills is not a strong predictor. Although many ELLs acquire word recognition skills that either are or can be commensurate with those of their monolingual peers, a number of ELLs have difficulties in word recognition that resemble the reading difficulties of English monolingual students with reading disabilities.

Written Language Comprehension Skills

The Panel's findings (August & Shanahan, 2006) on the written language comprehension skills of ELLs are not as optimistic as those on their word recognition skills. Specifically, ELLs rarely reach the levels accomplished by their monolingual peers. Furthermore, the written English comprehension skills of ELLs are strongly associated with second-language status and oral English proficiency, for example, vocabulary knowledge, listening comprehension, syntactic skills, oral storytelling skills, and metalinguistic skills.

Related to their second-language status, the metalinguistic skills of ELLs include: 1) the unitary view of reading across the native language and English; 2) use of prior knowledge across the two languages; 3) use of cognate strategies in recognizing unknown vocabulary (Note: *cognates* are words in different languages with common ancestral roots that are similar in form and meaning, for example, *excellent* in English vs. *excelente* in Spanish); 4) use of code-switching (i.e., switching between languages at the sentence level to assist comprehension); and 5) use of translating (i.e., use of one language to figure out what was read in the other), particularly, paraphrased translating, which is more effective than direct or word-to-word translating (Garcia, 2000).

Other factors that contribute to the development of English written language comprehension include: 1) exposure to print; 2) opportunities to learn and quality of literacy instruction; 3) native-language literacy development; 4) ability to navigate complex text and to utilize prior knowledge to draw inferences; and 5) use of cross-linguistic transfer strategies (see also Garcia, 2003).

Figure 9-3 provides a summary on predictors of written language comprehension skills of ELLs.

Vocabulary knowledge has long been recognized as one of the most important predictors of reading comprehension for both native and non-native English speakers (see the review in Taffe, Blachowicz, & Fisher, 2009). The discrepancy in English vocabulary knowledge between English monolingual speakers and ELLs plays a significant role in accounting for the difference in their English reading performance, even when the ELLs possess strong native-language vocabulary knowledge. Two dimensions of diversity have been shown to make a difference in vocabulary development, also known as factors for the *vocabulary gap*: socioeconomic status (SES) (see also the discussion in Chapter 6) and English language proficiency (see Chapter 4). Even though they might be familiar with the vocabularies involving *basic interpersonal communication skills* (BICS), ELLs often have less exposure to and experiences with written English involving *cognitive academic language proficiency* (CALP) (Cummins, 1978, 1979, 1980, 1984). The fact that many ELLs are also from economically disadvantaged families further compounds the situation.

In general, ELLs know less about topics included in English text (Garcia, 2000) as well as the academic language used to express these topics (Birch, 2007). When differences in prior knowledge are controlled, the reading performance of ELLs and English monolingual learners showed no significant differences, although ELLs still scored significantly lower on questions that required inferential skills. Garcia (2000) suspected that the literal thinking skills of low- and average-performing ELLs might be related to the type of instruction that they had received. For example, Ramirez, Yuen, and Ramey (1991) found that regardless of the language of instruction, Spanish-speaking ELLs received passive teacher-directed instruction that did not promote the development of complex language

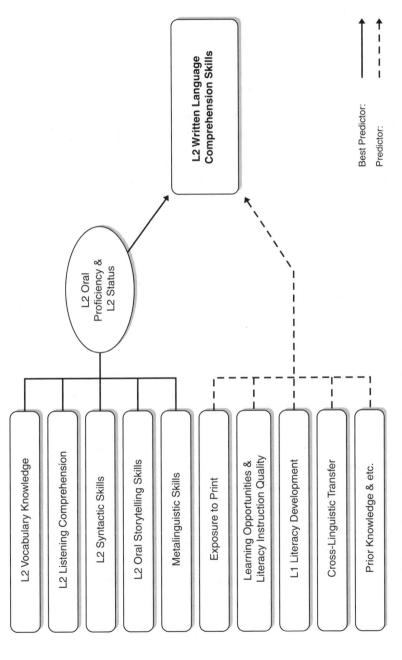

Figure 9-3. Predictors of written language comprehension skills of ELLs.

and higher order thinking skills (often related to the development of literate thought, see Chapters 1 and 2). Collier (1987) and other scholars (e.g., Birch, 2007) called for sustained instruction in academic English to prepare ELLs to comprehend conceptually complex texts, particularly for higher grades. Portes and Salas (2009) also proposed a developmentally sensitive and mediated learning approach for culturally and linguistically diverse students, particularly those who live in poverty, and stated that:

> . . . school-based activities need to be reorganized so that "basic skills" are not all that the child encounters: he or she also needs to learn higher-order skills. Too often we find that schooling, low expectations, and remedial classes fail to work within children's zone of proximal development and actually impede the development of their higher intellectual skills, motivation, and health. (p. 108)

With respect to reading strategies (see the types of cognitive and metacognitive strategies in Chapters 4–6), the general conclusion from the Panel (August & Shanahan, 2006) is that bilingual students who read strategically in one language also do so in their other language. It is difficult to conclude whether these students use exactly the same strategies across languages, however, because the use of strategies varies based on text genre, text difficulty, language dominance, and reading ability. Specifically, "text genre rather than language seemed to characterize their use of strategies; that is, the students demonstrated similar strategies while reading expository text compared to narrative text, regardless of the language" (Garcia, 2000, p. 823).

In sum, it is challenging for ELLs to achieve written language comprehension skills that are commensurate with those of English monolingual peers. Vocabulary knowledge, particularly school-based academic vocabulary, poses one of the biggest problems for ELLs. The best predictors of English written language comprehension skills of ELLs also include metalinguistic competence and other English oral proficiency variables such as listening comprehension, syntactic skills, and oral storytelling skills. Additional contributing factors include: exposure to print; learning opportunities and quality of literacy instruction; first-language literacy development; ability to navigate complex text and utilize prior knowledge to draw inferences; and use of cross-linguistic transfer strategies, particularly cognitive and metacognitive strategies. In many cases, particularly for ELLs coming from economically disadvantaged families, several factors interweave with each other and further aggravate the situation.

Motivational Factors

Motivation or the affective domain is an important but under-researched area in reading in English as a first language (i.e., as L1; see Mathewson, 2004; Miller & Faircloth, 2009). In fact, research on the effects of motivational factors on ELLs' reading comprehension is almost nonexistent (it was not one of the areas investigated by the Panel). Many issues can affect the motivation of ELLs, for example, lack of self-efficacy due to poor English language skills, lack of task value due to unchallenging or boring remedial activities, or limited prior knowledge of the topics and contents in reading materials (Rueda, Velasco, & Lim, 2008).

Guthrie, Rueda, Gambrell, and Morrison (2009) examined research on the roles of engagement, valuing, and identification in the reading development of students from diverse backgrounds. They hypothesized that engagement in reading, valuing reading achievement, and identification with reading achievement may be associated with competence/achievement in reading and with each other. Thus far, no strongly designed scientific investigations have verified these assertions; however, it is highly possible that engagement in reading is one of the building blocks of reading achievement.

Conclusion

It appears that the script or print literacy development of ELLs is qualitatively similar to that of English monolingual learners. That is, whether learning English as a first- or second- language, children need to acquire good decoding and orthographic skills before they can progress with accurate and fast word recognition skills, which are the prerequisites for subsequent adequate levels of reading comprehension. The findings are consistent with those on the literacy development of children with language/learning disabilities (see Chapter 6), sensory disabilities (see Chapter 7), and developmental disabilities (see Chapter 8). In essence, the Qualitative-Similarity Hypothesis (QSH; see the discussions in Chapters 4 and 7) might be applicable to all children who are learning English, regardless of their sensory/cognitive abilities or cultural/linguistic backgrounds.

From another perspective, the cultural/linguistic backgrounds of ELLs are unique and deserve special attention. This section discussed the predictors of three major components of reading for ELLs—word recognition skills, written language comprehension skills, and motivational factors. Although the predictors of subsequent reading success are similar to those for reading English as a first-language, a few variables are closely related to the exclusive cross-language transfer skills of ELLs. ELLs are at a higher risk than their English monolingual peers to encounter difficulties in reading, particularly for those from economically disadvantaged families.

LITERACY INSTRUCTION, PROGRAMS, AND ASSESSMENT

Teachers, school districts, and states must provide literacy instructional strategies, policies, and assessments that meet the special developmental needs of ELLs. In this section, we focus on instruction, programs, and assessment.

Literacy Instructional Strategies

Despite limited data, the Panel (August & Shanahan, 2006) suggested that, similar to the case for first-language literacy, instruction that emphasizes key curricular components—such as phonemic awareness, decoding, oral reading fluency, vocabulary, reading comprehension and writing—has potential benefits. It is averred that the principal ordering of literacy instruction might be the same for ELLs as it is for English monolingual learners. In other words, greater attention should be devoted to teaching decoding skills in the early years with more direct and ambitious attention to comprehension later. The focus on developing vocabulary and prior knowledge should be intensive and extensive throughout the entire instructional period.

There should also be specific instructional considerations to meet the unique needs of ELLs. For example, given the fact that certain English phonemes and phoneme combinations are not present in Spanish, it might be critical to provide additional activities and allocate more time to these areas for ELLs than what is typically provided for English monolingual learners. Another example is to use individualized scaffolded instruction on cognate recognition so that ELLs can figure out unknown English vocabulary while reading (Garcia, 1996).

The Panel (August & Shanahan, 2006) reported that instructional strategies, deemed successful in first-language literacy, do not improve the literacy skills of ELLs as much as they do for English monolingual learners. For example, although there has been some success in teaching ELLs to develop decoding and spelling skills, their reading comprehension and vocabulary knowledge continue to lag behind their English monolingual peers. These findings led the Panel to suggest that literacy instruction for ELLs must focus on reading skills *while* fostering enriched oral English-language development in meaningful contents because teaching reading skills alone is not sufficient.

General exemplary vocabulary instruction can also produce beneficial effects for ELLs. For example, ELLs learn better when vocabulary is taught to them explicitly, including cross-linguistic relationships such as cognates and multimeaning words (Carlo et al., 2004). In addition, direct vocabulary instruction in conjunction with significant amount of reading practice is more productive than relying on extensive reading alone (Zimmerman, 1997).

After reviewing the research on vocabulary development for ELLs, Taffe and colleagues (2009) stated: "given the best instruction, they need *more* of it; they need it *sooner*; and they need it with more *intentional supports and scaffolds* [emphases added in original]" (p. 321). Specifically, these investigators suggested three research-based strategies for enhancing vocabulary knowledge: 1) building concept-rich, language-rich, and word-rich learning environments; 2) teaching individual words for deep understanding and lasting retention; and 3) teaching strategies for independent word learning such as the use of morphology, context, and the dictionary.

For reading comprehension (i.e., text comprehension), suggestions for instruction include: 1) practice on English oral proficiency with attention to building background knowledge and deep vocabulary understanding; 2) direct instruction in code-switching (i.e., alternate language at sentence boundaries), cognates, code-mixing (i.e., use words from one language while speaking or writing in the other), and cross-linguistic transfer; and 3) explicit and systematic phonics instruction embedded in the context of vocabulary and text comprehension instruction (Goodin, Weber, Pearson, & Raphael, 2009).

Taken together, the suggested literacy instructional strategies for ELLs are similar to those for English monolingual learners. They are related to the five components identified by the NRP (2000) for first-language literacy instruction: phonemic awareness, phonics, fluency, vocabulary, and text comprehension. In addition, teachers should also be familiar with the following principles of classroom instruction for motivation and engagement: 1) relevance for interest, 2) autonomy support for ownership, 3) success for self-efficacy, 4) thematic units for mastery learning goals, and 5) collaborative structures for social motivation (Guthrie et al., 2009).

Literacy Programs

The first U.S. bilingual education act was passed in 1968 to address the instructional challenges of ELLs. The landmark case of *Lau vs. Nichols* (1974) mandated that all school districts meet the needs of their ELLs. Bilingual/bicultural educational programs were also recommended (see the review of U.S. bilingual education policy in Garcia, 2000). By the late 1980s, programs with English-only instruction were accepted and funded.

At present, there are several different programs for ELLs (Office for Civil Rights, 2010). For example, *dual language programs*, also known as *two-way* or *developmental programs*, are bilingual programs in which the goal is for students to develop language proficiency in two languages by receiving instruction in English and another language in a classroom typically comprised of native English speakers and native speakers of the other language. *Transitional bilingual education programs*, also known as *early-exit bilingual education programs*, maintain and develop skills in the primary language and culture of ELLs while introducing, maintaining, and developing skills in English. The primary purpose is to facilitate the ELLs' transition to an instructional program in English-only while receiving academic subject instruction in the native language to the extent necessary. One of the criticisms of transitional bilingual education programs is that ELLs are separated from native English-speaking peers.

Structured English immersion programs involve teachers who have a bilingual education or ESL teaching credential or background and strong receptive skills in the students' primary language. All class instruction is in English. The goal of this program is the acquisition of English language skills so that ELL students can participate adequately in an English-only mainstream classroom. Alternatively, *submersion programs* place ELLs in a general English-only program with little or no support services, based on the hypothesis that they will pick up English naturally. *Newcomer programs* are separate relatively self-contained educational interventions for newly arrived immigrants. Typically, students attend these programs before they enter more traditional interventions such as English language development programs or mainstream classrooms with supplemental ESL instruction.

Table 9-1 summarizes several different programs for ELLs.

One of the consistent findings of the Panel (August & Shanahan, 2006) is that language-minority students who are literate (i.e., can read and write) in their first-language are more likely to be successful in English literacy acquisition. It is highly possible that ELLs learn to read best when taught in both their native language and English from early in the process of formal schooling because reading instruction in a familiar language serves as a bridge to English literacy proficiency, especially when the native language is Spanish or French, which entails a phonetic orthography similar to that of English. The decoding, sound blending, and generic comprehension strategies are clearly transferable between languages (see the discussion in the previous section of this chapter).

In a widely-cited longitudinal study of the academic performance of immigrant children in the United States, Collier and Thomas (1989) reported that non-English speaking immigrant children performed best in schools when they arrived in the United States at ages 8 and 9 with developed literacy skills in their native languages, as compared to younger children who arrived at ages 5 and 6 without literacy skills in their native languages. They confirmed Cummins' (1981, 1989) hypothesis that ELLs can often develop basic interpersonal skills in two to three years of

Table 9-1. Summary of Different Programs for English Language Learners

Program	English Instruction	L1 Instruction	Share Classrooms with Native English Speakers
Dual Language Program	Yes	Yes	Yes
Transitional Bilingual Education Program	Yes	Yes	No
Structured English Immersion Program	Yes	No	No
Submersion Program	Yes	No	Yes
Newcomer Program	Yes	Varies	No

Source: Office for Civil Rights (2010).

instruction in English, but additional time is needed to develop cognitive academic proficiency to comprehend and learn from English text. For example, Collier and Thomas found that it took more than five to seven years of instruction in the United States for the 8- and 9-year-olds to perform at grade level in English, whereas seven to ten years of instruction was needed for the 5- and 6-year olds.

The benefits of first-language literacy proficiency for subsequent English literacy acquisition of ELLs seem indisputable. Nevertheless, the Panel (August & Shanahan, 2006) asserted that, although there is no indication that bilingual instruction impedes academic achievement in either the native language or English, the current literature fails to provide guidance on how to make bilingual instruction maximally effective for ELLs. In addition, except for areas with condensed populations of language-minority families such as California and Texas, first-language instruction is often not an option in many schools where students speak multiple languages or the teaching staff is not able to provide first-language instruction.

Researchers (see the review in Jimenez & Teague, 2009) have reported mixed findings regarding the quality and usefulness of ESL programs, particularly at the secondary-level, some of which are termed *ESL ghetto* (Valdes, 1998, 2001). The reason that many ELLs do not receive high-quality reading instruction might be due, in part, to the fact that many of them are enrolled in underfunded districts and are often taught by teachers who are not certified (Garcia, 2003). Another contributing factor is the manner in which ELLs are perceived and treated at school. For example, following eight ELLs at an Alaskan high school for five years, Coulter and Smith (2006) concluded that the native cultures and languages of ELLs were typically devalued by the school. Specifically, ELLs: 1) were excluded from school functions and activities; 2) were not given the same types of classrooms and materials as mainstream students; 3) received lower quality instruction; 4) were tracked into remedial classes with lower expectations; 5) were isolated from native English speakers; and 6) were expected to assimilate.

Reeves (2004, 2006) studied 279 high school teachers in a southeastern U.S. school district regarding their attitudes and perceptions of ELLs in their classrooms. She found that, although the teachers expressed positive attitudes toward the inclusion of ELLs in their classes, their actual instructional practices revealed an assimilationist, English-only policy.

Furthermore, many teachers lacked experience with diverse students and were unwilling to change or seek additional professional development or even to recognize the need to modify instruction to better meet the needs of ELLs.

In evaluating ESL programs in general, Jimenez and Teague (2009) concluded:

> ESL programs can be either beneficial or detrimental, depending on how they are conceptualized and implemented. Strong programs do the following: employ highly-trained teachers, encourage learners to engage with challenging yet appropriately adapted materials and activities, find ways to include parents and students in decision making, monitor student progress, allow opportunities for interaction and feedback (including with native English speakers), and focus on the development of the types of oral and written language valued by academic institutions. (p. 125)

In short, the nature of literacy programs for ELLs is not research-based but rather politics-driven. Additional research, especially sound research, is needed to provide guidelines. Factors related to the quality of programs include the amount of funding, the education of teachers, and the conceptualization and implementation of the programs.

Literacy Assessment

The Panel (August & Shanahan, 2006) concluded that current literacy assessments for making placement decisions for ELLs are inadequate. Most of the measures do not assess development over time or predict the reading performance of ELLs. Garcia and Bauer (2009) identified the following problems with assessment:

1. Due to differences in the development of receptive (reading and listening) and productive skills (writing and speaking), ELLs often demonstrate more comprehension of English reading when they are allowed to respond in their dominant language.

2. Because ELLs tend to process text in their second language, and in some cases in both languages, more slowly than monolinguals, they may need more time than monolinguals to complete written tests.

3. Their limited English proficiency may mean that they will miss identifying the correct answers on a formal reading test due to unfamiliar English vocabulary in the test instructions or in the test items.

4. Their vocabulary knowledge sometimes is underestimated because they know some vocabulary concepts in one language and different vocabulary concepts in another language. (p. 239)

There are few diagnostic assessments on reading comprehension for ELLs, and little research is available for identifying older ELLs with learning disabilities. In addition, large-scale standardized assessments are repeatedly used to render placement decisions, particularly at the secondary-level, which results in the fact that ELLs are often overrepresented in low-track classrooms (Jimenez & Teague, 2009). For example, Callahan (2005) reported that approximately 98% of the ELLs in northern California high schools were never enrolled in courses that would prepare them for four-year colleges. Garcia and Bauer (2009) suggested that ELLs should take authentic assessments in their native language so that information which has been shown to predict their English reading performance can be obtained and used to evaluate progress; Examples include phonological awareness and reading level in the native language, a uniform view of reading across the two languages, and cross-linguistic transfer of knowledge and strategies.

Considering the unique linguistic and sociocultural factors of ELLs, Prater (2009) remarked:

> Researchers who view reading comprehension as a composite of abilities such as McCardle et al. (2005), and researchers who view reading comprehension as a socially constructed meaning-making activity such as Gee (2003), arrive at similar conclusions about assessment for English language learners from very different paths. A student's home language, culture, opportunity to learn, attitude, and aptitude combine in unique ways to impact achievement outcomes including reading comprehension. The complexity of reading comprehension in L2 cannot be captured by research methods that parse the composite abilities required to understand texts and do not account for the social, cultural, linguistic, and contextual variables that influence reading comprehension. We must develop research practices that untangle the intricate connections among the myriad of factors that impact academic achievement among English language learners while embracing the linguistic and sociocultural realities of English language learners. (p. 619)

In essence, current literacy assessments for ELLs have serious limitations. Future researchers should be more sensitive to the distinctive literacy development of ELLs such as the unbalanced relationship between receptive and expressive language skills, the slower processing speed, and the inadequate development of vocabulary knowledge. Instead of, or perhaps in addition to, standardized assessments, authentic assessments in their native language should also be used to provide a more complete picture of the literacy skills of ELLs.

Conclusion

There is a huge gap between what we know and what we need to know regarding the literacy instruction, programs, and assessment of ELLs. Current practices in the field are more politics-driven than data-driven. The quality of literacy instruction varies significantly from program to program and from teacher to teacher. What works for first-language literacy instruction should be the starting point for exploring effective practices for ELLs. Finally, special attention should be given to the distinctive linguistic and sociocultural background of ELLs, which is the focus of the next section.

SOCIOCULTURAL CONTEXTS AND LITERACY ACHIEVEMENT

The Panel (August & Shanahan, 2006) found little evidence for the impact of sociocultural variables on literacy development or achievement of ELLs, primarily due to the fact that relatively few studies have been conducted and that most available studies are descriptive in nature. This does not necessarily mean that sociocultural variables do not influence literacy achievement, however. This section is divided into two parts to examine the influences of 1) the home environment or culture and 2) the community.

Influence of Home Environment or Culture

The Panel (August & Shanahan, 2006) suggested that bridging home-school differences in interaction patterns or styles can improve ELLs' engagement, motivation, and participation in classroom instruction, but no causal links to literacy achievement or development can be established, based on the limited available data. This means that the impact of parental involvement on children's literacy achievement is surprisingly limited. In addition, the family experiences of ELLs are diversely shaped not only by culture but also by highly personal attributes, so it will be naïve to overgeneralize their literacy achievement based on nominal group (e.g., cultural or ethnic) membership.

The Panel (August & Shanahan, 2006) proffered three conclusions about the role of home environment. 1) Parents express willingness and often have the ability to help ELLs succeed academically; however, their interest, motivation, and potential contributions are often underestimated and underutilized by schools. 2) A larger number of home literacy experiences and opportunities are, by and large, associated with better literacy outcomes. 3) The relationship between home language use and the children's literacy outcome is inconclusive or not understood sufficiently to provide a basis for policy and practice recommendations.

Cultural conflicts often occur between U.S. teachers and the parents of ELLs regarding the expectations for the children and the parents' responsibilities (Garcia, 2000). For example, in the ethnographic study conducted by Valdes (1996), immigrant Mexican parents did not understand why U.S. teachers wanted their children to learn the English alphabetic system because learning the sounds of key syllables is far more important in Mexican reading instruction. Spanish is a transparent language in which phoneme–grapheme correspondence is much more reliable than that of English. Learning the alphabetic system is considered meaningless in Spanish. The miscommunication or lack of communication between school and home might diminish parents' involvement or contribution to their children's academic success.

In sum, the influence of home environment or culture on the literacy achievement of ELLs is inconclusive due to lack of research data. Nevertheless, positive home literacy experiences and opportunities may improve engagement, motivation, and participation of ELLs in classroom instruction, which could result in better reading achievement. Equally as important, as discussed in the next section, is the contribution of the broader community in which ELLs and their parents reside.

Influence of the Community

Children with different cultural heritages and diverse life experiences have developed rich linguistic backgrounds that teachers can use to build both learning and literacy (Cummins, 2007; Heath, 1983; Lee, 1995; Moll,

Saez, & Doworin, 2001; Nocon & Cole, 2009; Snow, 2001). Many teachers ignore these potentially important areas, however. Nocon and Cole noted:

> Often this lack of interest reflects teachers' beliefs that home experiences of poor, minority group children are simply irrelevant to classroom learning. At other times, teachers actively seek to exclude from their classrooms what children have learned at home, because they devalue, stigmatize, or even pathologize the experiences of children whose cultures deviate from their own. This privileging of the norms of the teachers' culture is supported by public schooling, the values and practices of which in the United States are consistent with white, English-speaking, middle-class culture. (p. 13)

The question is this: How should we teach *other people's children* (Delpit, 1996)? Moll and Gonzalez (Gonzalez et al., 1995; Moll, 1990; Moll & Gonzalez, 1994) proposed a two-step culturally responsive pedagogy to tap into and build on the *cultural funds of knowledge* (i.e., the knowledge and skills developed in families and communities that sustain the functioning and well-being of households) of working class, Latina/o (primarily Mexican) families: 1) teachers serve as ethnographers to investigate the funds of knowledge in children's families and community; and 2) teachers connect their literacy instruction to the cultural resources documented outside of the classrooms. Based on Ladson-Billings' (1995) notion of *culturally relevant pedagogy*, ways to connect the classroom with the surrounding areas outside of school include: providing community service projects, and including materials and texts from the community such as local newspapers, community center brochures, or the work of local writers and artists in the classroom (Guthrie et al., 2009).

Classrooms that offer a closer match to conditions with which students are familiar or comfortable can improve their engagement and produce better performance (Guthrie et al., 2009). For example, when classroom interaction was compatible with that of the native culture, Au and Mason (1981) found that Hawaiian students demonstrated higher levels of achievement-related behaviors in: 1) academic engagement; 2) ownership of reading; 3) topical and correct responses; 4) number of ideas expressed; and 5) logical inferences.

It should also be emphasized that, compared with the language of the material with respect to student proficiency in that language, culturally familiar reading material is a relatively weak predictor of reading comprehension; that is, students read better in the language they know better (August & Shanahan, 2006). Nevertheless, culturally familiar reading material can assist ELLs in producing extended discourse on the text and improving their inferential skills, which eventually can increase their reading engagement and participation (Jimenez, 1997).

Guthrie et al. (2009) suggested that the beginning of all good teaching is knowledge on what students and their families know and value and offered the following points on connecting classrooms with families and communities:

> To form positive interpersonal relationships with students, we need to understand their lives outside of school. Although the demographic composition of a particular classroom may vary from year to year, teachers may be fairly assured that the students in their classrooms will be somewhat reflective of the school's community. Knowledge of the surrounding community, its ethnic and socioeconomic characteristics, and the types of prevalent businesses and community events should indicate which cultural influences students bring to the classroom. Therefore, teachers are well advised to become familiar with the community and to be aware of the cultural influences that are displayed, particularly if they differ from the communities in which teachers live or were brought up. (pp. 210-211)

In essence, a good teacher should connect the artifacts and contents of ELLs' neighborhood community and culture with those associated with classroom instruction. Although culturally familiar reading material is not a direct predictor of reading comprehension, it can increase students' engagement and motivation by facilitating their production of extended discourse on the text and improving their inferential skills.

Conclusion

Research on the effects of sociocultural variables on reading achievement of ELLs is still in its infancy. Few studies have linked positive home literacy experiences and opportunities or culturally familiar reading materials with advanced reading achievement of ELLs. Nevertheless, the sociocultural context is too important to be ignored. Providing reading instruction within the sociocultural context that is familiar to ELLs can build on their prior knowledge and their inferential skills, which, as discussed previously in this chapter (and elsewhere in this book for literacy, see Chapters 4–8), is critical for developing written English comprehension. Finally, instruction within familiar sociocultural contexts can increase the engagement and motivation of ELLs in reading.

LITERATE THOUGHT AND ENGLISH LANGUAGE LEARNERS

Unlike children with disabilities discussed in the previous chapters, ELLs, except for those with disabilities, do not have biological conditions that impede their reading development. The reading difficulties of ELLs are mainly related to their unique linguistic and cultural experiences and opportunities. Although ELLs can develop adequate English reading skills, their content area learning often suffers because they are often exposed to unchallenging, boring reading materials. Multiple pathways, such as the New and Multiple Literacies (Chapter 3) and other techniques related to critico-creative thinking (Chapter 5), should be provided so that ELLs can simultaneously obtain content knowledge and develop literate thinking skills.

In previous chapters, we have discussed that children with disabilities can 1) obtain and utilize information in modes other than print; 2) apply the skills acquired in non-print modes to develop or improve their print literacy comprehension; and 3) benefit from the New and Multiple Literacies and critico-creative domains. These assertions are also relevant for ELLs.

The New and Multiple Literacies for ELLs refer to not only different modes of literacies but also to different languages. ELLs, who have acquired print (or script) literacy competency in their native languages, can obtain content area knowledge and develop literate thinking skills via reading books or Web sites in their native languages. ELLs who have yet to acquire literacy competency in their native languages can, most likely, access and utilize information in their native languages through audiobooks, video, or video/audio clips on the Internet. To acquire oral English proficiency, ELLs can use contextual cues in video-based English materials, such as the setting, body language, gestures, facial expressions, intonation, and a variety of others to help them understand the meaning (Drucker, 2003).

Technology and the New and Multiple Literacies

The advancement of technology (e.g., computers; Universal Design for Learning [UDL—see Chapter 3]; DVDs; etc.) has improved the accessibility and comprehension of information for ELLs. A number of studies have documented the effectiveness of incorporating technology in literacy instruction. For example, Blum et al. (1995) found that ESL first graders' reading fluency, monitoring, and motivation improved when they had repeated home readings supplemented by audiotapes. Without the audiotapes, there was limited progress.

The effects of digitally embedded special features of the Internet on literacy development have also been documented. For example, students can easily find and read texts in both their native language and English and also take advantage of online translators. Other Internet features, such as online chatting, blogging, or podcasting, create opportunities for ELLs to use English in meaningful social interactions, particularly informal social peer interactions, with native English speakers (Solomon & Schrum, 2007).

Leu et al. (2008) proposed a three-phase *Internet Reciprocal Teaching* model: 1) direct instruction of basic and essential online reading comprehension skills and online tool use; 2) problem-based learning to extend the development of online reading comprehension skills, which includes daily, small-group activities to encourage students to discover and exchange online reading comprehension strategies; and 3) inquiry projects in small groups to extend and share the development of newly-developed reading comprehension skills and strategies.

Solomon and Schrum (2007) suggested that the iPod be used as a *language lab* for ELLs, particularly middle-school ELLs, to improve their English oral proficiency. For example, when paired to conduct an English conversation in their community, ELLs can use an iPod in combination with a voice recorder to record vocabulary, generate questions, conduct practice conversations, check pronunciation, and store language exercises for instant replay. When satisfied, ELLs can upload the product onto a computer for evaluation by their teachers.

In essence, the potential benefits of using technology for the development of literate thought are endless. The acquisition of content area knowledge and literate thinking skills should not be limited to the use of English print. ELLs should not wait until developing adequate English proficiency to be exposed to age-appropriate and challenging instructional materials. Technology such as the Internet can be particularly beneficial for many schools where there is no luxury of having teachers who are familiar with the native languages of ELLs. Without exposure to adequate instruction or enriching language and literacy materials, many ELLs might encounter learning difficulties due to cognitive impoverishment (see also, Chapters 1 and 2).

SUMMARY

This chapter highlights the challenges of developing literate language in ELLs and promotes the use of technology to facilitate the accessibility and utilization of information. The chapter concludes with specific implications for developing literate thought in multiple pathways.

The key points of this chapter are as follows:

- Several terms are associated with English language learners (ELLs). *Language Minority* (*LM*) refers to individuals from homes where a language other than a societal language is actively used. *Second-Language Learners* (*SLL*) are LMs whose second language (L2) proficiency is not yet developed to benefit from instruction solely in L2. An SLL whose second-language is English is called an *English language learner* (*ELL*), also known as *Limited English Proficient* (*LEP*). ELLs in traditional special education programs are referred to as *English as a Second Language* (*ESL*) learners or *English Speakers of Other Language* (*ESOL*).

- The best predictors of English word recognition skills of ELLs include phonological processing skills (in either their first language [L1] or in English) and concepts of print. There is evidence for cross-language transference of phonological awareness skills for ELLs, particularly for younger ELLs, during the early stages of learning English, or for ELLs whose first-language uses an alphabetic script.

- The best predictors of English written language comprehension skills of ELLs include vocabulary knowledge, metalinguistic competence, and English oral proficiency. Additional factors include: exposure to print; learning opportunities and quality of literacy instruction; first-language (L1) literacy development; ability to navigate complex text and utilize prior knowledge to draw inferences; and use of cross-linguistic transfer strategies.

- The best predictors of poor motivation in reading for ELLs include lack of self-efficacy due to poor English language skills or lack of task value due to unchallenging or boring remedial activities or limited prior knowledge.

- Effective literacy instructional strategies for ELLs are similar to those for English monolingual learners; however, special attention should be provided to explicit vocabulary and text comprehension instruction during meaningful, motivating literacy practice.

- Additional research is needed on the literacy programs of ELLs. Factors related to the quality of a program include amount of funding, the education of teachers, and conceptualization and implementation of the program.
- Few assessments are sensitive to the distinctive literacy development of ELLs. Authentic assessments in their native language (L1) should be used, at the least, to provide a more complete picture of the literacy skills.
- Positive home literacy experiences and opportunities can improve engagement, motivation, and participation of ELLs in classroom instruction, which could result in better reading achievement.
- Teachers should connect ELLs' neighborhood community and culture with the culture of the classroom by including community service projects, materials, and texts, and culturally familiar reading materials.
- Multiple pathways, such as the New and Multiple Literacies, including the incorporation of critico-creative thinking activities, should be provided for ELLs so that they can simultaneously acquire content area knowledge and literate thinking skills necessary for the development of literate thought.
- There have been some promising data on the effectiveness of using technology in literacy instruction for ELLs.

QUESTIONS FOR REFLECTION AND DISCUSSION

1. Describe the various terms associated with English language learners.

2. With respect to the literacy development of English language learners, what are the major highlights for a) word recognition, b) written language comprehension, and c) motivational factors?

3. Is there sufficient evidence to argue that the Qualitative-Similarity Hypothesis also pertains to English language learners? Why or why not?

4. Define and describe the major issues regarding literacy instruction, programs, and assessment of ELLs.

5. What are the educational implications for the development of literate thought for ELLs? How are these implications similar to or different from those discussed in previous chapters?

REFERENCES

Adams, M. (1990). *Beginning to read: Thinking and learning about print.* Cambridge, MA: The MIT Press.

Au, K., & Mason, J. M. (1981). Social organizational factors and learning to read: The balance of rights hypothesis. *Reading Research Quarterly, 17*(1), 115-152.

Aud, S., Hussar, W., Planty, M., Snyder, T., Bianco, K., Fox, M., Frohlich, L., Kemp, J., & Drake, L. (2010). *The condition of education 2010* (NCES 2010-028). Washington, DC: National Center for Education Statistics, Institute of Education Sciences, U.S. Department of Education.

August, D., & Shanahan, T. (Eds.). (2006). *Developing literacy in second-language learners: Report of the National Literacy Panel on language-minority children and youth.* Mahwah, NJ: Erlbaum.

Birch, B. (2007). *English L2 reading: Getting to the bottom* (2nd ed.). Mahwah, NJ: Erlbaum.

Blum, I. H., Koskinen, P. S., Tennant, N., Parker, E. M., Straub, M., & Curry, C. (1995). Using audiotaped books to extend classroom literacy instruction into the homes of second-language learners. *Journal of Reading Behavior, 27*(4), 535-563.

Callahan, R. M. (2005). Tracking and high school English learners: Limiting opportunity to learn. *American Educational Research Journal, 42*(2), 305-328.

Cardenas-Hagan, E., Carlson, C., & Pollard-Durodola, S. D. (2007). The cross-linguistic transfer of early literacy skills: The role of initial L1 and L2 skills and language of instruction. *Language, Speech, and Hearing Services in Schools, 38*(3), 249-259.

Carlo, M. S., August, D., McLaughlin, B., Snow, C. E., Dressler, C., Lippman, D. N., et al. (2004). Closing the gap: Addressing the vocabulary needs of English-language learners in bilingual and mainstream classrooms. *Reading Research Quarterly, 39*(2), 188-215.

Chall, J. S. (1983). *Stages of reading development.* New York: McGraw-Hill.

Chall, J. S. (1996). *Stages of reading development* (2nd ed.). New York: McGraw-Hill.

Collier, V. P. (1987). Age and rate of acquisition of second language for academic purposes. *TESOL Quarterly, 21*(4), 617-641.

Collier, V. P., & Thomas, W. P. (1989). How quickly can immigrants become proficient in school English? *Journal of Educational Issues of Language Minority Students, 16*(1-2), 187-212.

Coulter, C., & Smith, M. L. (2006). English language learners in a comprehensive high school. *Bilingual Research Journal, 30*(2), 309-335.

Cummins, J. (1978). Educational implications of mother tongue maintenance in minority language groups. *Canadian Modern Language Review, 35,* 395-416.

Cummins, J. (1979). Linguistic interdependence and the educational development of bilingual children. *Review of Educational Research, 49*(2), 222-251.

Cummins, J. (1980). The crosslingual dimensions of language proficiency: Implications for bilingual education and the optimal age issue. *TESOL Quarterly, 14*(2), 175-187.

Cummins, J. (1981). The role of primary language development in promoting educational success for language minority students. In California State Department of Education (Ed.), *Schooling and language minority students: A theoretical framework* (pp. 3-49). Los Angeles: Education, Dissemination, and Assessment Center, California State University.

Cummins, J. (1984). *Bilingual and special education: Issues in assessment and pedagogy.* San Diego, CA: College Hill Press.

Cummins, J. (1989). *Empowering minority students.* Sacramento, CA: California Association for Bilingual Education.

Cummins, J. (2007). Pedagogies for the poor: Realigning reading instruction for low-income students with scientifically based reading research. *Educational Researcher, 36*(9), 564-572.

Delpit, L. (1996). *Other people's children: Cultural conflict in the classroom.* New York: The New Press.

Drucker, M. J. (2003). What reading teachers should know about ESL learners. *The Reading Teacher, 57*(1), 22-29.

Durgunoglu, A., Nagy, W. E., & Hancin-Bhatt, B. J. (1993). Cross-language transfer of phonological awareness. *Journal of Educational Psychology, 85,* 453-465.

Garcia, G. E. (1996, December). *Improving the English reading of Mexican-American bilingual students through the use of cognate recognition strategies.* Paper presented at the National Reading Conference, Charleston, SC.

Garcia, G. E. (2000). Bilingual children's reading. In M. L. Kamil, P. B. Mosenthal, P. D. Pearson, & R. Barr (Eds.), *Handbook of reading research, Volume III* (pp. 813-834). Mahwah, NJ: Erlbaum.

Garcia, G. E. (2003). The reading comprehension development and instruction of English-language learners. In A. P. Sweet & C. E. Snow (Eds.), *Rethinking reading comprehension* (pp. 30-50). New York: The Guilford Press.

Garcia, G. E., & Bauer, E. (2009). Assessing student progress in the time of no child left behind. In L. M. Morrow, R. Rueda, & D. Lapp (Eds.), *Handbook of research on literacy and diversity* (pp. 233-253). New York: The Guilford Press.

Gonzalez, N., Moll, L., Tenery, M. F., Rivera, A., Rendon, P., Gonzales, R., & Amanti, C. (1995). Funds of knowledge for teaching in Latino households. *Urban Education, 29*(4), 443-470.

Goodin, S. M., Weber, C. M., Pearson, P. D., & Raphael, T. E. (2009). Comprehension: The means, motive, and opportunity for meeting the needs of diverse learners. In L. M. Morrow, R. Rueda, & D. Lapp (Eds.), *Handbook of research on literacy and diversity* (pp. 337-365). New York: The Guilford Press.

Guthrie, J. T., Rueda, R., Gambrell, L. B., & Morrison, D. A. (2009). Roles of engagement, valuing, and identification in reading development of students from diverse backgrounds. In L. M. Morrow, R. Rueda, & D. Lapp (Eds.), *Handbook of research on literacy and diversity* (pp. 195-215). New York: The Guilford Press.

Heath, S. B. (1983). *Ways with words: Language, life, and work in communities and classrooms*. Cambridge, UK: Cambridge University Press.

Hill, J., & Flynn, K. (2006). *Classroom instruction that works with English language learners*. Alexandria, VA: ASCD.

Jimenez, R. T. (1997). The strategic reading abilities and potential of five low-literacy Latina /o readers in middle school. *Reading Research Quarterly, 32*, 224-243.

Jimenez, R. T., & Teague, B. L. (2009). Language, literacy, and content: Adolescent English language learners. In L. M. Morrow, R. Rueda, & D. Lapp (Eds.), *Handbook of research on literacy and diversity* (pp. 114-134). New York: The Guilford Press.

Kindler, A. L. (2002). *Survey of the states' limited English proficient students and available educational programs and services. 2000-2001 summary report*. Washington, DC: National Clearinghouse for English Language Acquisition.

Ladson-Billings, G. (1995). Toward a theory of culturally relevant pedagogy. *American Educational Research Journal, 32*(3), 465-491.

Lau v. Nichols, 515 U.S. 563 (1974). U.S. Supreme Court Center. Retrieved January 19, 2011 from http://supreme.justia.com/us/414/563/

Lee, C. D. (1995). Signifying as a scaffold for literacy interpretation. *Journal of Black Psychology, 21*(4), 357-381.

Leu, D. J., Coiro, J., Castek, J., Hartman, D. K., Henry, L. A., & Reinking, D. (2008). Research on instruction and assessment in the new literacies of online reading comprehension. In C. C. Block & S. R. Parris (Eds.), *Comprehension instruction: Research-based best practices* (pp. 321-346). New York: Guilford Press.

Liow, S. J. R., & Poon, K. K. L. (1998). Phonological awareness in multi-lingual Chinese children. *Applied Psycholinguistics, 19*(3), 339-362.

Mathewson, G. (2004). Model of attitude influence upon reading and learning to read. In R. Ruddell & N. Unrau (Eds.), *Theoretical models and processes of reading* (5th ed.) (pp. 1431-1461). Newark, DE: International Reading Association.

McGuinness, D. (2004). *Early reading instruction: What science really tells us about how to teach reading*. Cambridge, MA: The MIT Press.

McGuinness, D. (2005). *Language development and learning to read: The scientific study of how language development affects reading skill*. Cambridge, MA: The MIT Press.

Miller, S., & Faircloth, B. (2009). Motivation and reading comprehension. In S. Israel & G. Duffy (Eds.), *Handbook of research on reading comprehension* (pp. 307-322). New York: Routledge.

Moll, L. C. (1990, February). *Literacy research in community and classroom: A sociocultural approach*. Paper presented at the conference on Multi-disciplinary Perspectives on Research Methodology in Language Arts, National Conference on Research in English, Chicago.

Moll, L. C., & Gonzalez, N. (1994). Critical issues: Lessons from research with language-minority children. *Journal of Reading Behavior: A Journal of Literacy, 26*(4), 439-456.

Moll, L. C., Saez, R., & Doworin, J. (2001). Exploring biliteracy: Two student case examples of writing as a social practice. *Elementary School Journal, 101*(4), 435-449.

National Early Literacy Panel (NELP). (2008). *Developing early literacy: Report of the National Early Literacy Panel.* Washington, DC: National Institute for Literacy: Available at http://www.nifl.gov/earlychildhood/NELP/NELPreport.html

National Reading Panel (NLP). (2000). *Report of the National Reading Panel: Teaching children to read – An evidence-based assessment of the scientific research literature on reading and its implications for reading instruction.* Jessup, MD: National Institute for Literacy at EDPubs.

Nocon, H., & Cole, M. (2009). Relating diversity and literacy theory. In L. M. Morrow, R. Rueda, & D. Lapp (Eds.), *Handbook of research on literacy and diversity* (pp. 13-31). New York: The Guilford Press.

Office for Civil Rights. (2010). *Developing programs for English language learners: Glossary.* Retrieved January 18, 2011 from http://www2.ed.gov/about/offices/list/ocr/ell/glossary.html

Perfetti, C. A. (2003). The universal grammar of reading. *Scientific Studies of Reading, 7*(1), 3-24.

Portes, P., & Salas, S. (2009). Poverty and its relation to development and literacy. In L. M. Morrow, R. Rueda, & D. Lapp (Eds.), *Handbook of research on literacy and diversity* (pp. 97-113). New York: The Guilford Press.

Prater, K. (2009). Reading comprehension and English language learners. In S. E. Israel & G. G. Duffy (Eds.), *Handbook of research on reading comprehension* (pp. 607-621). New York: Routledge.

Ramirez, J. D., Yuen, S. D., & Ramey, D. R. (1991). *Executive summary: Final report: Longitudinal study of structured English immersion strategy, early-exit and late-exit transitional bilingual education programs for language minority children.* San Mateo, CA: Aguirre International.

Reeves, J. (2004). "Like everybody else": Equalizing educational opportunity for English language learners. *TESOL Quarterly, 38*(1), 43-66.

Reeves, J. (2006). Secondary teacher attitudes toward including English language learners in mainstream classrooms. *Journal of Educational Research, 99,* 131-142.

Rueda, R., Velasco, A., & Lim, H. J. (2008). Comprehension instruction for English learners. In C. C. Block & S. R. Parris (Eds.), *Comprehension instruction: Research-based best practices* (2nd ed.) (pp. 294-305). New York: The Guilford Press.

Short, D., & Fitzsimmons, S. (2007). *Double the work: Challenges and solutions to acquiring language and academic literacy for adolescent English language learners – A report to Carnegie Corporation of New York.* Washington, DC: Alliance for Excellent Education.

Snow, C. (2001). Literacy and language: Relationships during the preschool years. In S. W. Beck & L. N. Olah (Eds.), *Perspectives on language and literacy: Beyond the here and now* (pp. 161-186). Cambridge, MA: Harvard Educational Review.

Snow, C. (2006). Cross-cutting themes and future research directions. In D. August & T. Shanahan (Eds.), *Developing literacy in second-language learners: Report of the*

National Literacy Panel on Language-Minority Children and Youth (pp. 631-652). Mahwah, NJ: Erlbaum.

Solomon, G., & Schrum, L. (2007). *Web 2.0: New tools, new schools.* Eugene, OR: International Society for Technology in Education.

Taffe, S. W., Blachowicz, C. L. Z., & Fisher, P. J. (2009). Vocabulary instruction for diverse students. In L. M. Morrow, R. Rueda, & D. Lapp (Eds.), *Handbook of research on literacy and diversity* (pp. 320-336). New York: The Guilford Press.

Valdes, G. (1996). *Con respeto: Bridging the distances between culturally diverse families and schools: An ethnographic portrait.* New York: Teachers College Press.

Valdes, G. (1998). The world outside and inside schools: Language and immigrant children. *Educational Researcher, 27*(6), 4-18.

Valdes, G. (2001). *Learning and not learning English: Latino students in American schools.* New York: Teachers College Press.

Zimmerman, C. (1997). Do reading and interactive vocabulary instruction make a difference? An empirical study. *TESOL Quarterly, 31*(1), 121-140.

FURTHER READING

Crawford, J. (1999). *Bilingual education: History, politics, theory, and practice* (4th ed.). Los Angeles: Bilingual Education Services.

Garcia, G. E. (2001). *Understanding and meeting the challenge of student diversity* (3rd ed.). Boston: Houghton Mifflin.

Garcia, G. E. (2005). *Teaching and learning in two languages: Bilingualism and schooling in the United States.* New York: Teachers College Press.

Rhodes, R. L., Ochoa, S. H., & Ortiz, S. O. (2005). *Assessing culturally and linguistically diverse students: A practical guide.* New York: The Guilford Press.

Zentella, A. C. (Ed.). (2005). *Building on strengths: Language and literacy in Latino families and communities.* New York: Teachers College Press.

CHAPTER 10

Literate Thought in A Brave New World

Thinking is not so much an act as a way of living or dwelling. . . . It is a remembering who we are as human beings and where we belong. It is a gathering and focusing of our whole selves on what lies before us and a taking to heart and mind these particular things before us in order to discover in them their essential nature and truth. Learning how to think can obviously aid us in this discovery. . . . The nature of reality and of man is both hidden and revealed; it both appears and withdraws from view, not in turn but concomitantly. Only the thinking that is truly involved, patient, and disciplined by long practice can come to know either the hidden or disclosed character of truth.

Gray, 1968, p. xi

Are we living in a brave new world? Two of Aldous Huxley's famous works are *Brave New World* and *Brave New World Revisited* (for both books, see Huxley, 2005). In *Brave New World*, Huxley attempted to portray the future effects of living in a fast-paced, rapidly changing society whose ideas, mores, and habits are molded by the processes and products of technology. This *negative utopia* anticipates advanced developments of mass productive and reproductive technology and, subsequently, one can see a demeanor in individuals that favors materialism, instant gratification, and narcissism. With overpopulation, forms of population control, and the use of drugs within his purview, in *Brave New World Revisited*, Huxley concluded that the world was becoming like a *Brave New World* much faster than he had originally imagined.

Fast forward to the beginning of the twenty-first century. Are we preparing students and others to live in a brave new world? According to one scholar (Bauerlein, 2008), our students—adolescents and young adults—may turn out to be the *dumbest generation*. Despite all the technological advances and accessibility to information, much of the time and energy seem to be spent on social networking and discovering shortcuts with respect to obtaining knowledge and understanding. In fact, Bauerlein as well as others (Blackburn, 2005; Specter, 2009) remarked that most of today's youth (and even a number of adults) exhibit a blatant disregard for deep, serious reading and reflective, rational thinking.

Admittedly, we might be overstating the situation because it is difficult to verify or falsify the above assertions via the use of systematic, scholarly methods. In other words, we seem to be posing *hard problems*, which cannot be resolved to everyone's satisfaction. Nevertheless, it is critical to address these and other problems by focusing on an *education for thinking* (e.g., Kuhn, 2005) or, in our view, an education for literate thought. This might move us closer to an understanding of the *nature of reality* and ourselves, as mentioned in the passage at the beginning of this chapter.

In this final chapter, we summarize a few major points and offer steps to extend further the development of the concept of literate thought. We explore a few of the fallacies associated with the concept of *functional literacy* and its close cousin, the *vocationalization of education*. Finally, for living in a brave new world, we propose an *education for literate thought* within the instruction of all content areas or disciplines.

MAJOR TENETS OF LITERATE THOUGHT: REDUX

Literate thought can and should be developed in both non-captured (i.e., face-to-face; through-the-air) and captured (e.g., print, audio/sign books, etc.) venues. The demands and constraints of the captured information venues are quite different from those of the non-captured ones. Indeed, these venues represent different modes of thought.

The captured mode permits reflection upon information that does not burden the individual's cognitive capacity in the same manner as does reflection on information in the extemporaneous non-captured mode. The captured mode thus has led to the development of a type of thinking manifested by models and theories as opposed to the type of thinking shaped by immediate or long-term memory and observation or apprenticeship (e.g., Olson, 1994; Rubin, 1995).

Whether the advances of technology and literate texts in society are a consequence or an epiphenomenon or something else of print (i.e., script literacy) is an open question. Nevertheless, the juxtaposition of print and sophisticated technologies and stored knowledge cannot be dismissed or left unexamined. Our understanding of this juxtaposition has been influenced, in part, by our exploration of the relationship between orality and literacy.

Relationship Between Orality and Literacy

The relationship between a specific captured mode (e.g., script literacy) and its non-captured counterpart (e.g., speech) is reciprocal and facilitative. Consider the evidence for the reciprocal relations between the spoken and written forms of English (Cain & Oakhill, 2007; McGuinness, 2004, 2005). It has been averred that the knowledge and use of English script literacy skills exert a pervasive influence on the manner in which words are organized in an individual's mental lexicon (i.e., in the mind). For example, reading skills can contribute to an understanding (and appreciation) of the phonological and morphological properties of spoken English. This understanding leads to the development of advanced reading skills because of the increased and growing awareness of the alphabetic system, the system upon which literacy is based.

The implication of the foregoing discussion seems to be biased— namely, that there is a relationship between literate thought and only print literacy. This implies that only script literacy skills are necessary for the concomitant or subsequent development of abstract, reflective thought. The dictum of Francis Bacon can be invoked here for partial support: "Reading maketh a full man, conference a ready man, and writing an exact man" (Beck, 1980, p. 181).

As we have argued in this book, these assertions are not supported by either theoretical or empirical evidence (Olson, 1989, 1994; Rubin, 1995; see also, Chapters 1 and 2). First, the use of language (i.e., through-the-air or face-to-face) is the underpinning of the relationship between orality and literacy or any form of captured information. Granted, individuals do need to possess *access* skills for a specific captured form (e.g., understanding the alphabetic system for print in English). Nevertheless, writing and other forms of external representations are secondary products, based on mental activities and interactions involving the use of a verbal language (Carruthers, Laurence, & Stich, 2005, 2006; Chomsky, 2006; Pinker, 1994).

From another perspective, as emphasized by several scholars (e.g., Olson, 1994; Rubin, 1995), print literacy skills are intertwined with specific thinking skills required in educational settings and schools. It is difficult to separate these two broad domains, but their juxtaposition also masks the reality of the essential connection between orality and literacy—that is, a connection driven by language. In short, literacy skills are manifestations of individuals who can engage in logical or reasoning activities. Script literacy is only one avenue that individuals can use to demonstrate their ability to address complex topics and interactions involving areas such as law, philosophy, and science.

In our view, the most colorful clarification of the relationship between orality and literacy can be seen in the historical examples of Socrates and Homer and with the story of *readers* (Olson, 1989, 1994; see Chapter 2) in the period prior to and during the early days of the printing press. Modern-day *clarifications* include the accomplishments of individuals with severe dyslexia and those who have either visual or hearing impairment. In addition, we (the authors) have stories about individuals in our graduate programs who could not access the printed word, but who obviously possessed high levels of literate thought that enabled them to obtain their degrees (e.g., via the use of audiobooks, interpreters, etc.).

There are additional perspectives on the relationships between orality and print literacy that are much more complex than what we have presented in this book (e.g., see Olson, 1994; Ong, 1982). Even more interesting is the fact that there is a range of genres, from simple to intricate, in both the oral and print modes. This leads us to a few final remarks on the topic of *complexity* with respect to the quality and quantity of information in both modes.

Complexity of Orality Versus Print Literacy

We examined the issue of whether information presented in an *oral* or *conversational* (including signed) mode, non-captured or captured, is really as complex (e.g., abstract, layers of interpretations) as information that is captured in print (e.g., an alphabetic literacy). Research has revealed that written information is decontextualized, less redundant, and abstract, especially if one considers the use of complex and dense sentence structures used to express concepts or ideas (e.g., McGuinness, 2004, 2005; Olson, 1994). It thus has been argued that written language is not simply speech written down (or captured), and the ability to read and write requires a set of linguistic and cognitive skills that proceed beyond those needed for through-the-air (e.g., spoken or signed) language comprehension—even in a captured form as in videobooks or audiobooks and so on.

We (the authors) agree that written language requires more than the ability to comprehend through-the-air language. We have argued that this should be contextualized broadly, however; that is, any type of captured information (e.g., print, audio, sign) requires additional skills that proceed beyond the comprehension of the non-captured through-the-air counterpart. This is due to several factors but primarily that captured information in any mode is decontextualized and tends to place more demands on its users.

Much of the research on the complexity issue has focused on the structure of the language of print versus the type of language used in spoken discourses as well as the skills needed to comprehend information either orally or in print (Cain & Oakhill, 2007; Israel & Duffy, 2009; McGuinness, 2004, 2005). We averred that complexity should be measured by another variable: the quality and quantity associated with the *content* of the information.

The content of presenting or delivering information in the conversational or non-captured mode (speaking or signing) can be as complex and difficult as information presented in the written mode (Olson, 1989, 1994; Rubin, 1995). In addition, it has been argued that there is a range of genres in the oral mode (i.e., orality) similar to those that exist for print literacy (Denny, 1991; Feldman, 1991). In short, the complexity element of any mode has an array of difficulty factors, which proceeds beyond the mere capture or non-capture of information. In essence, this supports our call for a reconceptualization of literacy—that is, literacy, at the least, is a form of captured information (see also, Ellsworth, Hedley, & Baratta, 1994).

Reconceptualization of Literacy

It would be shortsighted to conclude that we are advocating the denigration of script (print) literacy or its importance for participating in a society. Rather, we support the broader view: the notion of literacy should be reconceptualized with a focus on the processes and components of literate thought, for example, as discussed in Chapter 3 on the New and Multiple Literacies and in the chapters on children with disabilities (Chapters 6–8) and those who are English language learners (Chapter 9). With the advent of advanced technologies, there are multiple paths to the promised land of developing high level literate thinking skills in children and adolescents, especially for those who struggle with print.

One difficult task is to convince educators and policymakers that information captured in the non-print modes (e.g., performance literacy) can be used to develop literate thinking skills, even at the expense of reducing the emphasis on script literacy. Part of the reason for this reluctance is due to the widespread and traditional use, not to mention prestige, of script literacy in learned professions such as medicine, law, science and industry, and, of course, education.

There is also the perception of *permanency* to script or print literacy. One can refer to the information in print periodically and as often as necessary because it is captured on paper (or electronically). Furthermore, learned, scholarly discussions and debates seem to evolve about information presented in print materials—albeit, such endeavors typically can occur in spoken (or signed) groups discourses as well.

As we attempt to demonstrate in this book, the availability and ease of modern technology has pervasively challenged our traditional views of literacy. There are a number of venues for representing and working with learned information and discourse that are just as efficient and effective as information in print. Indeed, alternatives to print might be preferred by many individuals. Several scholars have argued that a fixed medium such as print is not sufficient for meeting the complex challenging needs of society often associated with the calls for educational reform (see discussions in Bloome & Paul, 2006; Ellsworth et al., 1994; Montague, 1990).

In our view, it should be possible for individuals to develop high levels of critical and reflective thinking skills without having adequate skills in script literacy. These individuals can be exposed to the same amount and diversity of learned, complex information as that available in print. Scholarly debates, discussions, and instruction can be organized around information presented in any captured mode (Paul & Wang, 2006a, 2006b). Individuals can access and reflect on the information and become engaged in meaningful discussions.

Let us accept the argument that literate thought is possible to develop with the use of information in any captured mode—assuming that quantity and quality are roughly equivalent. We surmise that at least two major questions can be raised as well as several secondary questions. 1) Is it cost efficient to duplicate everything that is already available in print; that is, to present *all* information in several captured forms—print, video and/or audio recordings, Braille, and sign? Along the lines of this question, we can inquire: If there are bilingual education programs, does this mean that all information has to be duplicated by translation into the home language of the students? What about the presence of a variety of languages within a society? Is it feasible and desirable to present information in different languages or in a variety of captured modes? What would this do to the emphasis on developing the majority language of society?

The second major question (and subquestions) may be more critical for many scholars. 2) Is literate thought, without print literacy skills, sufficient for participation in a scientific, technological society such as the United States (and others)? That is, is it really possible for individuals to possess the necessary skills to compete, develop, and participate fully in a society that is heavily dependent on and developed by the use of print? If the development of cognition (and deep thinking skills) is independent of the mode of captured information, does this become an equity and diversity issue or, perhaps, an oppression issue if only print literacy is required in educational settings (e.g., see Freire & Macedo, 1987, for an interesting perspective)?

Addressing these and other questions related to the reconceptualization of literacy requires more space than we have here. Nevertheless, we contend that, for individuals with script literacy problems (see Chapters 6–9), the choice of mode basically can be construed as an accessibility issue. We understand the importance and value of developing script literacy skills, but not at the expense of developing literate thought. We find it problematic to compel the use of only a script-literacy mode if it is clear that the same individuals could have reached high literate thought levels via the use of conversational (face-to-face; through-the-air) information and other information captured by the use of audio and video media.

FUNCTIONAL LITERACY: AN AMBIGUITY

Our call for the reconceptualization of literacy also means a reexamination of another traditional concept, *functional literacy*, which is problematic and can lead to the *vocationalization* of education. The term, functional literacy (i.e., in a narrow sense), has been applied only to script or print literacy. In fact, the lack of functional literacy is often considered to be associated with the ills of society that include poverty, crime, or an uneducated and uninvolved populace (Olson, 1994; Rubin, 1995). Use of this term can be traced to a widely-adopted description (Hunter & Harman, 1979):

> A person is literate when he has acquired the essential knowledge and skills which enable him to engage in all those activities in which literacy is required for effective functioning in his group and community and whose attainments in reading, writing, and arithmetic make it possible for him to continue to use these skills toward his own and the community's development. (p. 14)

Functional literacy is often considered to be one of the main goals of education, especially for children with disabilities. In addition, it is possible to argue that the overuse and misapplication of this concept engender an overreliance on the development of functional curricula (e.g., the instruction and development of functional, daily living, or life skills) (e.g., see discussion in Heward, 2009 for children with disabilities).

We caution that there might be another consequence of the idea of functional literacy: an overemphasis on the vocationalization of education for many individuals with difficulties in script literacy. That is, there is a tendency to assume that such individuals should be *tracked*, as early as possible, in vocational programs during the latter stages of their compulsory education period (e.g., in middle or high school). A corollary is the belief that a major goal of education is to prepare individuals for a specific *vocation*, which seems to call into question the value of a liberal arts education either in kindergarten to grade 12 or in the first two to four years of a college or university education (see related discussions in deMarrais & LeCompte, 1995; McLaren, 1994; Rippa, 1997).

The traditional concept of functional literacy implies that individuals are illiterate if they cannot access and interpret information captured in print orthographies. In short, the real issue is not the inability to access information in print. Rather, it is the comprehension and application of learned information, regardless of the manner in which it is presented or delivered. We have emphasized that there is a separation between the mode of information—captured or non-captured (through the air)—and one's comprehension or interpretation of it. There are levels of literacy influenced by the richness or layers of interpretations proffered by individuals (Olson, 1989, 1994; Robinson, 1990; Rubin, 1995). This richness is also dependent on what individuals bring to the social interactive situations and practices. Perhaps the focus should be on educational literacy, not functional literacy.

EDUCATIONAL LITERACY

In essence—and we recognize that this is controversial—educational literacy refers to an awareness or knowledge in the academic content areas, particularly, but not limited to, the great or accumulated works in literature, history, and science (for a related discussion on *educational justice*, see Michael & Trezek, 2006; and see, the notion of cultural literacy, Hirsch, 1987; Hirsch, Kett, & Trefil, 2002). In Chapter 4, we attempted to demonstrate that an improvement of discipline knowledge (e.g., knowledge of mathematics, science, etc.) requires an understanding of the epistemology of the discipline. The lack of or poorly-developed literate thought, however can mean that, even with this awareness or knowledge, individuals are still unable to think reflectively, logically, or creatively with respect to solving problems or answering questions. That is, individuals may not develop the ability to think like a mathematician, a scientist, or a historian (e.g., Donovan & Bransford, 2005; Phillips & Soltis, 2004).

Perhaps the crux of the matter is that there is a lack of a functional level of literate thought. It is important to relate a range of literate thinking abilities to a specific content discipline or topic. To say that someone is simply a good literate thinker requires a context. A good literate thinker of what? This is analogous to other questions such as: A good reader of what? A good writer of what? (see discussions in Israel & Duffy, 2009; Paul & Whitelaw, 2011; Pearson, 2004).

We certainly do not mean to imply that developing a *functional level* of literate thought is the end goal of education—rather, it is the bare minimum. We harbor no illusion that this is an easy feat for children and adolescents, particularly those with disabilities or for who are English language learners (as discussed in Chapters 6–9). Nevertheless, we believe that this has not always been the main focus in education, including education for children with disabilities.

FUTURE RESEARCH ON LITERATE THOUGHT

For us (the authors), literate thought is predominantly a cognitive activity involving a reflection on thoughts in the mind and on input from outside the mind (i.e., social artifacts, practices, intercourses). We have drawn from several major research disciplines to explicate this model of literate thought—namely, comprehension, and print (script, reading, writing) and oral literacy (Chapters 1 and 2), the New and Multiple Literacies (Chapter 3), cognitive and disciplinary structures (Chapter 4), and critico-creative thinking (Chapter 5).

We have discussed the development of literate thought in children with disabilities (Chapters 6–8) and those labeled as English language learners (Chapter 9). Much of our focus in those chapters was guided by research on the development of print (script) literacy in these children. The ability to access, interpret, and use print (i.e., reading and writing) dominates the activities of schools. We hope it is clear, however, that print is only one avenue for developing high-level thinking skills. And, unfortunately, it might not be the best or most feasible mode for a number of these children and adolescents.

We are interested, of course, in the development of critical, logical, and reflective thinking for all individuals. Research and theorizing on literate thought is in its infancy, albeit there certainly have been scholarly debates on the various components. Progress will always be slow, laborious, and challenging due to ongoing discussions on the nature and extent of epistemology (e.g., Bernecker & Dretske, 2000; Phillips & Soltis, 2004; Pring, 2004), including the nature and extent of cognition (e.g., Bruning, Schraw, Norby, & Ronning, 2004; Jarvis, 2000).

It should be highlighted that literate thought does not involve the use of only the scientific method. The scientific method is valuable but so is the use of speculative and creative thought, intuition, and even *wild* or imaginative (out-of-the-box) thinking (e.g., Beveridge, 1980; Heidegger, 1968). To prepare students and others for a *brave new world*, bombarded by the explosion of a range of technologies and varying social and cultural perspectives, it is important to develop and enhance a positive, assertive attitude toward reflective and creative thought. This involves the use of synthesis and even syncretism. In particular, such an attitude is necessary to evaluate positions critically and to tolerate differences in opinions, beliefs, ideologies, theories, philosophies, religions, modes of thought, and so on. Whatever the approach, our contention is that all students should be encouraged to dialogue with themselves (i.e., metacognitively) and others and, most importantly, to develop their own views on and understanding of a wide range of topics within a number of venues based on the use of literate thinking skills.

It is difficult to conduct research on literate thought without the use of complex research methodologies similar to those used in the emerging research on script literacy, particularly the New and Multiple Literacies. Future researchers should focus on examining in depth the processes and components of literate thought as well as its implications for diversity and inclusiveness. A few general questions include the following:

1. What are the language, cognitive, social, and affective requisites for developing literate thought?

2. Does the research on comprehension, critical thinking, and the New and Multiple Literacies contribute to our understanding of literate thought?

3. What access and interpretation skills are associated with the various types of literacies, including the New and Multiple Literacies?

4. What are the issues in evaluating the quality of literate thinking skills in individuals?

5. What are the implications of understanding the research on disciplinary structures and the development of literate thought?

6. How is literate thought related to the notions of openness, prejudice, bias, and other types of consciousness?

FINAL REMARKS

In our brave new world of the twenty-first century, we have floating brains and brains in a vat (Davis, 2002), multiple realities (Blackmore, 2004), multiverse (Hawking & Mlodinow, 2010), and virtual realities (Heim, 1993). From one perspective, a number of arguments focus on the value of the humanities—or to reconceptualize this—on the value of applying ideas, approaches, and questions posed in the humanities to all scholarly endeavors. In our view, these activities reflect, at the least, some of the components and processes of literate thought. In any case, we are convinced that literate thought is important for a participatory democracy, the development of critical and imaginative thinking skills, and an appreciation of perspectives, cultures, as well as *our own humanity.*

SUMMARY

In this final chapter, we reiterate our major points regarding the modes, components, and processes of literate thought. We explore the constraints of terms such as functional literacy and its close cousin, vocationalization, proposing instead a focus on educational literacy. After delineating a few future research questions, we boldly argue that there should be an education for literate thought to prepare individuals for living in the twenty-first century—the updated version of the *brave new world.*

A few major points are:

- Literate thought can and should be developed in both non-captured (i.e., face-to-face; through-the-air) and captured (e.g., print, audio/ sign books, etc.) venues.
- The relationship between a specific captured mode (e.g., script literacy) and its non-captured counterpart (e.g., speech) is reciprocal and facilitative.
- The use of language (i.e., through-the-air or face-to-face) is the underpinning of the relationship between orality and literacy or any form of captured information.
- Any type of captured information (e.g., print, audio, sign) requires additional skills that proceed beyond the comprehension of the non-captured through-the-air counterpart. This is due to several factors, the primary one being that captured information in any mode is decontextualized and tends to place more demands on its users.
- Literacy should be reconceptualized with a focus on the processes and components of literate thought. There are multiple paths, including the use of technology, to the promised land of developing high level literate thinking skills in children and adolescents, especially for those who struggle with print.
- Future researchers should focus on examining in depth the processes and components of literate thought as well as its implications for diversity and inclusiveness.

QUESTIONS FOR REFLECTION AND DISCUSSION

1. What are the major highlights in the section on the tenets of literate thought?

2. What is the basis for the argument that literacy should be reconceptualized?

3. What is *functional literacy* and why is it a problematic notion?

4. What is meant by the phrase *educational literacy*?

5. In your view, is literate thought sufficient for living in a *brave new world*? Why or why not?

REFERENCES

Bauerlein, M. (2008). *The dumbest generation: How the digital age stupefies young Americans and jeopardizes our future (or, don't trust anyone under 30)*. New York: Penguin.

Beck, E. (1980). (Ed.). *Familiar quotations: A collection of passages, phrases, and proverbs traced to their sources in ancient and modern literature: John Bartlett*. Boston, MA: Little, Brown, & Company.

Bernecker, S., & Dretske, F. (Eds.). (2000). *Knowledge: Readings in contemporary epistemology*. New York: Oxford University Press.

Beveridge, W. (1980). *Seeds of discovery*. New York, NY: W.W. Norton & Company.

Blackburn, S. (2005). *Truth: A guide*. New York: Oxford University Press.

Blackmore, S. (2004). *Consciousness: An introduction*. New York: Oxford University Press.

Bloome, D. & Paul, P. (Guest Editors). (2006). *Theory into Practice: Literacies of and for a diverse society, 45*(4).

Bruning, R., Schraw, G., Norby, M., & Ronning, R. (2004). *Cognitive psychology and instruction* (4th ed.). Upper Saddle River, NJ: Pearson/Merrill/Prentice Hall.

Cain, K., & Oakhill, J. (Eds.). (2007). *Children's comprehension problems in oral and written language*. New York: The Guilford Press.

Carruthers, P., Laurence, S., & Stich, S. (Eds.). (2005). *The innate mind: Structure and contents*. New York: Oxford University Press.

Carruthers, P., Laurence, S. & Stich, S. (Eds.). (2006). *The innate mind: Volume 2: Culture and cognition*. New York: Oxford University Press.

Chomsky, N. (2006). *Language and mind* (3rd ed.). New York: Cambridge University Press.

Davis, K. (2002). *Don't know much about the universe: Everything you need to know about outer space but never learned*. New York: Perennial.

deMarrais, K. B., & LeCompte, M. (1995). *The way schools work: A sociological analysis of education*. New York: Longman.

Denny, J. P. (1991). Rational thought in oral culture and literate decontextualization. In D. Olson & N. Torrance (Eds.), *Literacy and orality* (pp. 66-89). New York, NY: Cambridge University Press.

Donovan, M., & Bransford, J. (Eds.). (2005). *How students learn: History, mathematics, and science in the classroom*. Washington, DC: The National Academies Press.

Ellsworth, N., Hedley, C., & Baratta, A. (Eds.). (1994). *Literacy: A redefinition*. Hillsdale, NJ: Erlbaum.

Feldman, C. (1991). Oral metalanguage. In D. Olson & N. Torrance (Eds.), *Literacy and orality* (pp. 47-65). New York, NY: Cambridge University Press.

Freire, P., & Macedo, D. (1987). *Literacy: Reading the word and the world*. South Hadley, MA: Bergin & Garvey.

Gray, J. G. (1968). Introduction. In M. Heidegger, *What is called thinking?* (pp. vi-xvi). New York: Harper & Row. [Translated by J. G. Gray].

Hawking, S., & Mlodinow, L. (2010). *The grand design*. New York: Bantam Books.

Heidegger, M. (1968). *What is called thinking?* New York: Harper & Row. [Translated by J. G. Gray].

Heim, M. (1993). *The metaphysics of virtual reality*. New York: Oxford University Press.

Heward, W. (2009). *Exceptional children: an introduction to special education* (9th ed.). Upper Saddle River, NJ: Merrill/Pearson.

Hirsch, E. D. (1987). *Cultural literacy: What every American needs to know*. Boston, MA: Houghton Mifflin.

Hirsch, E. D., Kett, J., & Trefil, J. (Eds.). (2002). *The new dictionary of cultural literacy* (3rd ed.). Boston, MA: Houghton Mifflin Company.

Hunter, C., & Harman, D. (1979). *Adult illiteracy in the United States: A report to the Ford Foundation*. New York: McGraw-Hill.

Huxley, A. (2005). *Brave new world and brave new world revisited*. New York: HarperCollins.

Israel, S., & Duffy, G. (Eds.). (2009). *Handbook of research on reading comprehension*. New York: Routledge.

Jarvis, M. (2000). *Theoretical approaches in psychology*. Philadelphia, PA: Routledge.

Kuhn, D. (2005). *Education for thinking*. Cambridge, MA: Harvard University Press.

McGuinness, D. (2004). *Early reading instruction: What science really tells us about how to teach reading*. Cambridge, MA: The MIT Press.

McGuinness, D. (2005). *Language development and learning to read: The scientific study of how language development affects reading skill*. Cambridge, MA: The MIT Press.

McLaren, P. (1994). *Life in schools: An introduction to critical pedagogy in the foundations of education* (2nd ed.). New York: Longman.

Michael, M., & Trezek, B. (2006). Universal design and multiple literacies: Creating access and ownership for students with disabilities. *Theory into Practice, 45*(4), 311-318.

Montague, M. (1990). *Computers, cognition, and writing instruction*. Albany: State University of New York Press.

Olson, D. (1989). Literate thought. In C. K. Leong & B. Randhawa (Eds.), *Understanding literacy and cognition* (pp. 3–15). New York: Plenum.

Olson, D. (1994). *The world on paper*. Cambridge, UK: Cambridge University Press.

Ong, W. (1982). *Orality and literacy: The technologizing of the word*. London: Methuen.

Paul, P., & Wang, Y. (2006a). Multiliteracies and literate thought. *Theory into Practice*, *45*(4), 304-310.

Paul, P., & Wang, Y. (2006b). Literate thought and deafness: A call for a new perspective and line of research on literacy. *Punjab University Journal of Special Education* (Pakistan), *2*(1), 28-37.

Paul, P., & Whitelaw, G. (2011). *Hearing and deafness: An introduction for health and educational professionals*. Sudbury, MA: Jones & Bartlett Learning.

Pearson, P. D. (2004). The reading wars. *Educational Policy, 18*(1), 216-252.

Phillips, D., & Soltis, J. (2004). *Perspectives on learning*. New York: Teachers College Press.

Pinker, S. (1994). *The language instinct: How the mind creates language*. New York: William Morrow & Company.

Pring, R. (2004). *Philosophy of educational research* (2nd ed.). New York: Continuum.

Rippa, S. A. (1997). *Education in a free society: An American history* (8th ed.). White Plains, NY: Longman.

Robinson, J. (1990). *Conversations on the written word: Essays on language and literacy*. Portsmouth, NH: Boynton/Cook.

Rubin, D. (1995). *Memory in oral traditions: The cognitive psychology of epic, ballads, and counting-out rhymes*. New York: Oxford University Press.

Specter, M. (2009). *Denialism: How irrational thinking hinders scientific progress, harms the planet, and threatens our lives*. New York: The Penguin Press.

FURTHER READING

Eacker, J. (1983). *Problems of metaphysics and psychology*. Chicago: Nelson-Hall.

Harris, J. (1992). *Against relativism: A philosophical defense of method*. LaSalle, IL: Open Court.

Hofstadter, D., & Dennett, D. (2000). *The mind's I: Fantasies and reflections on self and soul*. New York: Basic Books. [Note: Composed and arranged by authors].

Nagel, T. (1986). *The view from nowhere*. New York: Oxford University Press.

Olson, D. (2004). The cognitive consequences of literacy. In T. Nunes & P. Bryant (Eds.), *Handbook of children's literacy* (pp. 539-555). Boston, MA: Kluwer Academic Publishers.

Taylor, R. (1983). *Metaphysics* (3rd ed.). Englewood Cliffs, NJ: Prentice-Hall.

INDEX